Blood Vessel Wall and Thrombosis

Volume I

Editor
Raymund Machovich, M.D., Ph.D., D.Sc.
2nd Institute of Biochemistry
Semmelweis University Medical School
Budapest, Hungary
and
Hematology Research
Mayo Clinic
Rochester, Minnesota

CRC Press, Inc.
Boca Raton, Florida

Library of Congress Cataloging-in-Publication Data

Blood vessel wall and thrombosis.

Includes bibliographies and index.
1. Thrombosis—Etiology. 2. Blood-vessels.
3. Endothelium. 4. Hemostasis. I. Machovich,
Raymund, 1936- . [DNLM: 1. Blood Vessels—
physiopathology. 2. Endothelium—physiopathology.
3. Hemostasis. 4. Thrombosis—blood. WH 310 B6556]
RC694.3.B56 1988 616.1'35 87-24298
ISBN 0-8493-5624-5 (set
ISBN 0-8493-5626-1 (v. 1)
ISBN 0-8493-5627-X (v. 2)

Direct all inquiries to CRC Press, Inc., 2000 Corporate Blvd., N.W., Boca Raton, Florida, 33431.

International Standard Book Number 0-8493-5624-5(set)
International Standard Book Number 0-8493-5626-2 (v. 1)
International Standard Book Number 0-8493-5627-X (v. 2)

Library of Congress Card Number 87-24298
Printed in the United States

PREFACE

Thrombosis is one of the most serious medical problems of our time. The mechanisms by which thrombosis develops have been studied extensively for many decades. Attention has always been centered on the role of the blood vessel wall and its interaction with the platelets, the coagulation factors, and their inhibitors. More details are known about the intricate interactions among the multiple factors operative in thrombus formation and lysis. We have, as yet, been unsuccessful in finding the crucial determinant for effective prevention and treatment of this number one killer in the developed world.

The purpose of these multiauthor volumes is to present the latest, authoritative information on the regulatory role of the blood vessel wall on the process of hemostasis in health and disease. From this point of view, blood vessel wall and circulating blood can be considered as an indivisible system. Such an interpretation is also supported by the fact that pathological changes in hemostasis are not only involved in intravascular thrombus formation and bleeding from thc injured vessel wall, but also contribute to various pathological injuries of the vessel wall e.g., in atherosclerosis, hypertension, diabetic angiopathy, immunopathology alterations, and tumor metastasis.

The regulation of hemostatic interactions involves a delicate balance of pro- and anticoagulant forces. Our knowledge of the structure and function of the blood vessel wall as well as of cellular and humoral factors of blood involved in hemostasis has logarithmically increased during the past few years. For specialists and nonspecialists these two volumes provide an easier survey of the vast range of the accumulated knowledge in this fascinating field of biomedicine.

Susan R. Hollán, M.D.
May 1986

THE EDITOR

Raymund Machovich received his M.D. degree from Semmelweis University Medical School (Budapest) in 1961 and subsequently specialized in internal medicine. He obtained the Ph.D. degree in 1972 for his work in the laboratory of Professor B. F. Straub on the biosynthesis of pancreatic enzymes. His research on thrombosis and hemostasis began in 1973, and he was awarded the D.Sc. degree in 1978 for his thesis, ''Regulation of Thrombin Inactivation''.

He spent 1 year (1970) in the laboratory of Professor E. Knox (Harvard Medical School) working with Dr. O. Greengard on the activation of thymidine kinase in tumor cells. Eight years later, he received the Canadian Heart Foundation Award and attended McMaster University for 1 year studying the role of heparin in hemostasis. In 1982, he spent 6 months at the Centre National de Transfusion Sanguine in Paris.

In addition to his research activities, he teaches a course in biochemistry at the Semmelweis University Medical School, Budapest, Hungary.

Dr. Machovich has published about 70 papers and has edited a two-volume book *The Thrombin,* (CRC Press, 1984). He was an editor of *Thrombosis Research* from 1981 to 1985 and is currently a member of the editorial board of *Excerpta Medica.*

Presently, he is working at the Mayo Clinic in Rochester, Minnesota.

ACKNOWLEDGMENT

I wish to express my sincere gratitude to Mrs. Ildikó Machovich for her helpful criticisms and participation in the preparation of the manuscript.

I am also indebted to the director and staff of CRC Press, Inc.

CONTRIBUTORS

Róza Ádány, M.D.
Assistant Professor
Department of Clinical Chemistry
University Medical School
Debrecen, Hungary

J. Dawes, M.A., D.Phil.
Director
Scottish National Blood Transfusion Service
Edinburgh, Scotland

Elisabetta Dejana, Ph.D.
Vascular Physiopathology Unit
Istituto Mario Negri
Milan, Italy

Laurence A. Erickson, Ph.D.
Research Scientist
Atherosclerosis and Thrombosis Research
The Upjohn Company
Kalamazoo, Michigan

Avrum I. Gotlieb, M.D.
Associate Professor
Vascular Research Center
Toronto General Hospital
Toronto, Ontario, Canada

B. Lowell Langille, Ph.D.
Associate Professor
Department of Pathology
University of Toronto
Toronto, Ontario, Canada

Lucia R. Languino, M.D.
Vascular Physiopathology Unit
Istituto Mario Negri
Milan, Italy

Raymund Machovich, M.D., Ph.D.
Semmelweis University Medical School
2nd Institute of Biochemistry
Budapest, Hungary
Hematology Research
Mayo Clinic
Rochester, Minnesota

Jozsef Mandl, M.D., Ph.D.
Assistant Professor
Semmelweis University Medical School
1st Institute of Biochemistry
Budapest, Hungary

László Muszbek, M.D., Ph.D.
Professor and Head
Department of Clinical Chemistry
University Medical School
Debrecen, Hungary

D. S. Pepper, B.Sc., Ph.D.
Scottish National Blood Transfusion Service
Edinburgh, Scotland

Frederick J. Walker, Ph.D
Indiana University School of Medicine
Terre Haute Center for Medical Eduation
Terre Haute, Indiana

TABLE OF CONTENTS

Chapter 1

HEMOSTASIS

Raymund Machovich

TABLE OF CONTENTS

I. INTRODUCTION

The term hemostasis refers, on the one hand, to the ability of blood to arrest bleeding from an injured part of the blood vessel wall, and on the other hand, to prevent thrombus formation inside the blood circulation. The balance between these two extreme states is rigorously controlled, i.e., various functions of endothelial cells, smooth muscle cells, liver cells, and platelets, as well as several molecular components of the blood coagulation-fibrinolytic system are involved in the regulation of hemostasis. Any disorganization in the processes of hemostasis may lead to hemorrhagic or thromboembolic diseases. Thrombus formation, however, is one of the most serious medical problems of our time.

The crucial questions in thrombosis are the following: (1) What is/are the trigger(s) causing initiation of plug formation in a nonappropriate part of the blood vessel wall and (2) how does a failure of stop-signal(s) for blood coagulation develop? Although several factors, both cellular and molecular, may participate in thrombus formation, one of the most essential components is certainly the blood vessel wall, especially the endothelial cells.

The purpose of this chapter is to give an overall view on hemostasis, to show the inherent features among the cellular and molecular components of it, and to discuss the role of blood vessel wall in hemostasis. Details about the cellular and molecular factors and their morphological and functional changes under pathological conditions are described in the appropriate chapters.

II. STRUCTURE AND FUNCTION OF BLOOD VESSEL WALL

Almost all types of human cells communicate with the external environment indirectly. Without blood vessels they are not able to exist and to accomplish their biological roles. Endothelial cells supply and, at the same time, limit, hormones, nutrients, oxygen, etc. for the metabolism of other cells. Even the regulation of the various cell functions occurs through the endothelium. Its most important roles are to maintain blood pressure and to direct blood-tissue exchange via both permeability and barrier functions. These functions, however, depend on the thromboresistant nature of the endothelial cells.

A. Morphology of Artery, Vein, and Capillary

The size of blood vessels varies according to their functions. When the inner diameter of a vessel is over or under 100 μm, it is called macro- or microvasculature, respectively.[1] The microvasculature includes the capillary, which is less than 7 μm in the diameter of lumen.

The structure of vessel walls, the macrovasculature in general terms, is described as intima, media, and adventitia.[1,2] The innermost stratum of the vessel wall consists of the intima, which is built up from endothelial monolayer on the subendothelial zone. The subendothelial zone is composed of basement membrane, elastin, and microfibrils. The intima is divided from media by the internal elastic lamina. The media is organized mainly of smooth muscle cells. The outermost layer of the blood vessel walls, the adventitia, is separated from the media by the external elastic lamina. The adventitia contains fibroblasts, extracellular connective tissues, small blood vessels, lymph vessels, and nerves. Artery, vein, and capillary differ not only in size, but also in the components and structure of blood vessel wall (Figure 1 and Figure 2).

Arteries can be found from the heart to the capillaries with a steadily diminished caliber. Since the total cross-sectional area of the arterial system expands to the capillaries, the rate of blood flow decreases also continuously.[3]

Blood is carried from the capillaries by the veins, with increasing caliber, toward the heart, and the blood flow is slow in veins compared to arterial flow. As for the histology of veins, in general, the media is poorly developed (or even absent in smaller veins), whereas the adventitia is several times as thick as the media in veins.

Capillaries, the greatest surface of the vasculature, are the principal vessels of the entire circulatory system. Practically, they consist of endothelial cell monolayer and basal lamina (basement membrane) with a lumen diameter of 7 μm or less. The extracellular connective

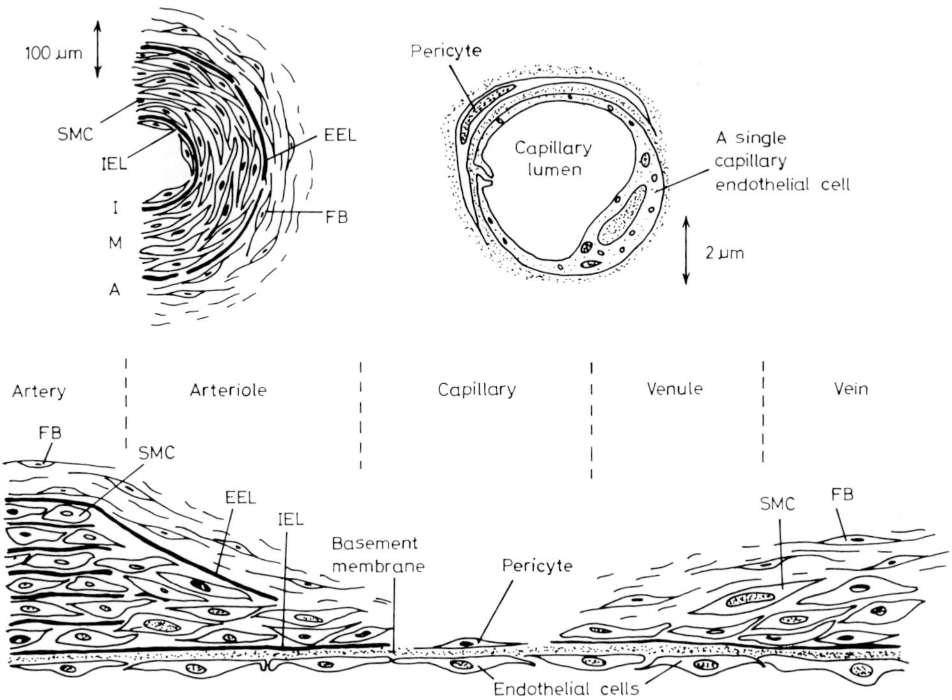

FIGURE 1. Schematic diagram of blood vessel walls. The main structure components of arteries and veins and their relative distributions are symbolized. Cross-segment of an arteriole and capillary are shown separately with indication of approximate sizes. Abbreviations: I, intima; M, media; A, adventitia; IEL, internal elastic lamina; EEL, external elastic lamina; SMC, smooth muscle cells; FB, fibroblast.

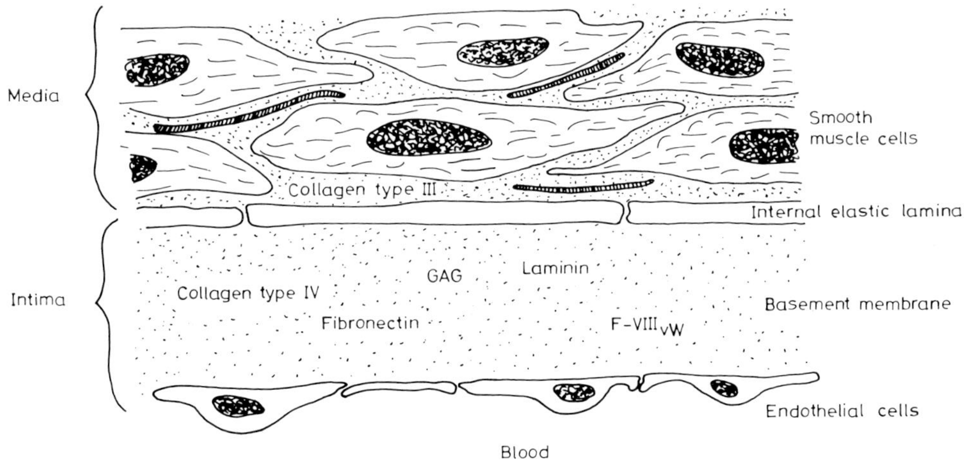

FIGURE 2. Structure of intima. Abbreviations used: GAG, glycosaminoglycans of vessel wall, mainly heparan sulfate, dermatan sulfate, chondroitin-4 sulfate, and chondroitin-6 sulfate; F-VIII$_{vw}$, F-VIII$_{vw}$.

tissue, produced primarily by endothelial cells, refers to collagen type IV, glycosaminoglycans, Factor VIII$_{\text{von Willebrand}}$ (F-VIII$_{vW}$), and glycoproteins such as fibronectin, laminin, and entactin[4] (Figure 2).

Two major types of capillaries can be distinguished: continuous and fenestrated.[5] The continuous capillaries of skeletal muscle, connective tissue, and CNS contain endothelial cells with a thick area around the nucleus and thin cytoplasm covering the remainder of the luminal surface. Fenestrated capillaries of renal glomeruli, endocrine glands, and intestine have extremely attenuated endothelium penetrated by pores approximately 90 nm in diameter. These fenestrae are closed by thin diaphragms with a probable function of rapid exchange of molecules between blood and tissue.

1. Cellular Components of the Blood Vessel Wall

The occurrence of different cellular elements of the blood vessel wall depends on its function in blood circulation. In the capillary, the wall consists virtually of endothelial cells with a few pericytes. Large vessels, like arteries and veins, contain additional types of cells. In the subendothelial space of these vessel walls, mast cells can be found. The media is mainly a build-up of smooth muscle cells, whereas adventitia consists of fibroblasts, adipocytes, and rarely of some mast cells. The structural and functional integrity of a given vessel wall depends upon the integrity of its cellular components and of the extracellular matrix synthesized by these cells.[6]

a. Endothelial Cells

Almost all tissues live on blood supply, and this supply depends on endothelial cells. They form an adaptable life-support system;[7] without endothelium, the metabolism of the various cells, energy supply, hormonal control, immunological protection, and tissue growth and repair would be impossible. Endothelium at different vascular sites and organs displays individual peculiarities[8] in size and shape depending on the various predominant biological functions. Indeed, endothelial cells are continuously adapting to the composition of blood, to the pulsatile hydrostatic pressure, to the biologically active materials, etc. They also change according to their main functions, i.e., oxygen transport, gas and water exchange, metabolic equilibrium, and protein production for or removal from blood circulation. No matter how their roles are specialized, a common task for all endothelial cells is the thromboresistance under normal conditions. Since these are the stipulations of blood circulation, endothelium is discussed in this chapter, first from this viewpoint.

Endothelial cells are approximately 40 μm in diameter and 3 μm thick, forming a monolayer over every vessel basement membrane. They have three surfaces: cohesive, adhesive (abluminal), and nonthrombogenic (luminal).[5] The cohesive site adjoins endothelial cells to one another by means of cell junctions serving for transport processes, and these junctions show various morphologies depending on the localization of the vessel.[9] The abluminal surface of endothelial cells adheres to the connective tissue of the subendothelial zone. The surface that faces the lumen is the nonthrombogenic one and this thromboresistant nature of the membrane is further supported by factors synthesized and secreted by these cells.

From a morphological aspect, endothelial cells, like other types of cells, have nucleus, mitochondria, microtubules, microfilaments, pinocytotic vesicles, etc.[10] In addition, endothelial cells contain unique organelles, vesicles, and components characteristic for these cells:

1. Weibel-Palade body,[11] a rod-shaped tubular organelle with ca. 3-μm length and 0.1-μm diameter, derived from the Golgi apparatus,[12] probably serving as a storage vesicle for $F\text{-}VIII_{vW}$
2. Small, approximately 80-nm vesicles[10] for transport by endocytosis at the luminal surface and by exocytosis at the external surface or vice versa
3. $F\text{-}VIII_{vW}$ antigen
4. Type IV procollagen
5. Angiotensin converting enzyme
6. A characteristic glycocalyx

These can be considered as characteristic components of the endothelial cells.

b. Smooth Muscle Cells

The media of the blood vessel wall consists of elongated smooth muscle cells having a single nucleus and containing thick as well as thin filaments aligned with the long axis of the cells.[13]

The main functions of these cells are (1) contraction to control blood flow, (2) synthesis of various connective tissue elements, and (3) lipid uptake, synthesis, and turnover.[13,14]

1. Although the mechanism of contraction of smooth muscle cells of blood vessel is fundamentally the same as in skeletal muscle,* it differs functionally in two aspects: (a) the level of ATP-ase activity is lower in smooth muscle than in skeletal muscle cells and is subjected to a direct calcium regulation and (b) the myosin of smooth muscle cells is able to interact with actin molecule when its light chain is phosphorylated.[16] The cascade of reactions, by which the contraction of smooth muscle cells is activated, is triggered by the increase of Ca^{2+} level inside the cell. The effect of Ca^{2+} is mediated by calmodulin. The calmodulin-Ca^{2+} complex formed activates myosin light-chain kinase and as a consequence myosin is phosphorylated and becomes active.[17] The enzyme reaction that follows Ca^{2+} binding to calmodulin is relatively slow to activate smooth muscle cell contraction. As a result, smooth muscle cells rarely undergo quick contraction, but enable the vessel wall to maintain a constant tension with great efficiency.
2. Smooth muscle cells are able to synthesize and secrete collagen and elastin as well as glycosaminoglycans.
3. Lipid synthesis is stimulated in smooth muscle cells of blood vessels when the cell medium contains lipid-free serum, whereas it is inhibited when exogeneous lipid is present.[18] Human arterial smooth muscle cells preferentially bind and take up low-density lipoproteins (LDL) and very low-density lipoproteins (VLDL). This type of cells also incorporates oleic and linoleic acids and participates in the synthesis and removal of different cholesterol esters.[19]

c. Other Cells

While intima contains endothelial cells and media contains smooth muscle cells, the main cellular components of adventitia are fibroblasts and mast cells.[5,20] Fibroblasts are useful for the synthesis of collagen type I and III, fibronectin, glycosaminoglycans, lipids, elastin, and molecular components with a procoagulant nature. Furthermore, fibroblasts, together with smooth muscle cells, are able to accumulate LDL and cholesterol, forming ''foam cells'' in the arterial wall, thereby playing a role in atherogenesis.[21] Mast cells, on the other hand, can produce and store heparin, histamine, serotonin, and hyaluronic acid.[22] The secretion of heparin may contribute to the nonthrombogenic character of the blood vessel wall.

2. Extracellular Components of the Blood Vessel Wall

Cells of the blood vessel wall synthesize and secrete several kinds of macromolecules (Table 1**) forming extracellular matrix, which in turn determines the mechanical properties of the blood vessel wall, contributes to the microenvironment of the cells, and influences

* Muscle contraction is a result of sliding of actin against myosin filaments. The head part of myosin undergoes an ATP dependent cycle by attaching to actin and detaching from that. The conformational change pulls one filament against the next. These functions are regulated by calmodulin and Ca^{2+}. When the Ca^{2+} level increases in response to neurogen stimulus, the myosin head is allowed to interact with actin, resulting in contraction.[15]

** A brief summary of the main components of hemostasis can be found in Table 1.

Table 1
SOME CELLULAR AND MOLECULAR COMPONENTS OF BLOOD AND BLOOD VESSEL WALL PARTICIPATING IN HEMOSTASIS

Origin	Component	Structure	Functions
Vessel wall (endothelial cells, smooth muscle cells, fibroblasts)	Collagen (several types)	Three-chain glycoprotein, with M_r approximately 300,000 daltons	Vascular structure, procoagulant
	Elastin	Insoluble, nonpolar amino acid rich, cross-linked protein	A network giving flexibility to vessel walls
	Glycosaminoglycans (GAGs)	Linear chain polysaccharides with various negative charges, with heterogeneous M_r	Structural part of vessels, transport processes, anticoagulant
	Lipoproteins LDL, HDL, VLDL	Complexes of proteins and lipids with various density and with heterogenous M_r, M_r from 300,000 up to 10^7 daltons	Transport for triglyceride and cholersterol, complex formation with GAG in vessel wall
	Fibronectin	A 2-chain glycoprotein with M_r 440,000 daltons	Cell-cell interactions
	Laminin	A 2-chain glycoprotein with M_r 850,000 daltons	Basement membrane structure for cellular-molecular interactions
	F-VIII_{vw}	Multimeric structure of a glycoprotein with M_r 220,000 daltons	Cell-cell interaction mainly for platelets and endothelial cells
	Tissue-factor	1-chain glycoprotein, M_r 52,000 daltons	Procoagulant in a complex of phospholipids
	Thrombomodulin	Insoluble membrane protein of endothelial cell, M_r 74,000 daltons	Cofactor for protein C activation, thrombin receptor
	Angiotensin converting enzyme	Endothelial cell membrane enzyme	Conversion of angiotensin I to II, inactivation of bradykinin
	Ecto-ADP-ase, adenosine	Endothelial cell membrane enzyme system	Adenosine formation from ADP (ATP, AMP) inhibition of platelet aggregation
	Prostacyclin (PGI_2)	Intermediate of arachidonic acid metabolism	Inhibitor of platelet aggregation
	Endothelium-derived relaxant factor	Unknown	Vascular relaxation

Platelets	Ca^{2+}	Stored, at very high conc., in dense granules, and released by TXA_2 into cytoplasm or by IP_3	An intracellular second messenger and a trigger for the contractile system inside platelet
	ADP	Stored in dense granules and secreted by platelet activation	A trigger for platelet activation
	Serotonin	Stored and secreted by dense granules	Vasoactive
	Platelet factor 3	Membrane phospholipids	Procoagulant (surface for blood coagulation acceleration)
	Platelet factor 4	A platelet specific single polypeptide chain, M_r 7,780 daltons with high affinity to heparin	Antiheparin activity
	Thrombospondin	A glycoprotein with M_r 450,000 daltons, synthesized also by endothelial and smooth muscle cells	"Lectin activity" in the platelet vessel wall interactions via collagen V, otherwise, its function is obscure
	Low affinity platelet factor 4 (LAPF4)	Single chain polypeptide consisted of 89 amino acid residues	Antiheparin activity, participating in inflammation, mitogen action
	β-Thromboglobulin	Single chain polypeptide, M_r 8,800 daltons, a plasmin induced proteolytic product of LAPF4	Antiheparin activity
	Platelet-derived growth factor (PDGF)	A 2-chain polypeptide, M_r 27,000 to 31,000 daltons, with near identity to a major portion of viral oncogene protein $p28^{r\text{-}sis}$	Mitogenic on various cells (fibroblasts, smooth muscle cells, endothelial cells) playing role in wound healing, tissue repair, arteriosclerosis, etc.
	Thromboxane A_2 (TXA_2)	An intermediate of arachidonic acid metabolism	Powerful inducer of platelet aggregation, smooth muscle cell contraction
Blood coagulation factors	Fibrinogen	2 × 3-chain glycoprotein, M_r 340,000 daltons, 3 mg/mℓ[a]	Sol-gel conversion by thrombin
	Prothrombin	Single chain glycoprotein, containing Gla residues, M_r 72,000 daltons, approximately 100 μg/mℓ	Proenzyme of thrombin
	Ca^{2+}	Present in blood plasma at m*M* conc.	To influence enzyme activities, to accelerate the conversion of zymogenes to enzymes on phospholipid surfaces

Table 1 (continued)
SOME CELLULAR AND MOLECULAR COMPONENTS OF BLOOD AND BLOOD VESSEL WALL PARTICIPATING IN HEMOSTASIS

Origin	Component	Structure	Functions
	F-V	Single chain glycoprotein, M_r 330,000 daltons, 7 μg/mℓ	A protein cofactor for prothrombin activation
	F-VII	Single chain protein, containing Gla residues, M_r 48,000 daltons, approximately 0.5 μg/mℓ	Enzyme and proenzyme for F-X activation
	F-VIII$_c$	A protein with M_r 240,000 daltons, 0.25 ng/mℓ	A protein cofactor for F-X activation
	F-IX	Single chain glycoprotein, containing Gla residues, M_r 57,000 daltons, approximately 5 μg/mℓ	Proenzyme for F-X activation
	F-X	2-chain glycoprotein, containing Gla residues, M_r 59,000 daltons, approximately 8 μg/mℓ	Proenzyme for prothrombin activation substrate for F-IXa or F-VIIa
	F-XI	2-chain glycoprotein, M_r 160,000 daltons, approximately 4 μg/mℓ	Substrate for F-XIIa, proenzyme of F-IX activation
	F-XII	Single chain glycoprotein, M_r 76,000 daltons, approximately 35 μg/mℓ	Proenzyme of the multifunctional proteinase F-XIIa
	F-XIII	A glycoprotein consisting of 4 polypeptide chains, M_r 320,000 daltons, approximately 15 μg/mℓ	A proenzyme, activated by thrombin, for cross-links formation in fibrin molecules
	Prekallikrein	A single chain polypeptide, M_r 82,000 daltons, approximately 30 μg/mℓ	Proenzyme of the proteinase kallikrein
	Protein C	A 2-chain glycoprotein, M_r 62,000 daltons, approximately 3 μg/mℓ	A precursor protein, activated by thrombin, with the capacity to inhibit thrombin formation and to initiate fibrinolysis
	Protein S	Single chain glycoprotein, M_r 69,000 daltons	A cofactor for F-Va and F-VIIIa inactivation by activated protein C

	High M_r kininogen (HMWK)	Single chain protein, M_r 110,000 daltons approximately 80 μg/mℓ	Procoagulant for F-XII, F-XI, and prekallikrein activation, substrate of kallikrein for the vasoactive bradykinin formation
Fibrinolytic system	Fibrin	Insoluble aggregate of fibrinogen molecules after loss of fibrinopeptide A and B	To stop hemorrhage, substrate for plasmin
	Plasminogen	A single chain glycoprotein M_r 90,000 daltons, approximately 180 μg/mℓ	Proenzyme form of plasmin, proteinase dissolving fibrin clot
	Plasminogen activator: urokinase-type	2 chain glycoprotein, M_r 54,000 daltons, synthesized by kidney, tumor cells, or endothelial cells	Induction of fibrinolysis via activation of plasminogen
	Plasminogen activator: tissue-type	A single and 2-chain polypeptide, M_r 70,000 daltons, synthesized by tumor and endothelial cells	Fibrinolysis initiation: after activation, 2-chain proteinase formed is a powerful activator of plasminogen bound to fibrin
Complement system	Clq	6-chain glycoprotein, M_r 410,000 daltons, approximately 160 μg/mℓ	Collagen-like protein bound to immune complex
	Clr	Single chain glycoprotein, M_r 83,000 daltons, approximately 50 μg/mℓ	Proenzyme of C1 macromolecular complex
	Cls	Single chain glycoprotein, M_r 83,000 daltons, approximately 50 μg/mℓ	Proenzyme in C1 macromolecular complex
	C2	Single chain polypeptide, M_r 110,000 daltons, approximately 15 μg/mℓ	Proenzyme, substrate for $\overline{\text{Cls}}$, resulting in C2a formation on erythrocytes
	C4	3-chain glycoprotein, M_r 206,000 daltons, approximately 500 μg/mℓ	Substrate for Cls, anaphylatoxic fragment release, cofactor for C4,2 in immune complexes
	C3	2-chain protein, M_r 180,000 daltons, approximately 1 to 2 mg/mℓ	Substrate for $\overline{\text{C2e}}$, phagocyte stimulation
	F-B	Single chain polypeptide, M_r 93,000 daltons, approximately 200 μg/mℓ	Proenzyme, substrate for F-D, chemotactic
	F-D	Single chain protein, M_r 24,000 daltons, approximately 1 μg/mℓ	Enzyme of C3b,B complex

Table 1 (continued)
SOME CELLULAR AND MOLECULAR COMPONENTS OF BLOOD AND BLOOD VESSEL WALL PARTICIPATING IN HEMOSTASIS

Origin	Component	Structure	Functions
	Properdin	A protein consisted of noncovalent tetramer subunits, M_r 200,000 daltons, approximately 20 μg/mℓ	Unknown
	C5	2-chain polypeptide, M_r 200,000 daltons, approximately 70 μg/mℓ	Substrate of C5 convertase, after cleavage, a complex of C5b,6,7
	C6	Single chain polypeptide, M_r 128,000 daltons, approximately 60 μg/mℓ	Binds to membrane, forming with C8 and C9 complement membrane attack complex, which initiates cell lysis
	C7	Single chain polypeptide, M_r 102,000 daltons, approximately 55 μg/mℓ	
	C8	3-chain protein, M_r 150,000 daltons, approximately 55 μg/mℓ	
	C9	Single chain protein, M_r 71,000 daltons, approximately 60 μg/mℓ	
Plasma proteinase inhibitors	α_2-Macroglobulin	Single chain glycoprotein, M_r 725,000 daltons, approximately 2.5 mg/mℓ	Inhibitor for trypsin, plasmin, thrombin, collagenase, plasminogen activators
	Antithrombin III	Single chain glycoprotein, M_r 68,000 daltons, approximately 300 μg/mℓ	Inhibitor for all serine proteinases of blood coagulation-fibrinolytic system, except of F-VIIa and activated protein C
	α_1-Proteinase inhibitor (α_1-antitrypsin)	Single chain glycoprotein, M_r 53,000 daltons, approximately 1 mg/mℓ	Inhibitor of trypsin, chymotrypsin, cathepsin G, elastase, collagenase, thrombin, plasmin, kallikrein, plasminogen activators
	Heparin cofactor II	Single chain glycoprotein, M_r 70,000 daltons, approximately 60 μg/mℓ	Inhibitor of thrombin
	Protein C inactivator	Glycoprotein, M_r 96,000 daltons	Inhibitor of activated protein C

	C1-inactivator (C1-INA)	Glycoprotein, M_r 100,000 daltons, approximately 170 μg/mℓ	Inhibitor of complement proteinase, Clr and Cls, F-XIa, F-XII, kallikrein, tissue-type plasminogen activator
	α_2-Antiplasmin	Single chain glycoprotein, M_r 68,000 daltons, approximately 60 μg/mℓ	Primary inhibitor of plasmin, besides inactivates thrombin, trypsin, F-Xa, F-XIa, tissue-type plasminogen activator
Polymorphonuclear cells	Platelet activating factor (PAF)	1-*O*-alkyl-2-acethyl-sn-glycerol-3-phosphorylcholine	Activator of platelet
	Leukotrienes	Intermediates of arachidonic acid metabolism	Chemotactic, especially in inflammations

[a] Concentrations mean blood plasma levels for all components indicated in this table: amount per milliliter of plasma.

cellular growth and differentiation. This extracellular matrix is synthesized mainly by smooth muscle cells, endothelial cells, fibroblasts, and mast cells and secreted in the form of soluble precursors. Collagen and elastin are processed to insoluble form and strengthened by cross-links in the extracellular space, while proteoglycans and fibronectins are insolubilized by self-association. The molecular bonds among matrix elements change from weak ionic association to stable covalent cross-links.

a. Collagen

Collagen is the most abundant structural protein of the mammalian body, and its synthesis and degradation are precisely controlled.[23] Several types of collagen, types I, II, III, IV, V, etc., have been identified.[24] (This nomenclature is based on historical methodology.) Types I and III, as well as IV, are the main components of collagen present in the blood vessel wall.

Each collagen molecule is composed of three α-chains.[25] The α-chain has an M_r of approximately 100,000 daltons with a right-handed helical conformation. Type I collagen consists of two α_1-chains and one α_2-chain, whereas type IV is built from trimers of identical α-chains.[26]

As to the structure of collagen, it forms a triple helix, and glycine is present in every third position in the α-chain, except at the end of the molecule.[27] The latter regions are intermolecularly cross-linked. Collagen also contains large amounts of proline, hydroxy-proline, and hydroxylysine, which are primarily responsible for the helical conformation of the α-chain. The modified amino acid residues also participate in the intra- and intermolecular cross-links and are responsible for the great strength of collagen fibers.

The α-chains of collagen molecules are synthesized in a precursor form of a higher molecular weight by approximately 55,000 daltons and are called pro-α-chain.[28] The post-translational modification of tyrosyl and prolyl residues by hydroxylases begins while the peptide chain is still bound to the ribosome.[29] Thereafter, the newly synthesized procollagen molecules are transported from the rough endoplasmic reticulum to the Golgi apparatus, stored in vesicles, and finally exported from the cell. Procollagen is soluble at physiological ionic strength and pH, however, after cleaving the extension peptides, the molecule is "insolubilized."[30]

The extracellular matrix can be degraded by neutral proteinases, mainly by collagenases synthesized by fibroblasts, macrophages, and leukocytes.[31] They are Ca^{2+}-dependent enzymes and cleave collagen at one site.[32] The two fragments released become more susceptible to proteolysis by other enzymes, namely by cathepsins. Internalization of collagen also occurs.[33] The extracellular and intracellular degradation of collagen is probably coordinated, but the manner is unknown at present.

b. Elastin

Elastin gives a rubber-like characteristic to the blood vessel wall, since it exhibits a high extensibility and capacity to regain the original size.[34] Elastin is present in the form of a network of coiled polypeptide chains joined at various angles by covalent cross-links, in an ordered fibril structure with helical arrangement.[35] A unique arrangement of hydrophobic amino acid residues and cross-linking domains via desmosine and isodesmosine, approximately 2 to 3/1000 amino acid residues, provides stability and flexibility of elastin.[36]

Nonpolar amino acids, glycine, alanine, valine, and proline, constitute approximately 70% of the total amino acid residues. No histidine, tyrosine, cysteine, or methionine and only 1% of hydroxyproline can be found.[14,37]

Elastin is synthesized in a soluble precursor form, called tropoelastin having an M_r of approximately 70,000 daltons.[38] Like collagen and other secretory proteins, the N-terminal part of tropoelastin synthesized on ribosomes contains a leader sequence. During post-translational modification, some lysine residues are oxidized to corresponding aldehydes by lysyl oxidase, a Cu^{2+} containing enzyme, resulting in cross-links and insolubilization of the molecules.[39] About 10% of prolyl residues of elastin are also hydroxylated in the post-translational processing.[40]

Regarding the degradation of elastin, it is refractory to most proteinases, except elastase. Nevertheless, during inflammation, an increased degradation of elastin can occur.

c. *Microfibrillar Proteins*

Microfibrils, with a diameter of approximately 20 nm, are present in the matrix of aortic tissues in association with elastin and perhaps with fibronectin.[41] When ascorbate is absent, microfibrillar proteins become the predominant components of the matrix.[42] Although they have been studied, due to their extreme insolubility, the chemical structure, the biosynthesis, and the secretion, as well as the degradation of the microfibrils, are not well known.

d. *Glycosaminoglycans*

Several kinds of glycosaminoglycans (GAGs) can be found in the blood vessel wall, partly as structure elements and partly as functional units.[43] In general terms, GAGs are linear chain polysaccharides of very heterogeneous molecular weights and with various negative charges. GAGs consist of repeated units of *N*-sulfated and *O*-sulfated or acetylated glucosamine, α-L-iduronic acid and unsulfated β-D-glucuronic acid, or galactosamine residues joined by 1-4 glycosidic linkage.[44] GAGs, except hyaluronic acid, are covalently linked to proteins forming proteoglycan monomers via either *O*-glycosidic bond between Ser and Gal-Gal-xylose, or *N*-glycosidic bond between *N*-acetyl glucosamine and the amide group of Asn, or *O*-glycosidic bond between *N*-acetylgalactosamine and the hydroxyl group of Thr or Ser.[45]

Several types of GAGs have been distinguished.[46] These are the following: chondroitin 4-sulfate and chondroitin 6-sulfate, keratan sulfate, hyaluronic acid, heparan sulfate, and heparin. The biosynthesis of the proteoglycans, mainly in smooth muscle cells as well as in endothelial cells, is a rather complex process. The core protein, approximately 8%, is synthesized as an approximately 370,000-dalton precursor; then posttranslational modifications take place, including the removal of the signal peptide resulting in an approximately 200,000-dalton protein.[47] GAG chains are formed by sequential addition of monosaccharide units in the Golgi apparatus.[48]

e. *Fibronectin*

Fibronectin ("cold insoluble globulin"), a glycoprotein with 2 chains of M_r 220,000 daltons each, can be found in two forms.[49] Both the soluble and the insoluble form are a dimer of the polypeptide chains.[50] The exact relationship between the two forms is not known at present, although their amino acid composition as well as their carbohydrate content have been documented.[51]

Fibronectin is synthesized by fibroblasts, smooth muscle cells, endothelial cells, platelets, and by several tumor cell lines.[49-54] Fibronectin contains various domains[53] for the binding of:

1. Collagen (primarily type III)
2. Heparin, heparan sulfate, and hyaluronic acid
3. Fibrin
4. Actin, microfibrillar proteins (binding via cell membrane)
5. Factor XIII
6. Thrombin
7. DNA
8. Foreign surface

These domains, generally, in several combinations with different other molecules (e.g., activated platelet has a common recognition site for the complex of fibrinogen-F-VIII_{vW}-fibronectin) participate in cell-cell and cell-extracellular matrix interaction. They are also involved in opsonization, covering a surface to make it available for phagocytosis, thereby playing a role in the adhesion and migration as well as in the proliferation of various cells.[54]

f. Laminin

Laminin, a high molecular weight glycoprotein with M_r 850,000 daltons, consists of two polypeptide chains joined by disulfide bonds.[55] It contains approximately 10% cysteine located in one third of the molecule.

Laminin can be found exclusively in the basement membranes of the blood vessel wall.[56] It may play a role in the attachment of some cell types, like aortic endothelial cells to the collagens of basement membrane.[57] Moreover, it can act as an adhesive protein for tumor metastasis.[58]

g. Factor VIII vW (F-VIII_{vW})

F-VIII_{vW} is a large glycoprotein with complex multimeric structure up to M_r 2×10^7 daltons, formed from variable numbers of a subunit of M_r 220,000 daltons.[59] The multimers, dimers, or tetramers, are built up from disulfide-linked subunits.[60] F-VIII_{vW} protein is synthesized mainly by megakaryocytes, stored in both membranes and granules of platelets,[61] and released by the stimuli of thrombin, collagen, or ADP.[62]

Endothelial cells also synthesize F-VIII_{vW}, first in the form of precursor with M_r 260,000 daltons which is slowly cleaved to its 220,000-dalton subunit.[63] Both the precursor and the subunit are glycosylated, thereafter stored in the specific organelles of endothelial cells, i.e., in the Weibel-Palade bodies.[64] It is released by stimulus, like thrombin binding.[65] The F-VIII_{vW} released from endothelial cells can be found in the matrix of the blood vessel wall. As to its localization in the matrix, data in the literature are controversial, namely, whether it is collagen dependent or not.[66] According to our present knowledge, the main function of F-VIII_{vW} is to mediate the binding of platelets to subendothelium after vascular injury.

3. Organization of Cellular and Molecular Components of the Blood Vessel Wall

The structure of blood vessel walls changes according to their function, namely artery, capillary, and vein differ in the ratio of their intima, media, and adventitia, as discussed earlier. These strata are built up mainly from endothelial cells, smooth muscle cells, and fibroblasts, together with their products, respectively.

Endothelial cells on the basal membrane are primarily responsible for the synthesis of the extracellular matrix in basement membrane;[10] collagen type IV, glycosaminoglycans, fibronectin, laminin, and F-VIII_{vW} are the main components of this layer.[67-71] Between the intima and media an acellular, fenestrated elastic structure called internal elastic lamina, can be found, consisting predominantly of elastin and collagen type I and III with powerful procoagulant nature. The latter are synthesized by the cells of media.

The mammalian aortic medial layer is characterized by a well-ordered structure in connection with the smooth muscle cells. Several single layers of smooth muscle cells alternate with concentric layers of elastin fibers. Elastin associated microfibrils, collagen, and proteoglycan also participate in this network. One layer of smooth muscle cells with the adjacent layer of extracellular macromolecules constitute the lamellar unit.[72] The lamellar unit serves as structural and functional requirements for the high tensile strength, appropriate distensibility, viscoelastic response to pulsating pressure, and uniform distribution of stress on the blood vessel wall. The arrangement of the extracellular matrix around the cells ensures the mechanical strength of the entire structure. The number of lamellar units in the media varies with the size of arteries and with the species.[73] Within one species, the amount of lamellar units is completed at birth and stays constant during growth; only the size of the units changes due to the increasing deposition of the extracellular matrix. The components of the extracellular matrix (12% soluble protein, 76% elastin, 12% collagen, and less than 1% of proteoglycans, fibronectin, and microfibrillar proteins) are synthesized by the smooth muscle cells.[74] Of the collagen, approximately 90% are types I and III. Proteoglycans of aorta consist of 65% chondroitin sulfate, 22% dermatan sulfate, 8% heparan sulfate, and 4% hyaluronic acid.[75] While chondroitin sulfate and dermatan sulfate are in association with collagen, heparan sulfate binds to elastin.[76] A spontaneous association of fibronectin, heparin, and collagen type II also occurs, resulting in an insoluble terner complex from which the glycosaminoglycan can be released in a biologically active form by plasmin. The structure of smooth muscle cells and the composition of the extracellular matrix change in various diseases.

The third layer of the blood vessel wall, the adventitia, is highly developed in the veins. Adventitia is separated from the media by the external elastic lamina. It is built up from a dense inner and a loose external part containing collagen, predominantly type I, and elastic fibers in longitudinal and helical organization, as well as glycosaminoglycans and lipids.[77] The cellular elements are fibroblasts, adipocytes, mast cells, and a few smooth muscle cells.

The presence of vasa vasorum, lymph vessel, and nerves is also characteristic of the adventitia, especially of arteries.[78]

B. Functions of Blood Vessel Walls

Practically all tissues and organs can communicate with the outside world through blood circulation and via endothelial cells. This means that the structure and function of the various organs are closely related to blood circulation. Blood supplies the various cells with oxygen, metabolites (carbohydrates, lipids, amino acids, nucleotides), vitamins, and hormones, and it also plays a role in the elimination of unnecessary or even unwanted materials. Blood takes an essential part in the defense mechanism of the organism by the immunological system, as well.

According to these considerations, the main function of blood circulation and blood vessel walls is the transport of the molecular and cellular components necessary for life. The precondition of these processes, however, depends on the maintenance and the regulation of the blood pressure in the circulatory system, as well as on the ability of blood to prevent the loss of its fluidity inside the vessels. Although the transport processes take place primarily in the capillaries and the maintenance of the circulation of blood is the function of the heart and the arterial venous system, the mechanism by which the circulatory system maintains hemostasis should be a common feature of all parts of the circulatory system.

1. Transport Processes via Blood Vessel Walls

Blood-tissue exchange means both permeability and barrier function of blood vessel walls. Capillaries, where these actions take place, are greater in number than 10^{10} in human beings.[3] The microvasculature is classified functionally as nutritive or operative, i.e., nutritive units are present in all tissues with a continuous flow, whereas operating units are present in some specialized organs, like the kidney, where flow is related to its excretory function.[3]

Endothelium is one of the most permeable tissues in the human body. In all probability, not only do cellular pathways exist for transport in capillaries, but extracellular ones exist as well. The main transport processes are the following:[3,10,80] molecules with M_r less than 60,000 daltons can cross the endothelium by diffusion through "pores" called also "intracellular clefts".[3] For passage of large molecules into interstitial tissues, lymph endothelium can form tight junctions. Fenestrae and transendothelial channels are also hypothesized to be involved in the transport of large molecules. Nevertheless, according to our present knowledge, the formation of vesicles is the major route for transporting macromolecules via

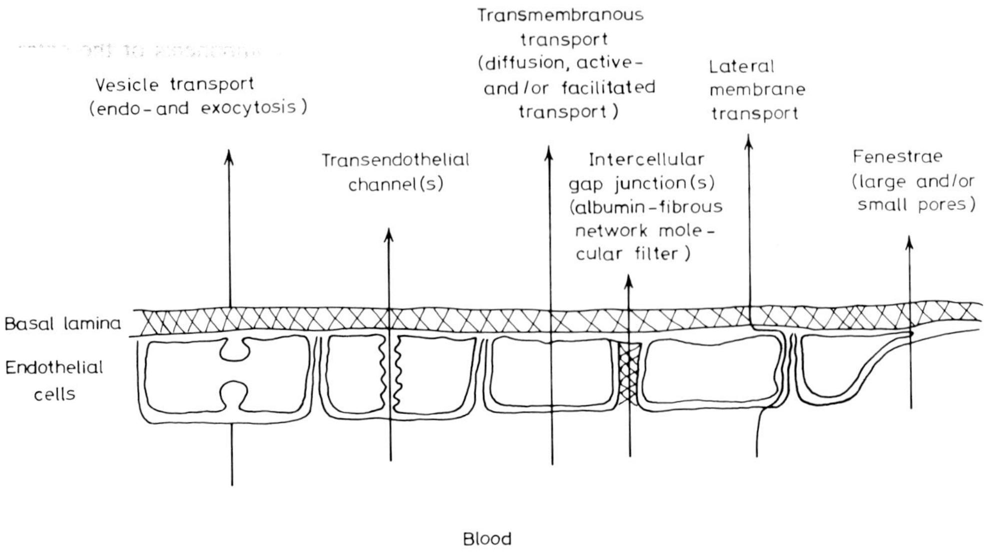

FIGURE 3. Transport process via endothelium. The possible transport mechanisms for large and small molecular components as well as for water are schematically summarized on the basis of References 3 and 10. Basement membrane, as an extracellular filter matrix, also contributes to the transcellular and/or intercellular transport processes.[79] The transendothelial channels may originate from vesicles. Fenestrae, single-layer diaphragms, may contain small and/or large pores with an approximate diameter of 9 or 60 nm, respectively. In the intercellular gap junctions, albumin is supposed to occupy space within the fibrous matrix by an electrostatic interaction between positively charged sites of albumin and negatively charged fibers, and the network formed determines the selectivity of this transport process.[80]

capillaries. As many as 75,000 vesicles have been estimated in a permeable endothelial cell.[3] These transport processes result in high selectivity of endothelium or conversely, a barrier function of the capillaries (Figure 3).

2. Role of the Blood Vessel Wall in the Maintenance of Blood Pressure

The function of the blood vessel wall, primarily of the arteries, is to distribute the blood from the heart-lung system to various tissues. The arteries are always exposed to high blood pressure. In elastic arteries, like the aorta and pulmonary arteries, blood flow is relatively constant, and it is maintained during diastole and systole by the structure of these vessel walls, i.e., largely by the medial elastic tissue.[3] On the other hand, the medium size arteries supply blood to the tissues according to the actual requirements. These requirements are met by the change of diameter of the lumen of the arterial walls.[81,82] Such a function is based on the medial smooth muscle cells. Furthermore, these arteries do not contain large elastic lamella called muscle-elastic units. Their function is controlled mainly by the nervous system.

Microvasculature has both continuous and intermittent blood flow, and these pressures are regulated by local or autoregulatory mechanisms.[83] Two mechanisms are generally mentioned: myogenic and metabolic.[3] Autoregulation may take place by the function of precapillary spincters, however, the involvement of vasoconstriction may also be considered.[3] Besides the function of smooth muscle cells in the modulation of blood flow in microvasculature, endothelial cells themselves can participate in it. Endothelial cells contain contractile systems which possibly enable these cells to oscillate, called ''vasomotion'', to make contraction-relaxation in a few seconds.[10,84]

In general terms, blood circulation is controlled by several neurogenic and/or metabolic factors, and in these processes smooth muscle cells and endothelial cells are highly in-

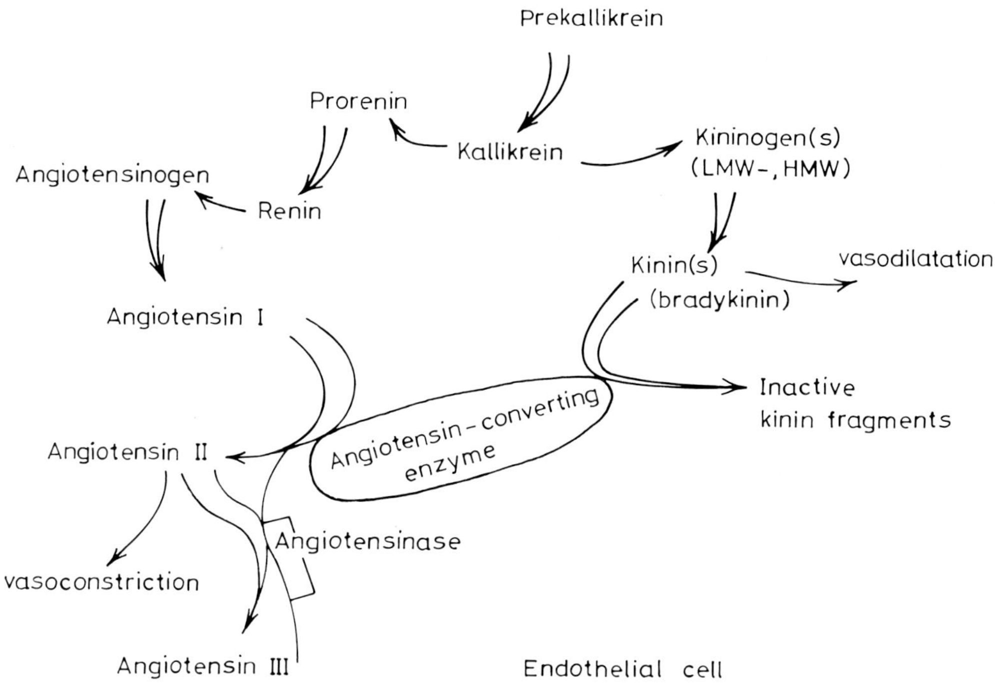

FIGURE 4. The renin-angiotensin and kallikrein-kinin system. When kallikrein is formed from prekallikrein by the action of F-XIIa or other enzyme(s) (also Figures 15 and 16), kallikrein, in turn, can activate plasma prorenin with M_r 56,000 daltons to renin, M_r 40,000 daltons, and/or release bradykinin from low molecular weight (LMW-) and high molecular weight (HMW-) kininogens. The renin formed converts angiotensinogen to angiotensin I, a peptide containing Asp-Arg-Val-Tyr-Ile-His-Pro-Phe-His-Leu, which is further hydrolyzed on endothelial cell surface by the angiotensin-converting enzyme, a dipeptidyl carboxypeptidase (EC 3.4.15.1). The resulting heptapeptide, designated as angiotensin II, has the capacity to induce vasoconstriction. Angiotensin II, however, may be inactivated by another endothelial surface enzyme, angiotensinase, leading to the formation of an inactive fragment called angiotensin III. Kinin(s) formed, on the other hand, initiates vascular dilation and increase of blood vessel permeability, but may be inactivated by the angiotensin-converting enzyme. Wide and narrow arrows denote conversion and action, respectively.

volved.[85,86] The activities of these cells are influenced by vasoactive peptides, hormones, and various intermediate metabolites, resulting in vasoconstriction, vasodilation, change in permeability, or, at least in the modulation of one of the effects mentioned. The factors involved in these processes are the following:[3,81,87] amines (histamine, serotonin, acetylcholine), catecholamines (epinephrine, norepinephrine, dopamine), PAF (platelet activating factor), angiotensin-renin and kinin-kallikrein system (angiotensin II, bradykinin), adenosine and adenin nucleotides, prostaglandins (thromboxane A_2 and prostacyclin), hormones (glucocorticoids, estrogens, oxytocin, vasopressin, glucagon, secretin, pancreozymin), and relaxant factor. Besides, many other conditions, such as a change in pH, hypoxemia, concentration of K^+, etc., can influence blood circulation. These actions, however, are beyond the scope of the present project.

Endothelial cells can influence blood vessel wall function via vasoactive peptides and other factor(s) synthesized by these cells.[87-89] Thus, angiotensin-converting enzyme, an endothelial cell surface associated enzyme, cleaves the terminal peptide from angiotensin I to form the vasoconstrictor angiotensin II. The same enzyme also has the ability to hydrolyse bradykinin, thereby resulting in the interruption of a vasodilating action. The reactions are briefly summarized in Figure 4.

Recently, an endothelium-derived vascular relaxing factor, "relaxant factor", has been found.[90] It has a short, species-dependent half-life between 5 and 50 sec.[91] It differs from prostanoids, being a ketone or aldehyde, and is not formed via the cyclooxygenase pathway.[91,92] Since endothelial cells are also able to synthesize leukotrienes,[93] their role in regulation of blood vessel contraction is not clear. Moreover, leukotriene, 15 HETE (15-hydroxy-5,8,11,13-eicosatetraenoic acid), is formed during inflammation, and it can be chemotactic. Its function in smooth muscle cell-neutrophil cell-endothelial cell "communication" is also possible. Regarding the formation and action of the relaxant factor, it is released by various stimuli, such as thrombin or acetylcholine, at a concentration of 10^{-7} *M* or less. At a higher concentration of acetylcholine, however, PGI_2 and PGE_2 are also released,[94] and the thrombin action shows species specificity.[528]

3. Endothelium as a Thromboresistant Surface

Whether a plug formation occurs at the appropriate time and place is determined by trigger(s) for the interaction of the blood vessel wall with platelets and with various factors of the blood coagulation-fibrinolytic system. In such an interaction, the subendothelium plays the essential role during injury, whereas the endothelial cells prevent thrombus formation under normal condition.

Endothelial cells can show both thrombotic and thromboresistant properties.[95] A procoagulant factor has been identified as thromboplastin, a tissue factor.[96] The synthesis of this component is inducible by endotoxin, tumor promoter phorbol ester, and by granulocytes and lymphocytes as well as platelets or their extracts.[97,98] Thromboplastin, a phospholipid-protein complex, is the most potent trigger of blood coagulation, although it cannot be in contact with blood without causing damage of cells. F-VIII_{VW}, synthesized by endothelial cells,[63,99] also plays an important role in the adhesion of platelets to the vessel wall.[100] Moreover, endothelial cells possess an enzyme that can activate F-XII by a specific cleavage. F-XII may be the main target for this enzyme, since neither F-XI nor prekallikrein is activated by this.[101] F-XIIa formed leads to activation of both coagulation and kinin-forming pathways.

Endothelial cells also have thrombotic tendency via inhibition of the fibrinolytic system.[102,103] Thrombin, plasmin, fibrinogen, F-X and -Xa, F-IX and -IXa, and prothrombin can bind to endothelial cells. Their exact role, especially in triggering blood coagulation, is not known at present, and if they have any role, it is that they may function during damage of the endothelium.[104] For example, F-IX[105] bound to bovine aortic endothelial cells can be activated by F-XIa or by F-VIIa without exogenous tissue factor when endothelial cells are exposed to phorbol ester.[106,107] The cell-bound F-IXa formed,[107,108] however, requires thrombin-treated F-VIII and Ca^{2+} without exogeneous phospholipid to activate F-X. Both F-X and -Xa can also bind to endothelial cells ($K_d \approx 10^{-9}$ *M*[108]) and the latter activates prothrombin on the aortic endothelial cells.[109] Thus, endothelial cells can promote the activation of F-IX, F-X, and prothrombin in the absence of platelets. Nevertheless, their significance in the initiation of blood coagulation, especially on normal endothelium, is questionable at present.[110]

The most important nature of the intact endothelial cells, however, is their nonthrombogenic character. This involves a specific surface structure, which modifies several biochemical reactions, primarily the activities of proteinases of the blood coagulation-fibrinolytic system and components synthesized and secreted by endothelial cells influencing platelet function as well as affecting the blood coagulation-fibrinolytic system.

a. Surface Structure of the Endothelial Cell Responsible for Its Anticoagulant Nature

Thrombin, the key enzyme of blood coagulation as well as a powerful trigger for platelet aggregation, can react with several molecular and cellular components of hemostasis. Among them, endothelial cells may be important targets for thrombin.

Binding of thrombin to endothelial cells — Thrombin shows high affinity for endothelium — approximately 100 times stronger than that for smooth muscle cells or fibroblasts.[111] Both the association and dissociation of thrombin with endothelial cells are rapid. The equilibrium between bound and free enzyme is attained within 1 min[111-113] and under this condition, thrombin binds to the cells with high and low affinity. Moreover, the active site of the enzyme is not involved in this initial step.[114] After the rapid and reversible binding, however, a slow interaction between enzyme and cell takes place. This second step is irreversible, active site specific, and associated with the formation of a covalent bond between thrombin and the membrane of the endothelial cell.[114]

Structure of thrombin necessary for binding — Thrombin, modified chemically at the active center, binds also to platelets and heparin.[115,116] Modification of arginine residues or of one lysine residue results in the loss of the heparin binding site of the enzyme.[117-119] Furthermore, the binding of thrombin to the endothelial cell is inhibited by heparin.[113,120] Although heparin also binds to endothelial cells[112,121] with high affinity, the K_d is approximately 3×10^{-7} *M*;[113] the inhibitory effect of heparin seems to be a consequence of the binding of the polysaccharide to thrombin rather than to the cells, since binding of heparin to the endothelial cell takes hours, while the thrombin-endothelial cell complex and the thrombin-heparin complex develop in minutes and seconds, respectively.[113,122] Experimental results with modified thrombins indicate that one lysine residue involved in the heparin binding site of the enzyme also participates in the binding of the enzyme with high affinity to endothelial cells.[113] Both interactions are tight; the K_d for thrombin-endothelial cell complex is approximately 10^{-8} *M*, whereas that for the thrombin-heparin complex is about 10^{-9} *M*.[113,118] The difference between the high- and low-affinity binding of enzyme is not clear at present in terms of cell receptors. The data mentioned above, however, suggest a model[115,123,124,525] for the heparin binding domain of thrombin and its relation to the binding domains for fibrinogen, platelets and the endothelial cells. Accordingly, the fibrinogen binding domain extends over a large portion of the enzyme surface overlapping with the low-affinity platelet binding domain. The high-affinity platelet binding domain overlaps with the heparin binding domain, which is involved, at least partially, in the high-affinity endothelial cell binding domain, as well. At present no reliable information is available about the localization of the low-affinity endothelial cell binding domain. The latter interaction may play a role under some pathological conditions, like inflammation or serious tissue damage, when there is enough time to develop a covalent bond between enzyme and cell.[114]

Endothelial cell receptors for thrombin — Endothelial cells have the capacity to bind about 3×10^4 thrombin molecules per cell with high affinity ($K_d \approx 3 \times 10^{-8}$ *M*) and approximately 3×10^6 molecules per cell with low affinity ($K_d \approx 2 \times 10^{-6}$ *M*).[113] These values change slightly depending on the origin of cells and thrombin molecules or even on the methods used for binding studies.[111,113,114,120] The low-affinity receptor for thrombin seems to be an endothelial cell protein with M_r 30,000 daltons, being responsible for the irreversible interaction between cell and enzyme.[114] The exact function of the high-affinity receptors, however, is not known at present. Both heparan sulfate and a specific protein receptor, thrombomodulin, may be the target for thrombin. The possibility that heparan sulfate is a thrombin receptor of the endothelial cell is supported by several data in the literature. Thrombin binding to endothelial cells can be prevented partially by heparitinase or chondroitinase ABC treatment of the cells and also by the presence of protamine or lipoprotein lipase, indicating that glycosaminoglycans of the endothelium may participate in the enzyme binding.[125-127] Endothelial cells are known to synthesize heparan sulfate,[128] and it is also known that several glycosaminoglycans of arteries have an anticoagulant nature.[118,129-131] Thrombin binding to a heparin-like molecule of endothelium is also supported by the finding that heparin inhibits the interaction of thrombin with endothelial cells, especially since thrombin binds to endothelial cells via its heparin binding site.[113,120,132] The role of glycosaminoglycans in the uptake of thrombin by endothelium has also been suggested by different methods.[133,134] Since both thrombin and antithrombin III bind to heparin and to heparin-like components,[135,136] a possible role of heparan sulfate of endothelium in thrombin and antithrombin III binding is suggested. Finally, the finding, that thrombin inactivation by antithrombin III is accelerated by the presence of endothelium, confirms also the role of heparan sulfate in thrombin binding.[113,136,137] Only one report in the literature argues that glycosaminoglycans are not involved in the reversible high affinity binding of thrombin to the vascular endothelium.[138] Thrombomodulin is the other candidate as a receptor for thrombin on the endothelial cell surface.[139] Thrombomodulin is an unusual protein with a M_r 75,000 daltons, having very high proline content and being exceptionally resistant to common denaturants.[140] It binds both thrombin and protein C, with a K_m of approximately 0.48 n*M* and 0.70 μ*M*, respectively, and in this complex, protein C activation by thrombin is accelerated by 1000-fold.[141] Thrombin bound to thrombomodulin, on the other hand, fails to clot fibrinogen to activate platelets or to cleave F-V,[142-144] and is inhibited in F-XIII activation.[145] The possible receptors of endothelial cell for thrombin are shown in Figure 5.

Importance of the interaction of thrombin with endothelial cells — In hemostasis, the most fundamental reactions are the conversion of fibrinogen to fibrin and the adhesion/aggregation of platelets, resulting in a sol-gel transformation of blood plasma. In both processes, thrombin plays an essential role. Besides, thrombin can react with several other molecules and with various cells. Although, thrombin is a multifunctional enzyme, it can react highly specifically with the molecular or cellular components of hemostasis. One of the most exciting questions at present is what determines the choice among the possible reaction routes catalyzed by thrombin? It seems to be an attractive hypothesis that factors, either endogeneous or exogeneous, present at the time and place of thrombin formation, modify the substrate specificity of thrombin. Briefly, thrombin formed from prothrombin may have various conformations depending on components bound to the enzyme. Thus, free thrombin formed in plasma reacts primarily with fibrinogen, F-XIII, F-V, F-VIII, and with platelets. These reactions result in thrombus formation and represent a positive feedback control mechanism. Free thrombin, however, can also react with plasma proteinase inhibitors, like antithrombin III, α_2-macroglobulin, heparin cofactor II, or even α_1-proteinase inhibitor, with the consequence of an enzyme-proteinase inhibitor complex formation, in which thrombin loses or changes its activity. These reactions, however, are relatively slow and take minutes, while clot formation by the fibrinogen-fibrin conversion occurs in a few seconds, thus, before thrombin inactivation blood plasma is coagulated. When heparin or heparin-like molecules are also present, thrombin reacts primarily with antithrombin III, and the reaction rate is so extremely accelerated that thrombin disappears in less than a few seconds. It means that blood plasma practically loses its ability to convert fibrinogen to fibrin. Accordingly, if thrombin binds to the endothelial cell membrane via heparin-like receptor(s), the inactivation of the enzyme is accelerated on the endothelium resulting in prevention of thrombus formation. Several data in the literature support this possibility.[113,126,127,137] The exact mechanism by which thrombin is inactivated by antithrombin III on endothelial cell surface is not clear at present. Antithrombin III also binds to endothelial cells at a different binding site as thrombin.[146,147] Since the concentration of antithrombin III in plasma is high, free antithrombin III can react with thrombin bound to endothelial cell membrane. However, the question of whether the binding of antithrombim III to endothelial cell is necessary for the enhanced inactivation rate of thrombin needs further investigation. If thrombin binds to another kind of receptor of endothelial surface, namely, to thrombomodulin, the conformation of the enzyme is modified in another manner. This form of thrombin reacts primarily with protein C, and the rate of activation of protein C is enhanced by at least 1000-fold.[141] Since activated protein C inactivates F-Va and F-VIIIa, as well as initiates fibrinolysis, the enhanced protein C activation on endothelium should be considered as a negative feedback control mechanism. Thus, thrombin, bound to thrombomodulin on the endothelial cell surface,

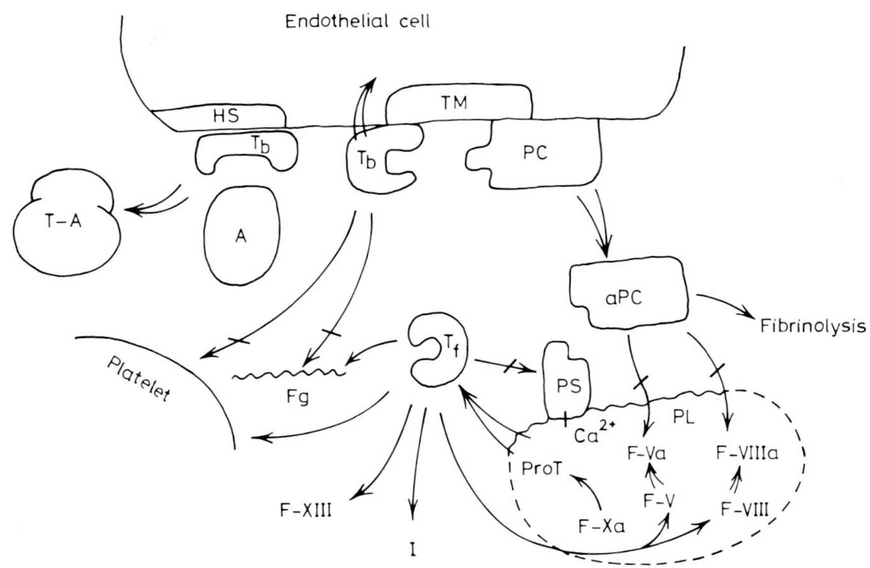

FIGURE 5. Changes in the possible functions of thrombin bound to endothelial cell surface. When thrombin (T_f) is formed during blood coagulation, the enzyme can convert fibrinogen (F_g) to fibrin, F-XIII to F-XIIIa, activate platelet, accelerate its own formation via positive feedback activation of F-VIII and of F-V, inactive protein S (PS), or it may be inactivated by plasma proteinase inhibitors (I), like antithrombin III $(A)_1$, α_2-macroglobulin, heparin cofactor II, or α_1-proteinase inhibitor. All of these reactions, however, promote thrombus formation, except the action with the inhibitor system. Thrombin bound to endothelial cell (T_b) may act in the opposite way, by either inhibiting its own formation from prothrombin (ProT) or being inactivated easily by A on the endothelial cell surface or taken up and digested by the cells directly. If thrombin binds to endothelial cell via heparan sulfate (HS), the rate of its inactivation by A may be extremely enhanced. If thrombin binds to thrombomodulin (TM), the enzyme reacts primarily with protein C (PC) resulting in an accelerated formation of activated protein C (aPC). In addition, thrombin bound to thrombomodulin loses its activity toward fibrinogen, platelet as well as F-V activation and F-XIII activation. aPC, a serine proteinase containing γ-carboxyglutamic acid (Gla), in turn, may initiate fibrinolysis, as well as inactivate F-VIIIa and F-Va, thereby decreasing the rate of activation of ProT by F-Xa in the prothrombinase complex. The action of aPC is facilitated by an additional Gla containing protein, protein S (PS), bound also to the phospholipid (PL) surfaces in the prothrombinase complex via Ca^{2+} bridges. The control of the choices among the possible reaction routes catalyzed by thrombin is not known at present.[525]

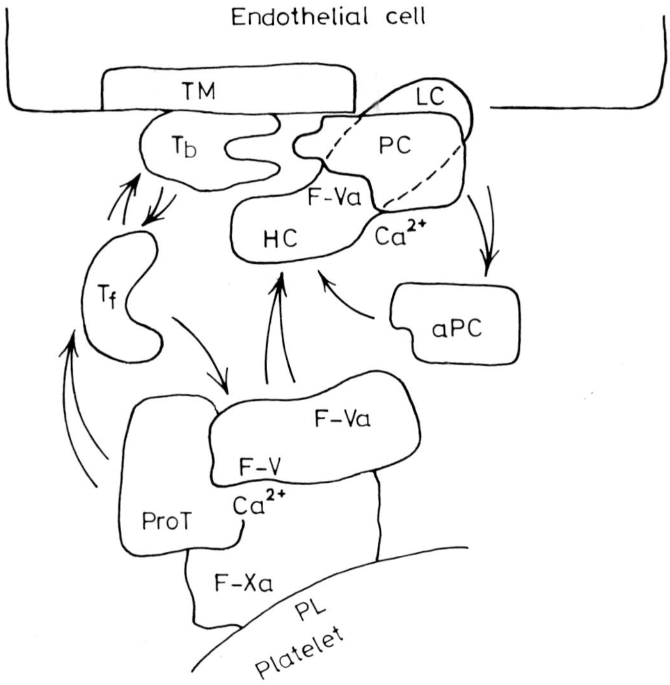

FIGURE 6. Role of F-Va in protein C activation by thrombin on endothelial cell surface. Thrombin (T_f), formed from prothrombin (ProT) in the prothrombinase complex containing F-Xa, F-V, and phospholipid (PL) or platelet membrane, can activate F-V or can bind to endothelial cell. Activated F-Va may also bind to endothelial cell through its light chain (LC). When thrombin binds to endothelial cell via thrombomodulin, it preferentially activates protein C, and this reaction is further accelerated by F-VaLC, up to 50 n*M* concentration. Over this level, however, F-Va as well as F-VaLC are inhibitory. In addition, activated protein C (aPC) also inactivates activated F-V. Thus, these reactions are ''self-controlled'' by positive and negative feedback regulations.

initiates a series of reactions resulting in inhibition of thrombus formation. In addition, thrombin bound to thrombomodulin loses its ability to clot fibrinogen and to activate platelets. The possible reactions of thrombin bound to the endothelial cell via thrombomodulin or heparan sulfate are summarized in Figure 5. The activation of protein C by thrombin on endothelial cell surface is more complicated (Figure 6), since the interaction of thrombin with protein C on endothelium is further influenced by F-V. The rate of thrombin catalyzed protein C activation on human umbilical vein endothelial cells is enhanced by F-Va, as well as by F-Va light chain, in a concentration up to 50 n*M*. Higher concentration of F-Va light chain, on the other hand, inhibits the acceleration of protein C activation on endothelium.[148] It is proposed that when thrombin is formed during vascular injury, thrombin binds to the endothelial cell via thrombomodulin, while F-V is also converted by thrombin to F-Va, containing the 110,000-dalton heavy chain and the 78,000-dalton light chain held together by Ca^{2+}. The endothelial cell bound F-Va further enhances the thrombomodulin accelerated protein C activation by thrombin. The activated protein C formed thereafter destroys F-Va, i.e., the latter loses its accelerating effect on prothrombin activation by F-Xa. The two chains of F-Va dissociate and only the light chain of F-Va remains bound to endothelium via thrombomodulin. Moreover, F-Va, at high concentration, prevents further protein C activation. Accordingly, F-Va, besides its direct action on platelets and blood coagulation, is also able to limit thrombin formation via enhanced protein C activation on endothelium and to increase prothrombin activation through inhibition of activated protein C formation.

Thus, thrombin, at low concentration, favors the inhibition of its own formation via protein C activation, resulting in prevention of thrombosis on normal endothelium. At high concentration, however, thrombin accelerates F-V activation, and as a consequence, both protein C activation is inhibited and prothrombin activation is enhanced directly as well as indirectly, resulting in increased fibrin formation during injury of the blood vessel wall.

b. Components of Endothelial Cells Influencing the Blood Coagulation-Fibrinolytic System, Platelet and Vascular Wall Function; Effects of Thrombin on Endothelium

Thrombin bound to endothelial cells results in reversible shape change of the cells. It is suggested that this alteration is mediated by energy-dependent processes and it is also supposed that extracellular Ca^{2+} influx is not required.[149] This action seems to have a connection with the low-affinity thrombin binding site, since it needs the active center of the enzyme and a relatively long incubation period.[150] The shape changes induced by thrombin, similar to histamine,[151] initiate gap formations in the endothelial monolayer. Although the gaps completely disappear within 24 hr, and their formation can be prevented by antithrombin III and heparin, a transient exposure of subendothelium may play a role in thrombosis and/or atherogenesis.

It is also concluded that normal endothelium of the jugular vein is not damaged by thrombin, and thrombin does not lead to deposition of platelets on the vessel wall, only if animals are pretreated with aspirin.[152] These data suggest that this effect is the result of prostanoid release induced by thrombin. Although it was proposed that while thrombin releases PGI_2 from veins, no such effect is demonstrable with aortas from the identical animal;[153] recent findings show that aortic endothelial cells are also able to synthesize PGI_2 and its release is accelerated by thrombin.[113,154-158]

Prostacyclin (PGI_2) is widely known as a potent inhibitor of platelet aggregation as well as a vasodilator of the blood vessel wall. Thus, PGI_2 may have a specific function relating to the regulation of platelet and vessel wall interactions as well as of vascular tone. The inherent capacity of the various cells present in the blood vessel wall to produce PGI_2 is different, i.e., in fibroblasts, smooth muscle cells, and in endothelial cells, it is low, intermediate, and high, respectively. The release of PGI_2 from the endothelial cells, but not from smooth muscle cells and fibroblasts, can be stimulated not only by thrombin, but by bradykinin, angiotensin II, and by histamine, as well.[159,160] These data mean that the angiotensin-converting enzyme of the endothelial cell surface works in close cooperation with the blood coagulation system.

Regarding the mechanism of PGI_2 stimulation, a thrombin-induced calcium influx and thereby phospholipase A_2 activation seems to be, at present, a reasonable explanation. PGI_2 production, however, cannot be stimulated continuously by thrombin. It is proposed that this process is regulated by different feedback mechanisms, e.g., PGI_2 synthesized inside endothelial cells increases endogeneous cAMP level, and in turn, it inhibits further PGI_2 production.[149,153] The arachidonic acid metabolism in endothelial cells, however, is rather complicated,[157] since endothelial cells have the capacity to synthesize not only PGI_2, but thromboxane A_2 (TXA_2), too, in a ratio of 10:1[149,156,161] leukotrienes,[93] as well as platelet activating factor (PAF).[162,163]

Moreover, nearly four to five leukocytes are reversibly associated with a single endothelial cell,[164,165] and this interaction is influenced by arachidonic acid metabolism. Furthermore, histamine, an inflammatory mediator released from mast cells, triggers PGI_2 production with a consequence of hypotension and plasma exudation. Since leukotrienes are also formed during inflammation and can be chemotactic, these data suggest that a very well-controlled communication system exists among endothelial cells, smooth muscle cells of the vessel wall, platelets, and the polymorphonuclear neutrophil cells.

Another possible mechanism by which endothelium defends against platelet adhesion/

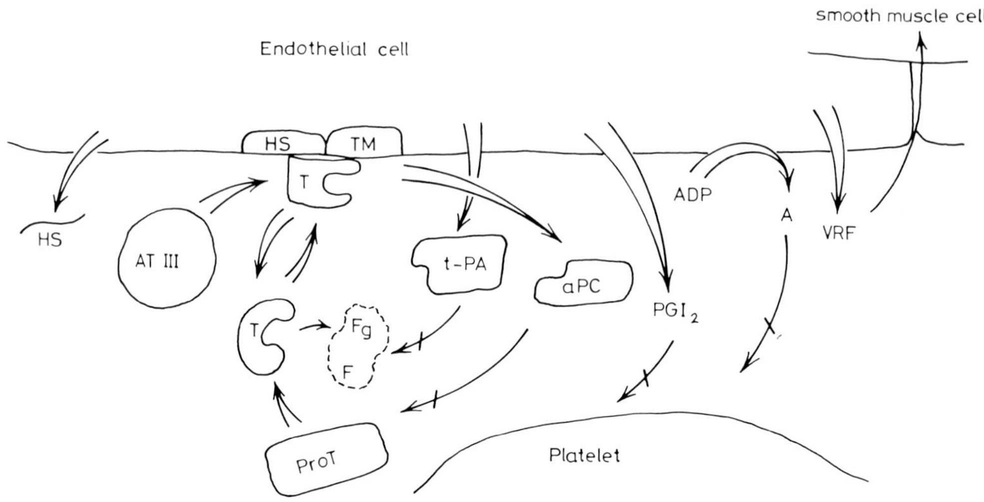

FIGURE 7. Antithrombotic nature of the endothelium. Native endothelial cell prevents thrombus (fibrin and platelet aggregate) formation by the nature of its surface, as well as by humoral components synthesized and secreted by this cell. On its surface, (1) thrombin (T) inactivation by antithrombin III (AT III) may be accelerated, (2) activation of protein C (aPC) is highly enhanced with the consequence of inhibition of prothrombin activation, and (3) the bound thrombin is inhibited toward fibrinogen conversion, platelet activation, F-XIII activation, and F-V activation (also Figure 5). Furthermore, endothelial cells are able to synthesize and secrete heparan sulfate (HS), with heparin-like activity in the thrombin-antithrombin III reaction. Endothelial cell produces and secretes tissue-type plasminogen activator (t-PA) with the capacity to activate plasminogen, primarily on fibrin where it is developed, thereby participating in the removal and dissolution of thrombus. A third way for endothelium to protect against thrombus formation is the inhibition of platelet adhesion/aggregation by (1) the synthesis and secretion of prostacyclin (PGI_2) and (2) by the conversion of ATP, ADP, and AMP (ADP) to adenosine (A) via an ecto-ADP-ase system. Both prostacyclin and adenosine are inhibitors of platelet activation. In addition, the release of a factor, designated vascular relaxant factor (VRF), by endothelial cells antagonizes the contraction of the smooth muscle cells of the blood vessel wall. All these components of endothelial cells contribute to the antithrombotic nature of the vascular wall.

aggregation is the adenosine formation. Endothelial cells require nucleosides for growth,[166] although they are also able to release adenine nucleotides when stimulated by thrombin,[167] and the ADP accumulated extracellularly would induce platelet aggregation. Endothelial cell surface, however, contains an ecto-ADP-ase system[168] which can degrade ATP, ADP, and AMP to adenosine. Adenosine, on the other hand, is a potent inhibitor of platelet aggregation as well as a vasodilator. Although adenosine is taken up by endothelial cells, it can be accumulated in the surrounding medium, since the rate of ADP hydrolysis is approximately 80-fold faster than adenosine uptake.[167]

Moreover, it has been found recently that thrombin stimulates the release of tissue plasminogen activator from endothelial cells.[169] This form of the plasminogen activator(s) (for details see later) shows high affinity to fibrin and the bound enzyme is a powerful activator of plasminogen. Plasmin formed, on the other hand, resolves fibrin, as well as activates the 1-chain tissue plasminogen activator ($M_r \approx 64{,}000$ daltons) to form a 2-chain, disulfide-bound, serine proteinase with the capacity to activate plasminogen to plasmin.[170] Thus, plasmin formed and bound to endothelial cells[171] can activate tissue plasminogen activator, resulting in a positive feedback mechanism of plasmin formation, thereby increasing fibrinolysis. Thus, endothelium participates very actively not only in the prevention of blood coagulation, inhibition of platelet aggregation, or in the regulation of blood vessel wall contraction, but it determines also the place and time of the activation of the fibrinolytic system. Accordingly, most, if not all, of these features discussed above emphasize the antithrombotic nature of the normal endothelium. These data are summarized in Figure 7.

III. STRUCTURE AND FUNCTION OF PLATELETS

Platelets are contractile as well as secretory cells. They can perform several functions in hemostasis by the storage and release of different biologically active molecules. The most important function of platelets, however, is their ability to lose their uniform distribution in blood plasma, forming aggregate and/or adhering to vascular surfaces.

A. Origin and Morphology of Platelets

Platelets, the anucleated cell fragments of bone marrow, megakaryocytes appear in blood circulation with a life span of 9 to 12 days in man.[172] They have discoid shape with a volume[173] of about 7 μm^3. Approximately 200,000 to 400,000 platelets per microliter of blood can be found in normal humans. If this number falls below 50,00 cells per microliter, petechial and purpural hemorrhages or excessive bleeding may develop in response to tissue injuries, and under 20,000 cells per microliter, spontaneous hemorrhage may occur.[174,175]

1. Megakaryocytes

Blood platelets originate from megakaryocytes of bone marrow,[176] whereas megakaryocytes develop from megakaryoblasts, which in turn originate from stem cells.[177] The megakaryocytes are polyploid with 4, 8, or 16 nuclear lobes, identified as 8N, 16N, or 32N types, respectively.[178] During maturation, the ratio of cytoplasm to nucleus increases, and at the last stage of development, megakaryocytes have a distinctly granular appearance, breaking up into platelets. Megakaryocyte maturation and the amount of platelets appearing in peripheral blood circulation may be under humoral control. Kidney and spleen are believed[179-181] to synthesize thrombopoietic stimulation factor(s), especially after hemorrhage, but the nature of such a factor has not yet been clearly identified.

2. Structure of Platelets

Platelet is the smallest cell type of mammalian blood. It lacks a nucleus like the red cell, but as a contractile and secretory cell, the platelet exhibits a variety of functions and a complexity of structure, reminding one of other tissues like nerve cells, specialized secretory organs, or smooth muscle cells.

To follow its functional activities, the complicated anatomy of platelet has been schematically divided into various regions.[182] The pheripheral zone, the sol-gel zone, the organelle zone, and the membrane system of the platelet are the major structural elements. The structural elements of the peripheral zone include the cell surface and the channels of the open canalicular system (OCS), representing invaginations of the plasma membranes, thereby resulting in a large surface area exposed to blood plasma. The peripheral zone consists of the exterior coat (glycocalyx), the unit membrane, and the submembrane region.

The exterior coat is composed of glycosaminoglycans, glycolipids, and various glycoproteins, i.e., Ia, Ib, Ic, IIa, IIb, III, IV, and V (for details, see Reference 529). They are generally responsible for the binding of the various agents inducing adhesion/aggregation and changes in the shape of platelets. The phospholipid membrane composes the platelet factor 3 (PF3) structure, which accelerates blood coagulation, although the mechanism by which it becomes available for the blood coagulation factors is not known at present.[183] The unit membrane provides the separation of intracelllular and extracellular constituents containing a Na/K ATP-ase and other cation and anion pumps which maintain the appropriate transmembrane ionic gradients. The submembrane region lies under the unit membrane and is built up from microfilaments participating in the maintenance of discoid shape in a close association with cell surface and with the microtubules of sol-gel zone.

The sol-gel zone represents a fiber system of platelets, and consists of the microtubules and the main contractile system, the microfilaments, which can be rapidly formed during platelet activation. In this zone, glycogen particles also occur with a possible energy supply. The rate of glycolysis is higher in platelets than in red cells or smooth muscle cells, and glucose is metabolized primarily to lactate.[184] Glycolysis is the main energy source of platelets providing for aggregation, secretion, and clot retraction functions.[185,186]

The organelle zone contains granules approximately 0.2 to 0.3 μm in diameter varying in electron density. The less electron dense, α-granules are round, oval, or irregular in form and are enclosed by unit membrane.[187] The most electron dense granules, the dense granules or dense bodies, are less numerous. Dense granules and α-granules, together with the lysosome-like organelles, are discharged during platelet release reaction. Mitochondria are also located in the organelle zone.

The internal membrane systems of platelets consisting of the open canalicular system (OCS) and the dense tubular system (DTS) cannot be found in other blood cells.[188] The OCS is formed by invaginations of surface membrane, tunneling into the cytoplasm like a serpent, and they serve as conduits for components secreted by platelets during the release reaction. The DTS originates from the rough endoplasmic reticulum of the megakaryocyte. Ca^{2+}/Mg^{2+} ATP-ase as well as cyclooxygenase are localized to DTS, suggesting that DTS is the place for prostaglandin synthesis as well as the storage site for calcium.[189] These two membrane systems, namely OCS and DTS, are not completely isolated from each other within the platelets.

B. Platelet Adhesion and Aggregation

Platelets show high propensity to adhere to almost any surface which is not normal, thus to surfaces formed by damage of endothelium or to artificial surfaces. The interaction of platelets with other cells or surfaces is called platelet adhesion. Platelets are also able to form aggregate when stimulated, thereby changing their homogeneous distribution in plasma. The platelet-platelet interaction, initiated by various triggers, is known as platelet aggregation. While in platelet adhesion F-VIII_{vW} is an essential "cofactor", in platelet aggregation fibrinogen and Ca^{2+} serve as accessory components.[190] Through these functions, platelets significantly contribute to hemostatic plug formation in order to prevent mortal hemorrhage, or, on the other hand, they are highly involved in thrombus formation under pathological conditions.

1. Morphological Changes of Platelets During Plug Formation

Normal platelets are disk-shaped, approximately 3 μm in diameter and 1 μm in thickness,[191] and this form is maintained by the submembrane filaments in cooperation with the circumferential microtubules of the sol-gel zone.[192] When platelets are exposed to agents inducing activation, the discoid shape can be changed. Platelets contain a contractile system as well, consisting of microtubules and microfilaments.[193] They are involved in the pseudopod extension, internal contraction, secretion of granular constituents, and in clot retraction.[194] The tubules themselves do not deliver contractile forces and do not affect platelet contraction and clot retraction,[195] but govern the internal architecture; namely organelles are moved to the center of the cell, in a proper orientation for facilitating secretory process. Since platelets are frequently exposed to various stimuli of the circulating blood, the microtubules may prevent an overwhelming secretory response and enable the incompletely activated platelets to recover their original form.[196]

The most important elements of the platelet contractile system, however, are the microfilaments of the sol-gel zone. Without stimuli, subunits of the microfilament proteins (actin and myosin) exist in a viscous state. After platelet stimulation, they are polymerized into filaments. Platelet filaments are approximately 5 nm in diameter and resemble actin-like structures, like in muscle. They act as muscle actomyosin with ATP-ase activity depending on Ca^{2+} concentration.[197] Increase of Ca^{2+} level by the action of thromboxane A_2 (TXA_2)

or by the phosphatidylinositol system leads to the actin-like molecules (thrombostenin B) to interact with the myosin-like structures of platelet (thrombostenin A). The ATP-dependent conformational change pulls one filament against the next, resulting in contraction. As a consequence, contents of granules of platelets are secreted. It is interesting that when several platelets are in adjacent position, the contraction is oriented toward the center of the cluster. The asymmetric location of contractile gel in aggregated platelets may be explained by the role of α-actin bound to the cytoplasmic side of the membrane,[198] which anchors the contraction of the platelet membranes in areas where platelets are adjacent. After discharge of the secretory organelles, the ring of the microtubules becomes fractured. If secretion does not take place, the aggregated or adhered cells recover their discoid form.[199]

When activation and secretion takes place, platelets become committed to participate in thrombus formation. The contents of storage organelles, released directly to the exterior, play various biological roles. The contractile system of platelets, however, has an additional function, namely serum is squeezed out of a blood clot during several hours, called clot retraction. Clot retraction involves a complex interaction between platelets and the fibrin meshwork of the clot.[186] Finally, platelet aggregate, together with fibrin network, may be incorporated into a thrombus, resulting in the normal or pathological occlusion of the wound or blood vessel wall, respectively.

2. *Components Released by Platelet Activation*

When platelets adhere to damaged vessel walls and/or form aggregate, as discussed earlier, they can release the content of their various granules.[200] Three subcellular structures, α-granules, dense granules, and lysosome-like granules, contain the main components participating in hemostasis, tissue repair, wound healing, and inflammation. These components may be released in different phases, depending on the stimuli:[201,202] first, α-granules; second, dense granules; and finally lysosomal enzymes, although these phases may overlap. Various stimuli trigger the release via different receptors, and each receptor initiates the release of certain amount of transmitters, like Ca^{2+}, stored at the membrane. The release reaction, an exocytosis, is ATP dependent.[201]

The most important constituents of platelet storage organelles are summarized in Figure 8. Their biological functions vary extremely. Briefly, while the components of dense granules play a role in the amplification of platelet activation, the hydrolytic enzymes of lysosome-like granules primarily influence the integrity of the blood vessel walls; the components of α-granules participate in the cellular interactions. Blood coagulation factors are involved primarily in the rate enhancement of thrombin formation. The components of granules are structurally, as well as functionally, very different. The heparin binding proteins, platelet factor 4, low affinity platelet factor 4, and β-thromboglobulin, act in the direction of increased fibrin formation by the neutralization of heparin action in the thrombin-antithrombin III reaction. Platelet-derived growth factor (PDGF), an approximately M_r 30,000-dalton polypeptide chain with extensive identity with the internal segment of the $p28^{sis}$ gene product of a sarcoma virus,[203] has mitogenic activity on various cells; thus smooth muscle cells, fibroblasts, and endothelial cells can be the target for these factors.* Whether the components of the granules are secreted by the platelet actively or they are liberated only by the damage of the cells is questionable at present. Their most significant function, however, besides influencing hemostasis, may be the stimulation of tissue repair, wound healing, or contribution to the development of blood vessel wall injury in atherosclerosis. Furthermore, the vascular permeability factor, bactericidal factor, and chemotactic factor, as well as serotonin, together with the lysosomal hydrolases, may play a role in inflammation. The possible roles of arachidonate metabolism will be discussed later.

* The receptor for the PDGF, also encoded by several tumor viruses, has M_r 180,000 daltons with tyrosine kinase activity.[203]

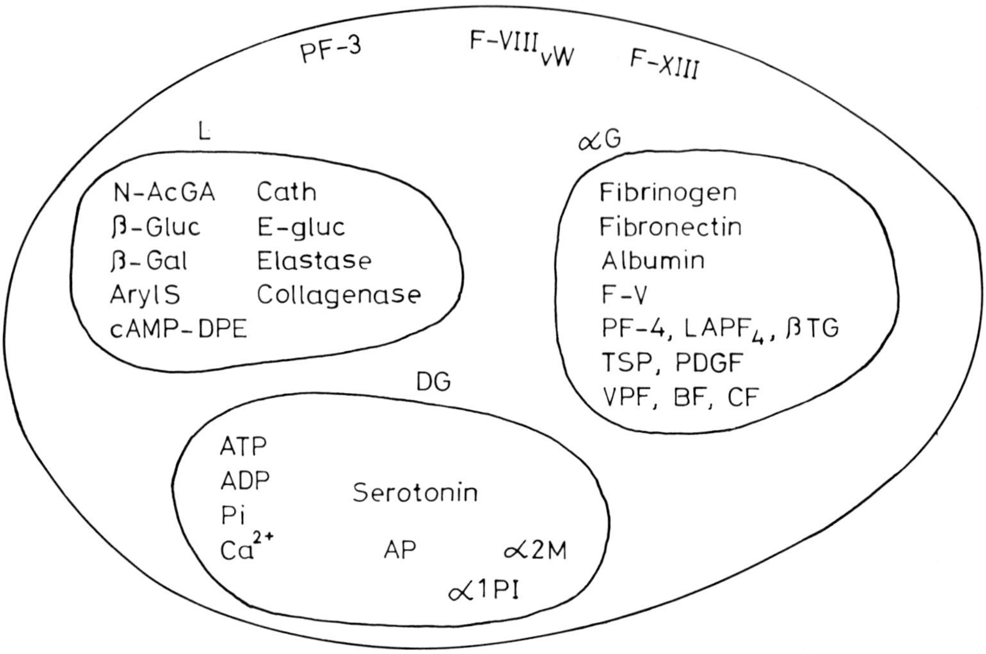

FIGURE 8. Components of platelet granules. Abbreviations: L, lysosome-like granule; DG, dense granule; α-G, α-granule; N-AcGA, N-acetyl glucosaminidase; β-Gal, β-galactosidase; ArylS, arylsulfatase; cAMP-DPE, cyclic 3′,5′-nucleotide diphosphoesterase; Cath, cathepsines; E-gluc, endoglucosidase; Ap, antiplasmin; α2M, α_2-macroglobulin; α1PI, α_1-proteinase inhibitor; PF4, platelet factor 4; LAPF4, low affinity platelet factor 4; β-TG, β-thromboglobulin; TSP, thrombospondin; PDGF, platelet derived growth factor; VPF, vascular permeability factor; BF, bactericidal factor; CF, chemotactic factor; PF3, platelet factor 3; F-V, Factor-V; F-XIII, Factor XIII; F-VIII_{vW}.

3. Surface Formation on Platelets for Acceleration of Blood Coagulation

As mentioned earlier, thrombin, an enzyme responsible for the most essential reactions in blood coagulation, does not exist in plasma under normal conditions. Thrombin is formed from prothrombin. The amount of thrombin formed, however, depends on the amount and activity of another proteinase, namely on F-Xa formed during the "cascade" of the blood coagulation system. The "cascade" involves the conversion of proenzymes to active enzymes, and in turn, they activate the next proenzyme, working as an amplifier. Moreover, these reactions take place in complexes, where, at each stage, zymogen activation rates are enhanced 10^4 to 10^5 times (for details, see Section IV).

Phospholipids provide the surface for coagulation factors via calcium bridges, primarily for vitamin K-dependent proteins containing Gla, and thus for prothrombin, F-X, F-IX, F-VII, protein C, and for protein S. Under normal conditions, the external surface of platelet membrane is not available for interaction with coagulation factors. During injury and/or membrane rupture, the inner phospholipid structure is exposed to the blood coagulation factors.[204] As a consequence, a positive feedback mechanism occurs between platelet stimulation and thrombin formation, resulting in additional acceleration of blood coagulation. For instance, during the damage to a vessel wall, collagen may be exposed to blood, triggering platelet activation. In the next step, activated platelet releases ADP, which induces activation of additional cells. The morphological change of the platelets makes phospholipids available for blood coagulation factors, primarily for prothrombin, F-X and F-IX. As a result, thrombin formation is accelerated. The thrombin formed, in turn, can attack directly additional intact platelets inducing further platelet aggregation and also activating F-V as well as FVIII.

Thereafter, activated F-V binds to prothrombin and F-Xa[205] on the phospholipid surface of activated platelet and the reaction rate of the prothrombin conversion is extremely enhanced.

Thrombin, on the other hand, can also bind to endothelial cells,[206] resulting in the activation of protein C.[207,208] The functions of activated protein C are the inactivation of F-Va[209,210] and F-VIIIa,[211] as well as the initiation of fibrinolysis.[212] The inactivation of F-Va in the prothrombinase complex on the platelet surface is also controlled by an additional vitamin K-dependent protein, i.e., protein S, bound to phospholipid surface, accelerates F-Va inactivation by activated protein C[213] by two to three orders of magnitude of rate enhancements.[214] These reactions involving proteins C and S, can be considered as a negative feedback regulation of thrombin formation (see also Figures 5 and 7). Moreover, activated platelets are able to interact with endothelial cells, and as a consequence, endothelial cell surface and components secreted by these cells further influence the reactions mentioned. Polymorphonuclear granulocytes generally also participate in these interactions with different functions. Thus, the exact interpretation of the importance of the various functions discussed earlier is far beyond our understanding.

C. Mechanisms of Platelet Activation

Although there is no direct evidence at present for the mechanism of activation of the contractile system of platelets, it is very probable that Ca^{2+} is the activator as well as the controller of the ultimate events of platelet activation-aggregation-release reactions. Since very different stimuli may lead to platelet aggregation, the most important question is how is Ca^{2+} mobilized inside the platelet?

According to our present knowledge, arachidonate and phosphatidylinositol metabolism are essential pathways for controlling the amount of Ca^{2+} acting on the contractile system. Besides Ca^{2+}, cAMP is also a transmitter between cell membrane and intracellular events. The two pathways, however, are not separated from each other.

Arachidonate metabolism, called also arachidonate cascade, starts with phospholipase A_2 activation by Ca^{2+} released from the platelet membrane.[215] Activated phospholipase A_2 thereafter splits arachidonic acid from membrane phospholipids. Cyclooxygenase converts arachidonic acid to endoperoxides (PGG_2, PGH_2) and the arachidonic acid oxygenated and cyclized is further modified by an enzyme in platelet, primarily by thromboxane synthetase resulting in thromboxane A_2 (TXA_2) formation. TXA_2 is considered an endogeneous calcium ionophore, responsible for the mobilization of Ca^{2+} from the dense bodies, where its concentration is unusually high. Finally, Ca^{2+} released activates the contractile system, and as a result, the release of the granules, containing aggregation inductors, is stimulated leading to the aggregation of additional platelets. The mechanism works as a positive feedback acceleration of platelet activation-aggregation. The overall processes are summarized in Figure 9.

1. Phospholipase A_2 Activation; the Ca^{2+}-Dependent Pathway

When a trigger initiates Ca^{2+} release, very probably via phospholipase C activation and an increase of inositol phospholipid turnover,[216,217] phospholipase A_2 is activated by this calcium and arachidonate becomes available for the cyclooxygenase system, As a result, thromboxan A_2 is formed with the consequence of the additional reactions discussed above. Besides, Ca^{2+} released by inositol triphosphate may activate directly the contractile system of platelets (Figure 9).

2. Inhibition of Adenylate Cyclase Activity; the cAMP-Dependent Pathway

Arachidonic acid metabolism is under a sophisticated control, and besides calcium, the cAMP level is also integrated in its regulation. For example, cAMP decreases TXA_2 formation through the inhibition of the activity of phospholipase A_2 and cyclooxygenase and

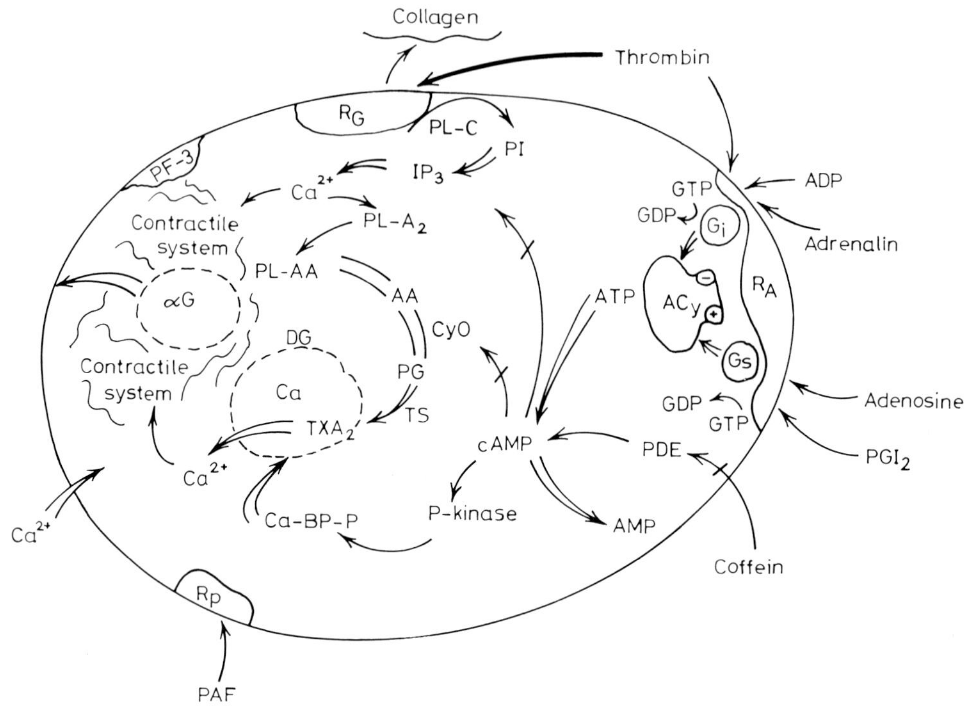

FIGURE 9. Mechanism of platelet activation and aggregation. Thrombin or collagen, bound to one kind of platelet receptor (R_G), initiates the activation of phospholipase C (PL-C), resulting in Ca^{2+} release from the endoplasmatic reticulum via the phosphatidyl inositol (PI)-inositol triphosphate (IP_3) system. The Ca^{2+} formed, in turn, may activate either phospholipase A_2 (PL-A_2) or the contractile system directly. The reaction routes of the Ca^{2+} action may be determined by calmodulin. By the action of PL-A_2, arachidonic acid (AA) is released from phospholipid (PL-AA) and converted to thromboxane A_2 (TXA_2) through prostaglandin endoperoxide(s) (PG) by the catalysis of cyclooxygenase (CyO) and thromboxane synthetase (TS). TXA_2 formed can mobilize Ca^{2+} from dense granule (DG), and the increased Ca^{2+} level further activates the contractile system of the platelet. As a consequence, phospholipids (PF-3) become available for blood coagulation factors and both α-granules (α-G) and DG are released. At a final stage, Ca^{2+} influx also contributes to the retraction of the platelet. The processes described are under the control of cAMP, i.e., cAMP inhibits calcium mobilization as well as TXA_2 formation. In addition, calcium pump (Ca-BP-P) is activated by protein kinase (P-kinase) phosphorylation in the presence of cAMP, resulting in the uptake of free Ca^{2+} by DG. Thus, intracellular increase of cAMP level inhibits platelet aggregation, whereas decrease of its level contributes to platelet activation. cAMP level, however, is regulated by adenylate cyclase (ACy) as well as phosphodiesterase (PDE) activities. Activation of ACy through Gs protein of another platelet receptor (R_A) by adenosine or PGI_2 as well as inhibition of PDE by caffeine, theophylline, papaverin, etc. result in cAMP elevation with protection against platelet aggregation. Epinephrine (adrenaline), ADP, or thrombin, on the other hand, are inhibitory for ACy activity via mobilization of Gi protein from the R_A receptor, thereby decreasing cAMP level, which, in turn, favors platelet aggregation. There exists a third way of platelet activation as well, i.e., a nonarachidonate-mediated initiation of platelet activation by platelet activating factor (PAF). Although this activation also involves calcium mobilization, the exact mechanism is unknown at present.

also decreases the intracellular calcium level via activation of the calcium-pump participating in Ca^{2+} reuptake by the pools.[218] Thus, when a membrane stimulus affects adenylate cyclase in such a way that the enzyme activity is inhibited, cAMP level decreases in the platelets; the enzymes involved in arachidonate metabolism are liberated from the inhibition, resulting in increased TXA_2 formation. Thus, release and aggregation proceed (Figure 9).

Antiaggregatory reactions can also develop either via the activation of adenylate cyclase or via the inhibition of phosphodiesterase involved in cAMP hydrolysis. In both cases, cAMP level increases and, as a consequence, TXA_2 formation decreases.

3. Platelet Activating Factor (PAF)

PAF, 1-*O*-alkyl-2-acetyl-*sn*-glycerol-3-phosphorylcholine,[219] is also a mediator of platelet aggregation.[220] In this mechanism, thrombin receptor, as well as TXA_2 and ADP are not involved.[221] PAF, released from leukocytes, is a very potent inducer of platelet aggregation and release reaction at a very low concentration, and it plays an important role in inflammation, in the interaction of platelet with leukocytes, and in vascular permeability changes.[222] The exact mechanism of its action is not known at present.

D. Triggers for Platelet Activation

Platelets are very sensitive to a variety of substances, which are endogenous and exogenous. Thus, collagen, ADP and its analogues,[223] thrombin, trypsin, papain, pronase,[224] fatty acids,[225,226] arachidonic acid,[227] bacterial endotoxins,[228,229] exotoxins,[230] heparin,[231] polylysine,[232] vasopressin,[233] dextrans,[234,235] hydrogen peroxide,[236] lectins,[237,238] snake venoms,[239] and several additional physiological as well as artificial components[240] have been reported to activate platelets. In this chapter, the survey of the possible triggers for platelet aggregation is restricted to the most important endogeneous agents playing the main role in physiological or/and pathological platelet aggregation.

1. Collagen

Collagens, being vascular constituents, may be in contact with circulating blood cells during damage of the blood vessel wall. Among the various collagens, type I and III are the potent inducers of platelet aggregation.[241] Different structural requirements for collagen are necessary to induce adhesion-aggregation. Thus, the native triple helix, the presence of lysine amino groups, and the degree of polymerization of collagen have been noted as requirements for being a trigger of platelet aggregation and release reactions. The mechanism by which collagen induces platelet activation is very probably the activation of phospholipase C (Figure 9).

2. Thrombin

Thrombin, formed during blood coagulation, is a powerful trigger for platelet activation and release reaction. The signal transmission may be initiated by the interaction of thrombin with at least two membrane receptors. Thus, phospholipase C activity can be stimulated, resulting in calcium release and/or a decrease of cAMP level mediated by the enzyme action on the adenylate cyclase receptor, which stimulates an increase in TXA_2 synthesis. Both ways, however, initiate the activation of the contractile system of platelets via action of Ca^{2+} released[242] (Figure 9).

3. ADP

ADP (but neither ATP nor AMP) is a secondary aggregating agent in the sense that it originates from platelets. For example, platelets accelerate their aggregation by releasing ADP from their dense granules, therefore this action is a positive feedback amplification. Approximately 8×10^4 binding sites for ADP exist on a platelet,[243] but ADP is not taken up by these cells.[244] Although the mechanism by which ADP induces platelet aggregation is not known exactly at present, the inhibition of adenylate cyclase by membrane bound ADP seems to be a possible explanation for the ADP-induced aggregation (Figure 9). Moreover, ADP may contribute to platelet aggregation by another mechanism as well. In platelet aggregate, the cells are bridged by Ca^{2+} and fibrinogen.[245,246] Under normal conditions, however, the receptors for these molecules are not available. ADP is considered to act by unmasking the Ca^{2+}-dependent fibrinogen receptors on platelets.[247]

4. Other Stimuli for Platelet Aggregation

The catecholamines, adrenaline and noradrenaline produce aggregation by the release of the granules of the platelet.[248,249] The exact nature of the receptor(s) is not known at present. Both α- and β-receptors have been suggested to participate in adrenaline-platelet interaction.[250,251] An action, via direct binding to thrombostenin,[252] has also been suggested as a possible mechanism for the platelet aggregation-release reaction.

Although serotonin is actively taken up and stored in the dense granules of platelet,[253] it can also yield platelet aggregation.[254] This response of the cells to serotonin, however, is only a single, reversible aggregation.[255] The physiological and/or pathological roles of serotonin in hemostasis and in pulmonary hypertension, and the function of platelets as merely transport vehicle for serotonin, are not clear at present.

Arachidonic acid added to platelets also induces platelet aggregation, being a substrate for TXA_2 formation. TXA_2 given extracellularly results in platelet aggregation.[256] The receptor(s) for PAF as well as the mechanism of platelet activation by PAF, as mentioned before, have not been documented yet.

E. Protection of Endothelium Against Platelet Adhesion and Aggregation

There can be no doubt about the criterion of endothelium to function as a nonthrombogenic surface to permit continuous blood circulation. There are several mechanisms by which endothelial cells, either by their products or by their surface properties, prevent platelet adhesion and aggregation.

1. Role of Prostacyclin (PGI_2)

Endothelial cells, both arterial and venous, produce PGI_2, and its synthesis-release is enhanced by various stimuli. Thus, thrombin formed and bound to endothelium induces increased PGI_2 release from native endothelial cells.[155] PGI_2 released activates adenylate cyclase, which increases cAMP formation, with the consequence of decreased TXA_2 synthesis. A decreased TXA_2 level, in turn, results in the inhibition of platelet aggregation (Figure 9).

2. Adenosine Formation

Endothelial cell surface contains an ecto-ADP-ase, which hydrolyses ATP, ADP, as well as AMP to adenosine.[167,168] Adenosine, on the other hand, is an inhibitor of platelet aggregation and is also a potent vasodilator. As a result of these reactions, platelet aggregation/adhesion is inhibited on normal endothelium (Figure 9).

3. Inactivation of Thrombin and Inhibition of Thrombin Formation on Endothelial Cell Surface

Thrombin is one of the most powerful triggers for platelet activation. On the other hand, when thrombin is bound to the endothelial cell via thrombomodulin, its activity on platelet surface is inhibited, but the activation of protein C is enhanced, resulting in a decrease in the rate of additional thrombin formation. Endothelial bound thrombin, however, is easily released, restoring its function on the platelet. Thrombin is also able to bind to the endothelial cell through heparin-like surface, very probably heparan sulfate, and this form of the enzyme may show a high sensitivity to antithrombin III, resulting in its accelerated inactivation by this inhibitor. Thus, the endothelial cell surface prevents platelet aggregation and thrombus formation (Figure 7).

IV. BLOOD COAGULATION

The most important feature of the circulating blood is its ability to lose its fluidity. This sol-gel conversion is based on the unusual character of a molecule in blood plasma, i.e., the fibrinogen. While fibrinogen is extremely soluble in water phase, after the loss of only two small peptides, it becomes insoluble. This reaction, the conversion of fibrinogen to fibrin, is the most crucial step in blood coagulation.

A. Conversion of Fibrinogen to Fibrin

Fibrin formation, however, is a very complicated process and involves several steps. Three phases, proteolysis, polymerization, and stabilization, can be distinguished during the conversion of fibrinogen to fibrin, although these steps are not separated in time from each other.

1. Structure of Fibrinogen

Fibrinogen, a glycoprotein with M_r 340,000 daltons,[257] is an elongated molecule[258] with considerable flexibility, having a length of approximately 450 Å and a cross-section[259] of 90 × 40 Å (Figure 10). It is synthesized and secreted by the liver and occurs in plasma at a high concentration, approximately 10 μM.[260]

Fibrinogen is composed of six polypeptide chains in the form of a symmetrical dimer, in which the chains as well as the dimer are held together by disulfide bridges.[261-263] The three types of polypeptide chains are designated Aα-, Bβ-, and γ-chain, containing 610, 461, and 410 amino acid moieties, respectively.[264] Thus, the entire molecule can be denoted as $(A\alpha, B\beta, \gamma)_2$ (Figure 10).

2. Molecular Mechanism of Fibrin Formation

The changes in fibrinogen molecule are initiated by the hydrolysis of four arginyl-glycine bonds, two on each of the Aα- and the Bβ-chains, respectively. The γ-chains are not involved in this process. After splitting of the specific peptide bonds, two kinds of peptides, fibrinopeptide A (FPA) and fibrinopeptide B (FPB), containing 16 and 14 amino acids,* respectively, can be released. The resulting molecule, the fibrinogen minus fibrinopeptides, is called fibrin monomer. Since fibrinogen is a dimer, four peptides can be hydrolysed. Thus, when one FPA, two FPA, or all four peptides are lost, the molecule is designated as des-A fibrin, des-AA fibrin, or des-AABB fibrin, respectively.

During the proteolytic phase, thrombin attacks the specific bonds, and the release of FPA is faster than that of FPB.[266] Regarding the kinetics of human fibrinopeptide release, a k_{cat}/K_m of 11 × 10^6 M^{-1} sec^{-1} for FPA and a k_{cat}/K_m of 3.9 × 10^6 M^{-1} sec^{-1} for FPB have been found.[267] It has also been suggested that the rate of release of FPB increases later in the reaction due to a conformational change in the des-AA fibrin oligomer.[268] For these actions of thrombin, a specific interaction between thrombin and fibrinogen is necessary. Both fibrinogen and thrombin are responsible for the high specificity. For instance, thrombin activity toward fibrinogen substrate can be lost, without decrease in proteolytic activity against small peptide substrate, indicating several intermolecular interactions.[269] For example, while fibrinogen is clotted by α-thrombin, fibrinogen is a poor substrate for β- or γ-thrombin, although these proteolytically modified enzymes retain their amidase and esterase activities.[270] Thus, the specificity of thrombin resides partly in the enzyme structure. The structure of fibrinogen, on the other hand, also contributes to the high specificity. The thrombin binding site of fibrinogen may be localized to the Phe8-Arg16, the Pro34-Lys44, as well as to the Cys45-Met51 sequences of the Aα-chain.[271,272] The localization of the thrombin binding site on Bβ-chain is not known at present.

During and after the limited proteolysis, however, another reaction, a nonenzymatic assembly process, with end-to-end and side-to-side interactions of fibrin monomers called polymerization takes place, resulting in the insoluble fibrin formation. In these reactions, several discrete steps serve different functions in the fibrin formation process[265] (Figure 10).

* The number of amino acid moieties of fibrinopeptides shows species specificity.

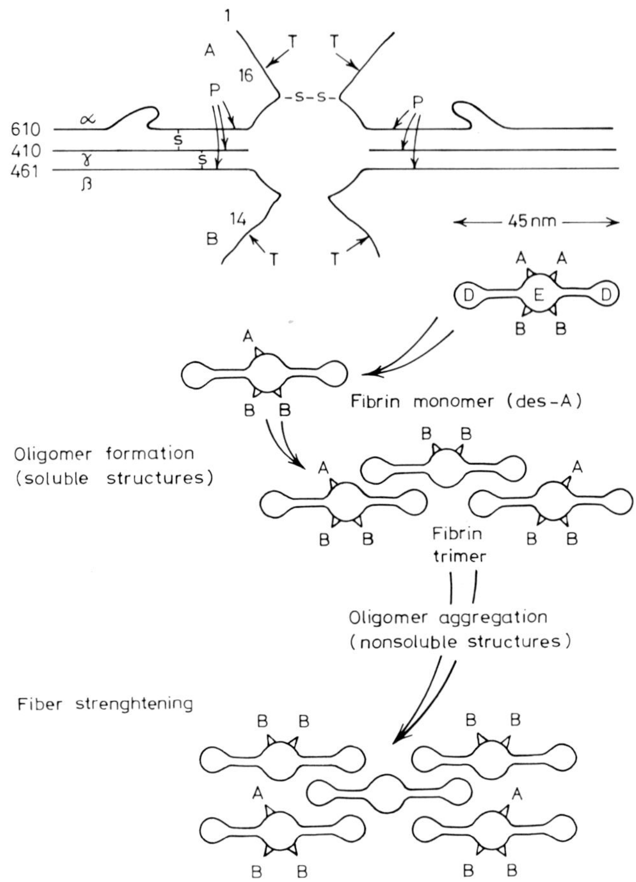

FIGURE 10. Structure of fibrinogen; actions of thrombin and plasmin. Fibrinogen consists of six polypeptide chains in the form of a covalently connected symmetrical dimer with M_r 340,000 daltons. In each half of the dimer, the three chains, designated Aα with an amino acid sequence of 1 to 610, Bβ of 1 to 461, and γ with an also known sequence of 1 to 410, are connected by disulfide bridges. The two halves of the dimer are also coupled with cystine links. There are a total of 29 disulfide bonds in the molecule. Thrombin splits two peptide bonds, i.e., between residues 16 and 17 of the Aα-chain and between residues 14 and 15 of the Bα-chain, resulting in the release of fibrinopeptide A (A) and fibrinopeptide B (B), respectively. On the basis of plasmin (P) digestion, other structural elements of fibrinogen can be distinguished, i.e., domain E (E) with M_r 51,600 daltons and domain D (D) containing 101 residues of α-, 327 residues of β-, and 347 amino acid residues of γ-chain, with an approximate M_r of 100,000 daltons. During fibrin formation, fibrinopeptide A and B are released by different rates. First, soluble fibrin oligomers are formed (for technical reasons, the processes are symbolized by E-D domain scheme, according to Reference 265). When several fibrinopeptides A are released, the assembly of fibrin oligomers forms aggregate, and the release of fibrinopeptide B is initiated with the consequence of strengthening of intra- and interoligomeric bonds resulting in water-insoluble fibrin formation. Finally, γ- and α-chains are cross-linked by F-XIIIa via lysine-glutamine covalent bonds (not shown in this figure).

The release of FPA by thrombin is the driving force for the fibrinogen conversion. The polymerization of the fibrin monomers into fibrin oligomers is immediate and irreversible, although this oligomeric bonding is not covalent. As thrombin continues its proteolytic action, larger oligomers are formed progressively. An additional assembly of fibrin oligomers into laterally associated fibrils and subsequent fiber, with network formation and gelation, occurs without the release of FPB. Thrombin can release FPB only from fibrin oligomeric structures, and as a consequence, the intraoligomeric bonds are strengthened, and also new interoligomeric interactions and strengthening of the interoligomeric bonds take place. Finally, cross-linkings are formed between Lys and Gln of antiparallel aligned γ-chains by the action of F-XIIIa, and this phase is called as stabilization. F-XIIIa, however, is also formed by the action of thrombin on the inactive zymogen molecule. From the tetrameric F-XIII (a_2b_2), an activation peptide is removed by thrombin from a_2 subunits containing the active sites, resulting in a modified tetramer molecule, designated as $a_2'b_2$. As a consequence, Ca^{2+} is able to induce an additional conformational change, necessary for the dissociation of a_2 and b_2 dimers, and the unmasking of active site SH groups (for more details, see References 273 and 274).

B. Control of Fibrinogen-Fibrin Conversion

The conversion of fibrinogen to fibrin is determined by the amount and activity of thrombin. Thrombin, however, does not exist in plasma, at least in a measurable amount. Thus, the rate of fibrinogen-fibrin conversion is controlled primarily by the rate of thrombin formation from prothrombin and by the rate of inactivation of thrombin by the action of plasma proteinase inhibitors. The actual conformation of thrombin, when formed in circulating blood, is also responsible for clotting fibrinogen, or for reacting with various cells and/or with different molecular components of blood plasma.

1. Amount of Thrombin Formed

Thrombin is formed from prothrombin by the proteolytic action of a serine proteinase, F-Xa. The activation requires cleavage of two peptide bonds in the prothrombin molecule.[204,275] The hydrolysis of the first peptide bond occurs at the middle of the prothrombin structure, resulting in two polypeptide intermediates, designated as Fragment 1-2 and Prethrombin 2 both with an approximate M_r of 36,000 daltons. The second attack of F-Xa takes place on Prethrombin 2 and leads to α-thrombin formation.[276] This enzyme consists of two chains, chain A and chain B, held together by a disulfide bridge, and the active site serine is located on chain B.

α-Thrombin is responsible for the conversion of fibrinogen to fibrin. Trypsin or α-thrombin, however, can also attack both the chain A and the chain B region of α-thrombin or Prethrombin 2, and as a consequence a three-chain (β-thrombin) and/or a four-chain (γ-thrombin) proteinase develop. The chains are bridged by disulfide bonds. These forms of thrombin lost their clotting activity.[277]

The activation of prothrombin by F-Xa, however, is more complicated than an enzyme-substrate reaction, i.e., several interactions with other components also take place during this limited proteolysis. Both prothrombin and F-Xa are bound to the phospholipid membrane surface of platelet by γ-carboxyglutamic acids (Gla) via Ca^{2+} bridge between the proteins and phospholipid. In addition, an accessory protein, F-Va bound to prothrombin, F-Xa, and to phospholipid, also participates in the acceleration of prothrombin activation reaction.[278] As a consequence, at least a 300,000-fold rate enhancement occurs in this prothrombinase complex (the prothrombinase complex is symbolized in Figure 11).

Accordingly, the rate of thrombin formation depends on (1) the activity of F-Xa, determined by the organization of the components of prothrombinase complex, influencing the rate of prothrombin activation, and (2) the amount of F-Xa, since under normal conditions, F-Xa does not exist (only its precursor form, the enzymatically inactive zymogen, can be found in blood plasma). F-X activation, on the other hand, depends on several reactions of the so-called "blood coagulation cascade", and there are also several levels of control mechanisms.

a. Amplifications and Rate Enhancements

The events leading to F-Xa formation are rather complicated, since they involve the conversion of several zymogens by limited proteolysis. These reactions are highly specific

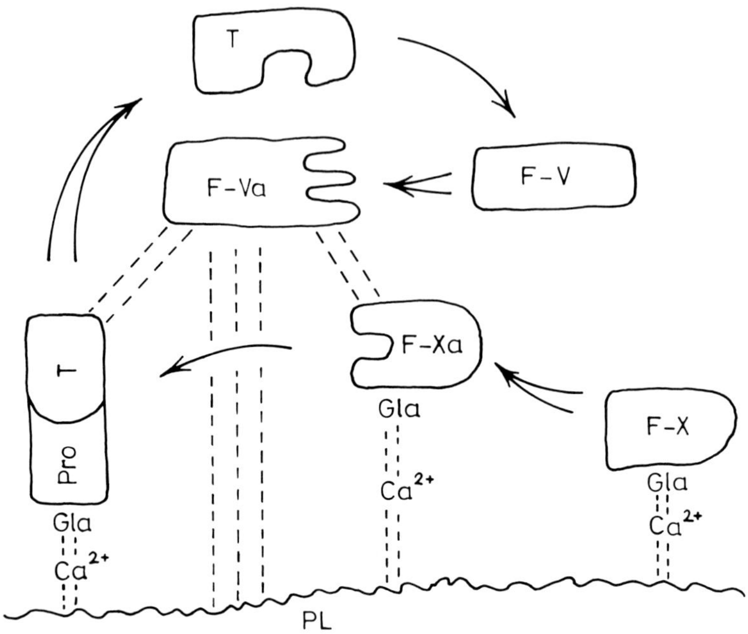

FIGURE 11. The prothrombinase complex. Prothrombin (ProT) is activated directly by the proteolytic action of the proteinase, F-Xa. This reaction is very slow in solution. Phospholipid surface (PL) formed from platelet membrane, however, extremely accelerates the reaction rate, and there is a further rate enhancement by the nonenzymatic procoagulant protein, F-Va. Both F-Xa and prothrombin are bound to the phospholipid surface via Gla-residues by Ca^{2+} bridges. F-Xa is formed from F-X by the action of F-VIIa or F-IXa. The conversion of prothrombin to thrombin (T) is under a positive feedback control mechanism, namely, F-V is transformed to F-Va by thrombin. In the prothrombinase complex, there is approximately a 2×10^5-fold rate enhancement in the conversion of prothrombin to thrombin by: (1) increase of local substrate and enzyme concentrations, (2) a favorable orientation of the protein molecules, (3) a conformational change in the enzyme (F-Xa) resulting in a more efficient proteinase, (4) labilization of the proenzyme (ProT), making it a more available substrate for F-Xa. These actions may decrease the apparent K_m and/or increase the apparent k_{cat}. The mechanism, detailed here, is valid not only for prothrombin activation, but for other proteinase activations in the blood coagulation cascade.

and irreversible and are influenced by additional factors: protein cofactors, Ca^{2+}, phospholipids, and other surface components[278] (Figure 12). When one of the blood coagulation factors, a proenzyme, is activated, it activates the next proenzyme, working as an amplifier in chain reactions. Thus, activation of a single molecule at an early step of the cascade induces the formation of a multitude of intermediate enzyme, the amount of which increases exponentially at each step.[280] The result is the appearance of high amount of F-Xa in the prothrombinase complex.

In each stage of the zymogen activation, protein cofactors (F-V, F-VIII, tissue factor, high molecular weight kininogen), phospholipids or other membrane surfaces, and Ca^{2+} participate in the reactions.[281] As a consequence, at each step of cascade system, zymogen activation rate is enhanced 10^4 to 10^5 times over that observed with proenzyme and proteinase alone[282] (Figure 12).

b. Feedback Mechanisms and Cross-Reactions

Both positive and negative feedback control mechanisms are involved in the regulation of the formation of F-Xa. Thrombin, the product of the action of F-Xa, may accelerate F-Xa development via activation of various components of the blood coagulation system, i.e., F-V, F-VIII, F-IX, and F-VII.[283] Thrombin can also activate protein C on the endothelial cell surface via thrombomodulin, and as a consequence activated protein C inactivates F-

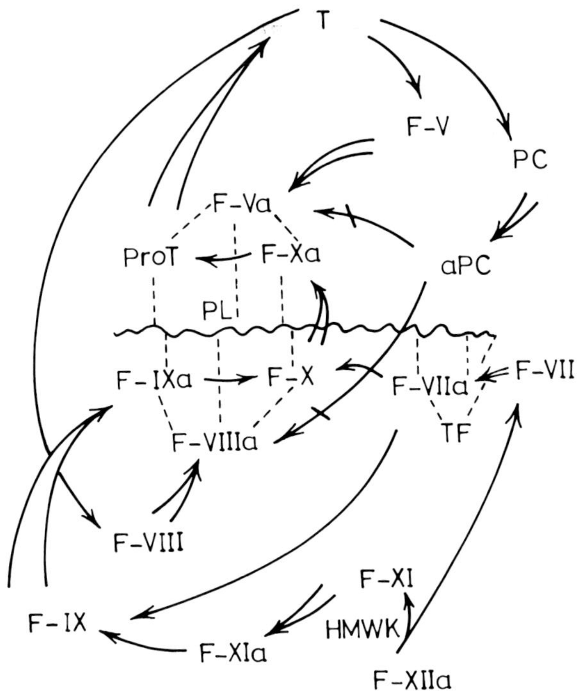

FIGURE 12. Blood coagulation cascade; amplification, rate enhancement, and feedback controls. Blood coagulation cascade can be described as a series of reactions in which inactive precursor proteins are converted into active forms, and these reactions are irreversible. When one factor, a proenzyme, is activated by limited and highly specific proteolysis, in turn, it activates the next proenzyme, acting as an amplifier in chain reactions. At the final stage, the increase in molecular numbers may be of several orders of magnitude. In addition, at each stage, zymogen activation rates are enhanced by 10^4 to 10^5 times in phospholipid-Ca^{2+}-proteins complexes (in which Gla residue containing proteins and the phospholipid membrane of platelets are participating) as well as in protein-protein-foreign surface complexes (contact phase activation). For more details see also Figures 14 and 15. The ultimate number of thrombin molecules formed, however, is influenced by various control mechanisms (not shown in this figure), i.e., (1) thrombin can accelerate its own formation via F-V and F-VIII activation, as a positive feedback control, (2) since protein C is activated by thrombin, and activated protein C in turn inactivates F-Va and F-VIIIa, this mechanism means a negative feedback control, and (3) the proteinases formed may be inactivated by plasma proteinase inhibitors, although in the complexes of coagulation cascade they are protected against inactivation. Abbreviations: wide arrows, conversion of zymogens; simple arrows, action of enzymes; crossed arrows, inhibitory actions; dotted symbols, complexes of phospholipid-Ca^{2+}-Gla-containing proteins; PL, phospholipid; F, factor; a, activated; ProT, prothrombin; PC, protein C; HMWK, high molecular weight kininogen; TF, tissue factor.

Va and F-VIIIa in the prothrombinase complex.[284] These actions of activated protein C result in decrease in both F-Xa and thrombin formation, indicating a negative feedback control mechanism (Figure 12).

Besides these reactions, some proteinases of the blood coagulation system are able to act not only on one, but on two or even more different zymogen molecules, resulting in cross-reactions in the cascade. Thus, F-VIIa can activate F-X directly as well as indirectly through the activation of F-IX, and F-IXa, in turn, activates F-X.[285] F-XIIa is able to activate F-XI as well as F-VII, and both F-VIIa and F-XIa initiate F-Xa formation (Figure 12). Furthermore, F-XIa acts not only in the direction of F-IX activation, but also may activate F-XII zymogen, resulting in positive feedback acceleration of F-XIIa formation. Moreover, F-XIIa is also able to activate prekallikrein, and the kallikrein formed either initiates the release of vaso-active peptides or acts as an activator of F-XII, resulting again in a positive feedback acceleration of blood coagulation. Since F-VII and the tissue factor system, as well as F-XII, the high molecular weight kininogens, and the kallikrein system may play important roles during the damage of the blood vessel wall, their structure and functions are discussed in depth separately.

c. Inhibitor System of the Proteinases of Blood Coagulation Cascade

Another important mechanism for the regulation of thrombin formation is the plasma proteinase inhibitor system of the circulating blood. Among the inhibitor molecules, antithrombin III, α_2-macroglobulin, heparin cofactor II and α_1-proteinase inhibitor are known to influence proteinases of the cascade.[286] Antithrombin III has a broad specificity toward the coagulation enzymes, inhibiting all proteinases except F-VIIa and activated protein C.[287] The physiological importance of these reactions, however, is questionable at present, since the accessibility of the proteinases for antithrombin III is limited when they are bound to the activation complex,[288] i.e., to the phospholipid-platelet membrane, Ca^{2+}, and accessory proteins, like F-Va or F-VIIIa. Only free enzymes seem to be sensitive to the inhibitor. Thus, among the blood coagulation enzymes thrombin is probably the most important target for antithrombin III.[289] Under some conditions, however, other proteinases may also be released from the activation complexes and become available for inhibitors. Heparin, a glycosaminoglycan, is supposed to act in such a way, especially under therapeutical application. Whether endogenous heparin or other heparin-like components of cells and/or cell membranes may function similarly is an interesting question at present.

The main problem with the reactions mentioned above, i.e., with the amplifications and rate enhancements, the feedback mechanisms, and cross-reactions, and the inhibitor system of coagulation proteinases, is that neither their relative importance, nor the factors influencing the choice among the possible reaction routes are known.

2. Activity of Thrombin

Besides the amount of thrombin formed in the blood coagulation cascade, the conversion of fibrinogen to fibrin is also determined by the actual conformation of this enzyme. Thrombin, as a multifunctional enzyme,[123,124, 290] may react with various cellular and molecular components of blood and blood vessel walls, resulting in modifications in its activity toward different substrates. Thus, thrombin binds to endothelial cell, platelet, fibroblast, hepatocyte, hepatoma cell, polymorphonuclear cell, heparin, and heparin-like surface, as well as activates F-XIII, protein C, complement system, F-V, F-VIII, F-IX, and it may react with plasma proteinase inhibitors.[124,289-294]

a. Bound and Free Thrombin

The interaction of thrombin with the various cellular elements of the blood, mainly with endothelial cells or platelets, can be reversible. Also, thrombin, as an enzyme, with or without its molecular substrates, like F-XIII, protein C, etc., is either in free or in bound form. Even in its reaction with proteinase inhibitors, thrombin does not necessarily lose its proteolytic activity, like in its interaction with α_2-macroglobulin.[295] Thus, thrombin, depending on its actual interaction with one of its targets, may lose its accessibility to a substrate, while its reactivity with another one may be increased, and vice versa.

Free thrombin, for example, reacts easily with fibrinogen, whereas thrombin bound to thrombomodulin loses its reactivity with fibrinogen, or F-V, or with platelet membrane.[142,296] On the other hand, this bound form of the enzyme has a favorable conformation to activate protein C. Furthermore, when thrombin is in the free form, it hydrolyses primarily the peptide bonds in fibrinogen molecules, whereas in a complex with heparin thrombin reacts essentially with antithrombin III.

b. Inactivation of Thrombin by Plasma Proteinase Inhibitors

Another way to control fibrinogen-fibrin conversion is the inactivation of thrombin. In circulating blood, a number of plasma proteinase inhibitors exist, and among them four inhibitors seem to be responsible for the majority of thrombin inactivation. These are antithrombin III, α_2-macroglobulin, heparin cofactor II, and α-$_1$-proteinase inhibitor.[289,297-299] Regarding their relative effectiveness, antithrombin III is responsible for about 70% of the total thrombin inactivating capacity of human plasma.[300,301] Considering that the reaction of thrombin with antithrombin III is extremely accelerated by heparin, whereas this glycosaminoglycan is rather inhibitory on the reaction between thrombin and α_2-macroglobulin as well as between thrombin and the α_1-proteinase inhibitor, the importance of antithrombin III in controlling thrombin activity is evident, especially since the blood vessel wall contains several heparin-like components. During the reaction of thrombin with antithrombin III, heparin cofactor II, or α_1-proteinase inhibitor, a 1:1 stoichiometric complex develops via a covalent bond between the hydroxyl group of active center serine of the enzyme and a carboxyl group of the inhibitor.[302,303] In these complexes, thrombin loses its fibrinogen clotting ability as well as all other proteolytic and esterolytic activities.[304] On the other hand, when thrombin reacts with α_2-macroglobulin, a covalent bond is formed between inhibitor and enzyme at a site that is different from the active center, via a thiol ester bridge.[305] In such a complex, thrombin loses its activity on fibrinogen substrate due to sterical hindrance, whereas its proteolytic activity, especially toward small molecular weight substrates, is preserved. Although thrombin may act as a proteolytic enzyme in a complex with α_2-macroglobulin, the possible biological functions of such a form of thrombin are not known at present.

c. Role of Heparin in Thrombin Inactivation and in Thrombin Formation

Heparin binds to different cells as well as to various molecules inducing several changes.[43,113,306-310] Among these interactions, the binding of heparin to endothelial cells, platelets, and to the enzymes and inhibitors of the blood coagulation-fibrinolytic system is important. Heparin influences hemostasis by the inhibition of blood coagulation, primarily via inactivation of thrombin, namely heparin facilitates the reaction between thrombin and antithrombin III. The mechanism by which heparin accelerates this reaction is the following:[123,289,522,523] Thrombin binds to a nonspecific binding site of heparin, resulting in a conformational change of the enzyme, as well as of heparin. This interaction renders the active center of thrombin more susceptible to its inhibitor. Antithrombin III, on the other hand, is bound to a specific binding site of heparin, resulting in a conformational alteration of the inhibitor molecule. In the ternary complex formed, an ordered structure of enzyme and inhibitor takes place. Thereafter, thrombin reacts with antithrombin III and the enzyme becomes inactive. Since the binding of thrombin-antithrombin III complex to heparin is less strong than that of the enzyme or inhibitor alone, the complex is released, and the free heparin can react again with a new thrombin and/or antithrombin III molecule, thereby acting as a catalyst. The reactions are summarized in Figure 13.

A similar reaction may take place between antithrombin III and other proteinases of the blood coagulation system. Since the other proteinases of blood coagulation are not available for antithrombin III in the phospholipid-Ca^{2+}-protein complex,[289,311] it is possible that heparin may have another function as well in these reactions: it releases proteinases from these complexes by destruction of the phospholipid-protein interaction. Thereafter, proteinases bound to heparin can react with antithrombin III in a thrombin-like manner.

C. Localization of Thrombus Formation

One of the main questions at present is that, besides the various factors influencing the formation and the sensitivity of thrombin to various substrates, what determines the site and the rate of thrombus formation?

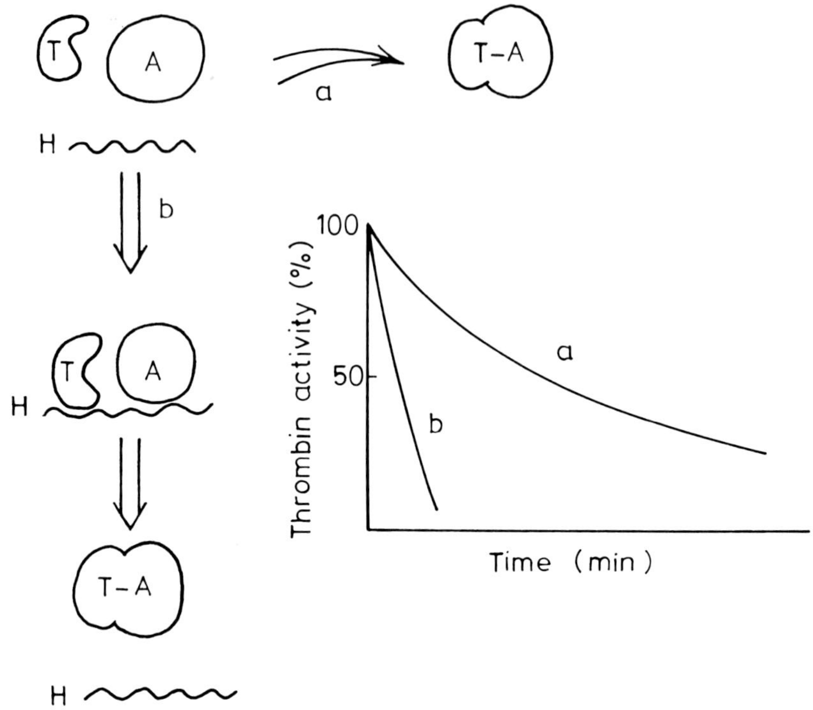

FIGURE 13. Mechanism of action of heparin in the reaction between thrombin and antithrombin III. Reaction route (a) symbolizes the relatively slow (a few minutes at physiological inhibitor concentration) interaction between thrombin (T) and antithrombin III (A). When heparin (H) is also present, the reaction (b) can be extremely accelerated (less than a few seconds) depending on the concentrations of the components. In this reaction route, both thrombin and antithrombin III bind to heparin, and in the ternary complex formed, thrombin reacts more easily with antithrombin III. Since the affinity of thrombin-antithrombin III-complex to heparin is less than that of the enzyme or inhibitor alone, the complex is released, and the free heparin can react again with a free thrombin and/or antithrombin III molecule, thereby acting as a catalyst (on the basis of References 123, 289, 522, and 523).

1. Tissue Damage; the Extrinsic Pathway

The coagulation of blood in plastic or siliconized glass tubes takes 25 min, whereas in the presence of tissue extracts blood is clotted in a few seconds.[312] This extreme acceleration of blood coagulation is the consequence of various components released by tissue damage.

These components are the following.[312,313]

1. Tissue factor, present in many types of organs, although with different specific activities; high activity is shown in brain, lung, or placenta, medium level is in kidney or spleen, and low or no activity is in muscle or platelets
2. F-VII, a vitamin K-dependent glycoprotein, synthesized in the liver and secreted into the blood circulation, having in its active center, serine residues with esterase and proteolytic activities, but with no effect on blood coagulation in the absence of tissue factor
3. Ca^{2+}

Accordingly, to initiate this ''extrinsic pathway'' of blood coagulation, tight cooperation between plasma proteins and tissue components is necessary (Figure 14).

The basic reaction in this pathway is the limited proteolytic activation of F-X by F-VII

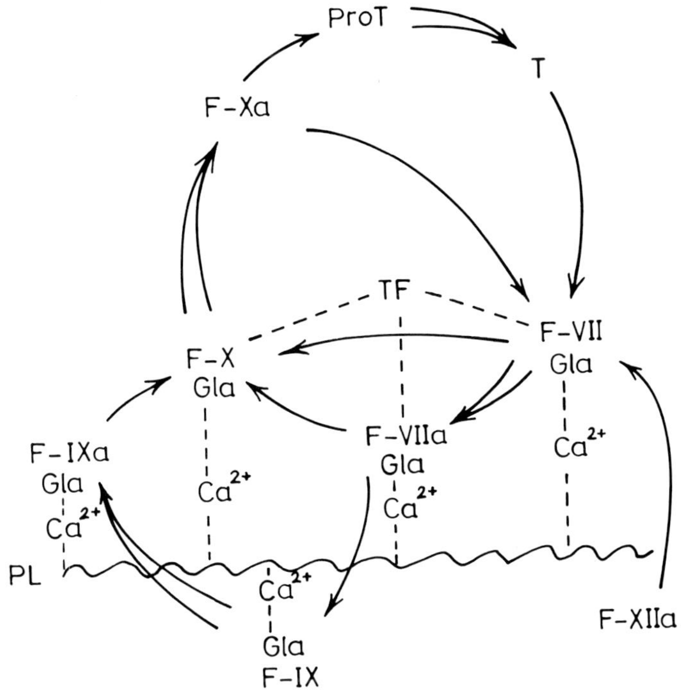

FIGURE 14. Tissue-factor pathway of blood coagulation. F-X can be converted to a serine proteinase (F-Xa) for prothrombin activation (ProT) in two ways. One is the extrinsic pathway. (The mechanism of prothrombin activation in the prothrombinase complex is not indicated here; for details see Figure 11.) When tissue damage occurs, F-VII, bound to phospholipid surface (PL) by Gla(s) of the protein via Ca^{2+} bridges, activates F-X. This reaction route is accelerated by tissue factor (TF). Although F-VII is a proteinase, it may be activated further by various proteinases, and the F-VIIa formed is more effective in F-X activation than F-VII. The conversion of F-VII to F-VIIa may be initiated by thrombin (T) or F-Xa, resulting in a positive feedback acceleration of thrombin formation, or by F-XIIa (not shown in this figure). F-VIIa formed, however, can convert not only F-X to F-Xa, but F-IX to F-IXa as well. The physiological or pathological significance of the latter reaction is not known (on the basis of References 280 and 312).

and in turn, the rapid conversion of prothrombin to thrombin by F-Xa resulting in fibrin formation. F-VII, without limited proteolysis, may function as an activator of F-X[314] in the presence of tissue factor. Namely, the conformation of F-VII in a complex with tissue factor is changed, similarly to plasminogen-streptokinase complex, or to prothrombin-staphylocoagulase complex, with the appearance of the active center serine. Thus, although the essential reaction is the limited proteolysis of F-X, i.e., its conversion to F-Xa by F-VII or F-VIIa, the trigger for this reaction is in the tissue factor release and phospholipid surface formation by the damage of the various cells of and around blood vessel walls.

F-VII consists of a single polypeptide chain, with M_r 48,000 daltons for human origin.[315] During limited proteolysis of an Arg-Ile bond by F-Xa,[316] or F-XIIa,[317] or F-IXa,[318] or by thrombin,[316] a two-chain proteinase, F-VIIa, emerges.[319] The activity of F-VIIa is higher by nearly two orders of magnitude than that of the single chain F-VII.[316] After additional attack by F-Xa, a second bond is hydrolysed on the heavy chain of F-VIIa, leading to the formation of inactive F-VIIa. The biological significance of the latter is not known at present.

The reactions, both F-Xa formation and F-VII activation, take place on phospholipid surface formed either by platelet or by endothelial cell destruction, via Ca^{2+} bridges between Gla of proteins and phospholipid of cell membranes. The most powerful trigger for F-VII and F-X activation, however, is the appearance of tissue factor. Tissue factor contains two components, an apoprotein, with a M_r of 56,000 daltons, and phospholipids.[320] It is devoid of any proteolytic activity and is insensitive to proteolytic activators.[321] Removal of phospholipids, however, results in the loss of biological activity.[322] Among purified phospholipids, phosphatidylethanolamine is the most effective, whereas phosphatidylserine, which is very active in other coagulation reactions, fails to restore tissue factor activity.[323] Regarding the mechanism of action of the apoprotein and phospholipid, it is very probable that similar to the prothrombinase complex, phospholipid serves as a surface for the binding of F-VII via γ-carboxyl glutamic acid and Ca^{2+} bridge, while tissue factor protein acts as a cofactor. Vitamin K-related proteins, however, show a different nature in the interaction with phospholipids, namely F-X and prothrombin form tight complexes, with a K_d of approximately 1 μM, whereas F-VII displays lower affinity, a K_d of approximately 15 μM.[324] Thus, the exact contribution of lipids to F-VII function is not clear yet.

2. Factor XII Activation; the Intrinsic Pathway

Blood coagulation can be also initiated by the variety of surfaces, negatively charged materials, like collagen, endotoxin, urate crystals, glass, kaolin, celite, etc.[325] The reactions involved in these blood coagulation processes, also called "intrinsic pathway" or "contact phase" of blood coagulation, are triggered by an enzyme, F-XIIa (Hageman factor). The reactions of contact phase activation are shown in Figure 15. F-XIIa is capable of activating F-XI and/or F-VII, which in turn activate F-IX and/or F-X, respectively.[326] Activated F-IX also activates F-X. Thus, F-XIIa, activating either F-XI or F-VII, initiates blood coagulation. This enzyme, however, does not exist in the blood plasma under normal conditions, only its precursor form, a single-chain glycoprotein with an M_r 76,000 daltons circulates in blood at a concentration of approximately 0.4 μM.[327]

This proteinase zymogen can be activated by limited proteolysis, without any change in molecular weight. A cleavage within the disulfide loop results in the formation of a disulfide-bridged two-chain active enzyme, designated α-F-XIIa. The 28,000-dalton carboxy terminal chain contains the enzymatically active site, whereas the heavy chain shows a high affinity to a negatively charged surface[328] (Figure 15). An additional proteolysis of α-F-XIIa results in the loss of the heavy chain with the formation of a small, approximately 28,000-dalton enzyme, designated β-F-XIIa.[329] α-F-XIIa binds to surfaces, whereas β-F-XIIa does not. Both α- and β-F-XIIa are prekallikrein activators, but only α-F-XIIa is a potent activator of F-XI, whereas β-F-XIIa acts on the conversion of F-VII to F-VIIa[317,330-332] (Figures 12 and 14).

The activation of prekallikrein and/or F-XI by F-XIIa is highly accelerated in the presence of a surface cofactor, the high molecular weight kininogen (HMWK). HMWK, present in human plasma at 0.7 μM concentration, is a single-chain protein with an approximate M_r of 110,000 daltons.[333] It contains an unusual amino acid sequence, rich in histidine, lysine, and glycine,[334] which is probably responsible for the binding of the molecule to negatively charged surfaces during contact activation.[335]

A conformational change of F-XII, rendering the surface-bound molecule much more sensitive to proteolytic activation by proteinases, like kallikrein, seems to be an essential step in the mechanism of F-XIIa formation.[336] Whether this conformational change of the proenzyme is enough for the development of the active center or a proteolytic attack is also necessary is questioned at present. Proteolytic enzymes, however, extremely accelerate F-XIIa formation with a mutual action of HMWK and the surface. Such a proteolytic enzyme may be liberated from endothelial cells during tissue damage, since endothelial cells contain a F-XII activating enzyme.[101] Moreover, additional enzymes may participate in F-XII activation. Thus, a reciprocal, positive feedback acceleration of F-XIIa formation can occur by the action of either kallikrein, formed from prekallikrein by F-XIIa, or by the action of F-XIa, generated from F-XI by F-XIIa (Figure 12).

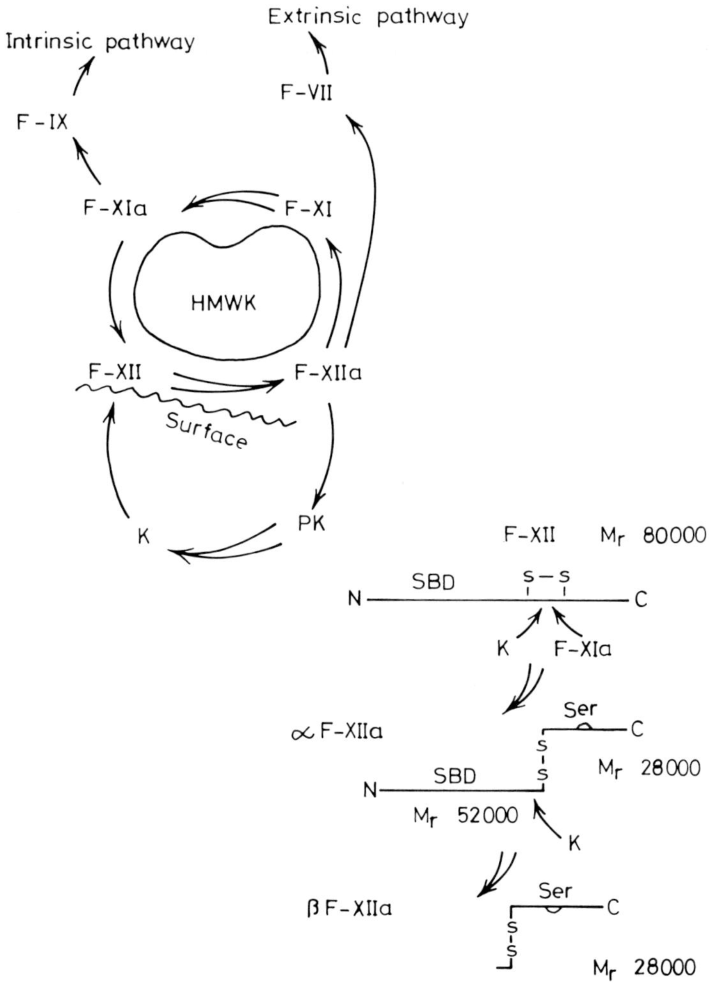

FIGURE 15. Contact phase of blood coagulation. F-XII, a single chain glycoprotein bound to a negatively charged surface, can be activated by the conformational change and proteolytic action of kallikrein (K) or F-XIa. The F-XIIa formed, primarily α-F-XIIa, consists of two chains held together by disulfide bridge with active center serine (Ser) on the light chain and the surface binding domain (SBD) on the heavy chain. The enzyme activates F-XI, or prekallikrein (PK), or Factor VII (F-VII), or other substrates (not shown here), thereby initiating blood coagulation and/or kallikrein formation and accelerating its own formation by positive feedback control mechanisms. The reactions are highly enhanced in the presence of the procoagulant high molecular weight kininogen (HMWK). α-F-XIIa, however, can be further modified by the proteolytic action of kallikrein, and (β-F-XIIa) formed loses its surface binding site, but preserves its active center (on the basis of References 326 and 327).

3. Fibrin Formation Induced by Factors Other than Factor VIIa or Factor XIIa

There are several diseases (cancer, infections, acute pancreatitis, etc.) which induce thrombosis via activation of blood coagulation factor(s) other than F-VII or F-XII. Although in these reactions the whole blood coagulation cascade, platelets, endothelial cells, and the fibrinolytic system may be involved, the trigger for initiation of blood coagulation emerges somewhere in the cascade without direct activation of F-XII or F-VII.

Fibrinogen can be converted directly to fibrin by the action of some proteinases of snake venoms, such as ancrod, batroxobin, or crotalase.[239] Another method of initiation of fibrin formation is a direct activation of prothrombin. A nonproteolytic activator, designated staphylocoagulase, emerges in a few infections, forms an active, 1:1 *M* ratio with intact prothrombin,[337] without change in the primary structure of prothrombin, but making the active center available for fibrinogen conversion to fibrin.[338] Again, some snake venoms contain enzymes with the ability to convert prothrombin to thrombin or thrombin-like enzyme, i.e., Taipan snake or tiger snake venom can activate prothrombin in a mechanism analogous to that of FXa in the prothrombinase complex.[339,340] Two other snake venoms, *Echis carinatus* and *Dispholidus typus,* activate prothrombin by another mechanism, through meizothrombin formation.[275,341-343]

The best-known mechanism for triggering blood coagulation, however, is F-X activation. During physiological activation, either by extrinsic or intrinsic pathway, the enzymatically inactive F-X, a glycoprotein with M_r 55,000 daltons,[344] is converted to a 2-polypeptide chain active proteinase by limited proteolysis with the loss of an activation peptide.[344,345] The reaction takes place on phospholipid surfaces, either on tissue phospholipid or platelet membrane, where the zymogen protein is bound by Ca^{2+} bridges via its light chain portion containing 12 Gla. In the complex, additional protein cofactors contribute to the extremely high rate enhancement of the limited proteolysis (Figure 12).

When the disulfide bridged two-chain proteinase is formed, the active center containing region is located on the heavy chain.[346] During activation, the enzyme is formed by the action of either F-IXa, a proteinase of the intrinsic pathway, or F-VIIa, a proteinase of the extrinsic pathway. F-X can also be activated by other enzymes via different mechanisms.[347-352] Thus, trypsin, cathepsin C, papain, or several kinds of snake venoms, like Russell's viper venom, *Bothrops atrox, Echis carinatus,* etc., can initiate blood coagulation, under various pathological conditions or by snake bites, respectively. A F-X activating cysteine proteinase has also been found in various malignant tissues.[353] This enzyme may play a pivotal role in tumor metastasis.

D. Multifunctional Role of Factor XIIa and Its Regulation

F-XIIa, similar to thrombin, plays various roles in hemostasis. It is involved in blood coagulation, fibrinolysis, the kinin-kallikrein system, and in the complement system (Figure 16).

1. Initiation of Blood Coagulation

As discussed earlier in detail, F-XIIa activates F-XI. F-XIa formed activates F-IX, leading to thrombin, and as a consequence, to fibrin formation, or F-XIa activates F-XII, resulting in a positive-feedback acceleration of blood coagulation. Activation of F-VII by F-XIIa may also initiate blood coagulation or participate in it, although the importance of this reaction is not known at present.

F-XIIa formation from F-XII, as a real trigger for blood coagulation, is also questioned at present, since "surface formation" on damaged endothelium, or the release of F-XII activating enzyme from endothelial cells, kallikrein (if formed), or plasmin developed during fibrinolysis may initiate F-XII activation (Figures 12 and 15).

2. Kinin-Kallikrein System

As mentioned earlier, F-XIIa, especially β-F-IIa, is a powerful trigger for the activation of prekallikrein, with the consequence of kallikrein formation. The activation process involves cleavage at a peptide bond of the single chain prekallikrein without change in the molecular weight of approximately 85,000 daltons. The two chains, heavy and light, are linked by disulfide bonds, and the active center serine is located on the latter.[354,355]

Kallikrein formed, in turn, may be involved in the acceleration of blood coagulation, initiation of fibrinolysis, activation of the renin-angiotensin system, and the complement system, via activation of F-XII, plasminogen, prorenin, and a direct reaction with the complement system.[291,356,357] The main function of kallikrein, however, is the formation of vasoactive peptides from plasma kininogens.

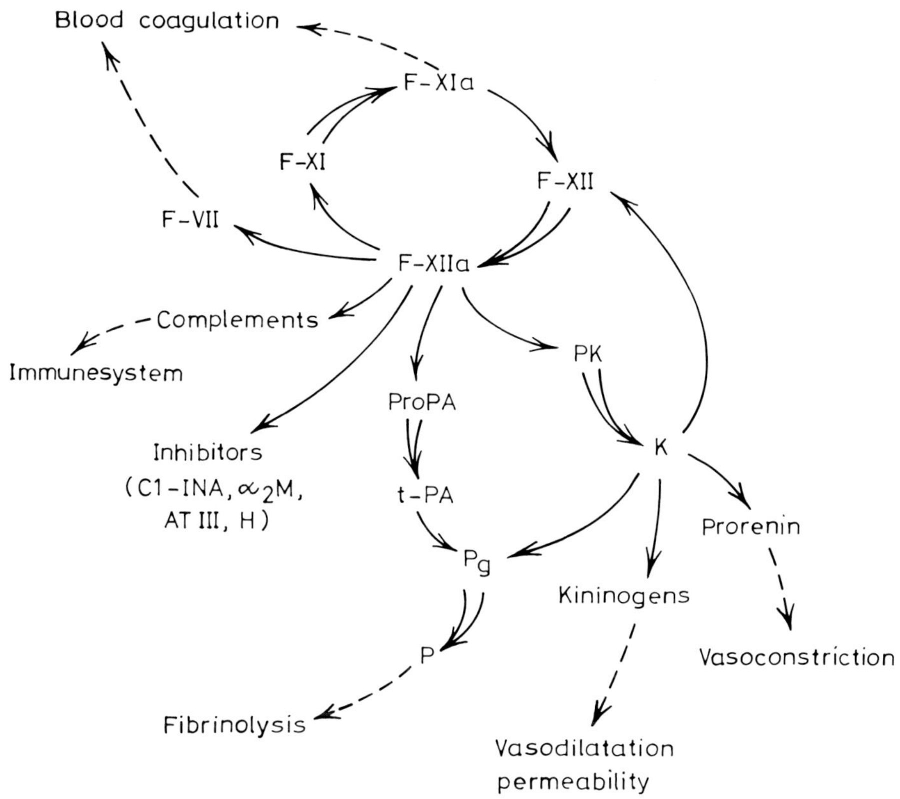

FIGURE 16. Multifunctional role of F-XIIa. F-XIIa has several biological functions via its actions on various substrates (see also Figure 15). Abbreviations: F, factors; a, activated; ProPA, proplasminogen activator; t-PA, tissue-type plasminogen activator; Pg, plasminogen; P, plasmin; PK, prekallikrein; K, kallikrein; C1-INA, C1-inactivator; α_2M, α_2-macroglobulin; AT III, antithrombin III; H, heparin.

Plasma kininogens, both the high molecular weight (HMWK), $M_r \approx 110{,}000$ daltons, and the low molecular weight (LMWK), $M_r \approx 60{,}000$ daltons, contain inactive kinins within their primary sequences.[358,359] They circulate in blood at a concentration of approximately 0.7 μM for HMWK and 2.8 μM for LMWK.[326,360] Although active kinins can be released from both HMWK and LMWK by either plasma kallikrein or tissue enzyme,[361] the main source for kinins seems to be the LMWK, whereas HMWK plays a central role in contact activation, being a nonenzymatic cofactor for the acceleration of activation of F-XI or prekallikrein by F-XIIa[362] (Figure 17; see also Figure 15).

Both HMWK and LMWK have a single polypeptide chain, but only HMWK contains an unusual region with high percentage of histidine, lysine, and glycine, which very probably is responsible for contact activation by forming the binding site to negatively charged surfaces.[363] During the attack of kallikrein, two peptide bonds are hydrolysed, either in HMWK or in LMWK with the liberation of vasoactive bradykinin. The two chains, heavy and light, formed in the molecule, are held together by a disulfide bridge[364] (Figure 17). The kinins increase permeability, cause dilation of blood vessels and hypotension, and are generally associated with inflammation.

3. Factor XIIa and Fibrinolysis

There is a reciprocal, direct as well as indirect, activation of blood coagulation and fibrinolysis via F-XII. Plasminogen can be activated directly by F-XIIa.[365,366] F-XIIa may also react, as indicated before, with F-XI or prekallikrein, and the activated enzymes in turn

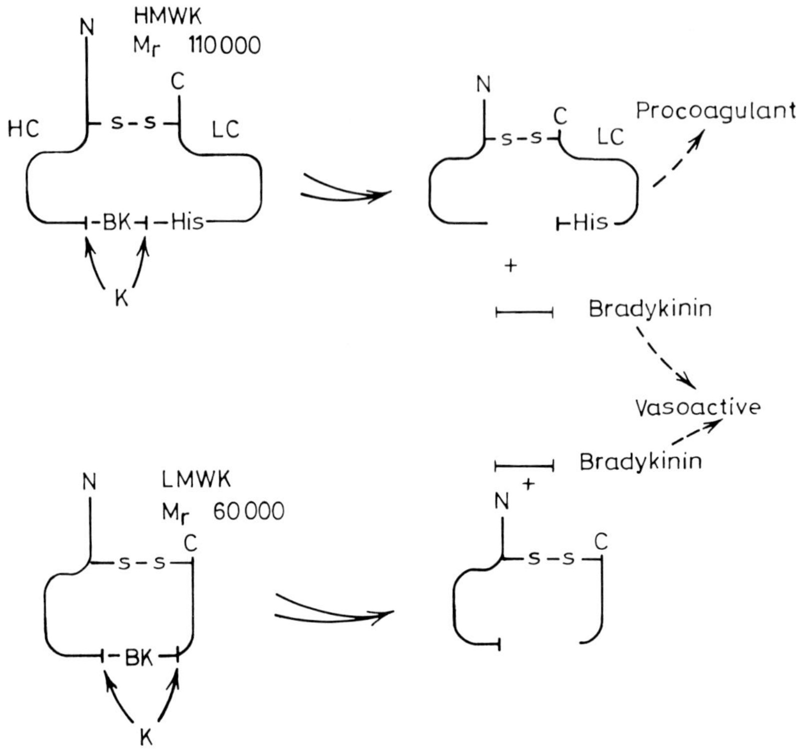

FIGURE 17. High and low molecular weight kininogens; bradykinin formation. High molecular weight kininogen (HMWK) contains sequences for both procoagulant and vasoactive functions. When kallikrein (K) splits two bonds in the parent molecule, bradykinin, the vasoactive peptide is released, and the HMWK becomes a two-chain molecule. The light chain (LC), containing a His-rich region responsible for the procoagulant action, is joined to heavy chain (HC) by a disulfide bridge. When kallikrein attacks low molecular weight kininogen (LMWK), bradykinin is also released, bu the parent molecule has no procoagulant function (on the basis of References 327 and 359).

activate plasminogen.[367-369] Moreover, thrombin, formed in the cascade of blood coagulation, activates protein C, and the proteinase generated initiates, indirectly, plasminogen activation via increase in both the urokinase and tissue-type plasminogen activator release by endothelial cells,[370] with the consequence of increased fibrinolysis.[371] In addition, thrombin, bound to endothelial cell, may accelerate the release of plasminogen activator from this cell.[169] All of these data also indicate that initiation of blood coagulation induces fibrinolysis. On the other hand, plasmin formed during the initiation of fibrinolysis can activate F-XII,[372] resulting in an activation of blood coagulation in the overall process.

4. Role of Factor XII in Complement Activation

Phagocytosis is one of the most important mechanisms to destroy pathogens. The lysis and/or destruction of pathogens is achieved by the presence of antigen-antibody complex, activating the proteins of the complement system. The complements, by developing a multimolecular, self-assembling system after activation, contain proteinases which are responsible for the immunopathologic events.[373] The complement proteins circulate in the blood in precursor forms. Following the activation, the complements interact sequentially to form active enzymes ($C\overline{1r}$; $C\overline{1s}$; $C\overline{4b,2a,3b}$; $C\overline{3b,Bb}$), two activated cofactors (C3b; C4b) with the ability to bind to membranes, five activation fragments (C2b; C3a; C4a; C5a; Ba), and a complex of C5b,6,7,8,9, with $M_r \geq 10^6$ which interferes with membrane integrity resulting in cell lysis. The conversion of complements to active constituents needs specific biochemical reactions, mainly limited proteolysis.[291,357] When the first component, Clqrs, interacts with an antigen-antibody complex developed with IgM or IgG1, IgG2, or IgG3 on the cell surface, a proteolytic enzyme, C1 esterase, is generated. The $C\overline{1}$ esterase, via activation of C4C2 components, leads to C3 activation by $\overline{C4b,C2a}$ convertase. As a consequence C3a, an anaphylatoxin, and $\overline{C3b}$ enzyme are formed. The latter, in turn, results in another anaphylatoxin, C5a, as well as $\overline{C5b,6,7}$ activation. Finally, C5b,6,7,8,9 complex is generated, leading to the lysis of cells. An alternate route of activation may occur by a direct activation of C3, initiated by the lipid region of bacterial lipopolysaccharides and IgA, IgE, or fragments of IgG. The reactions of the complement cascade can be controlled by at least two inhibitors: C1-inactivator (C1-INA) and C3b-inactivator. During the activation process, the intermediate components of complement system display various biological activities, i.e., chemotaxis for neutrophils, enhancement of phagocytosis, elaboration of anaphylatoxin, kinin actions on blood vessel walls, histamine release from mast cells, serotonin release from platelets, opsonization, cell membrane damages, acceleration of blood coagulation, etc.[291]

In tissue damage, the blood coagulation-fibrinolytic system influences the immunological reactions, complement activation, kinin formation, etc. Surface activation, the contact phase of blood coagulation, seems to play a major role in linking up a series of these processes primarily via F-XII. F-XIIa may influence the complement system directly on C1 component resulting in its activation;[291] the complement inhibitor factor, C1-INA, inhibits F-XIIa activity.[372,373]

Plasmin can cleave C1, in a Ca^{2+}-dependent manner, resulting in active $C\overline{1s}$,[374,375] whereas plasmin action on C3, C5, and C5b,6 yields fragments having anaphylactic and hemolytic activity.[376,377] Moreover, since plasmin can destroy the inhibitor protein C1-INA by direct enzymatic cleavage,[378] the apparent activation of C1 may be a consequence of the loss of control of C1 by C1-INA. Complement activation may also act in a reciprocal manner to promote fibrinolysis, since activated factor B of the complement system cleaves and activates plasminogen.[379]

Among blood coagulation factors, formed by the initiation of F-XIIa, thrombin influences the complement system through its action on C3 and C5, resulting in the formation of chemotactic fragments for polymorphonuclear neutrophils and biologically active C5a-like fragments, respectively.[380] A possible additional link between blood coagulation and complement system is protein S, which exists as a tight complex with C4 in a normal plasma.[381] Kallikrein, formed from prekallikrein by the action of F-XIIa, can also affect the complement system via C1 activation,[382] cleavage of C5 with the generation of a chemotactic factor for neutrophils,[383] and factor B proteolysis resulting in hemolytic activity.[384]

These data indicate that several proteinases of the blood coagulation-fibrinolytic system can mediate complement activation, and vice versa, with F-XII playing a central role. The significance and the relative importance of these complicated cross-reactions and feedback mechanisms under pathological conditions, however, is far from clear at present.

5. Inhibitor System of Factor XIIa

Among the various plasma proteinase inhibitors, antithrombin III and C1-inactivator (C1-INA) seem to participate in the inactivation of F-XIIa, since neither α_2-macroglobulin, α_1-proteinase inhibitor, nor α_2-antiplasmin inhibit this proteinase.[289,372,385-387] The mechanism by which antithrombin III inactivates F-XIIa is similar to the reaction between thrombin and antithrombin III, namely the inhibitor forms a stoichiometric complex with the proteinase via an irreversible ester bond between serine hydroxyl group of the active center of the enzyme and a carboxyl group of the inhibitor.[289,385] The reaction is accelerated in the presence of heparin.[388,389] Recent results, however, indicate that antithrombin III contributes to F-

XIIa inactivation in plasma only by approximately 2 to 4%.[390] Moreover, although heparin results in a rate enhancement of this reaction, the increase in the reaction rate is about fourfold even at a heparin concentration of therapeutical use.[391] Another inhibitor, the C1-inactivator, a glycoprotein with M_r 104,000 daltons, also occurs in plasma at a concentration of approximately 2 μM[386] and contributes to the F-XIIa inhibition in human plasma by approximately 92%.[390] This inhibitor, therefore, can be considered at present as the main regulator protein of F-XIIa. In addition, since C1-INA inhibits not only F-XIIa, but kallikrein and F-XIa as well,[372,378,392,393] this inhibitor seems to be involved in the control of the contact phase activation processes. Nevertheless, its role very probably is not essentially the stop signal for blood coagulation initiation, since congenital deficiency of C1-INA correlates with angioneurotic edema without thrombosis tendency.[386] Regarding other possible candidates for F-XIIa inactivation, an undefined protein has been found with a capacity to inhibit both F-XIIa and plasminogen activation.[394]

V. FIBRINOLYSIS

Fibrin, the end product of the blood coagulation process, is the substrate for plasmin, the ultimate enzyme of the fibrinolytic system. The fibrinolytic system, however, consists of a multicomponent assembly of proenzymes and inhibitors and is in a mutually compensating and balanced state with the blood coagulation system. For example, plasmin does not exist in plasma, at least in a measurable amount under normal conditions, but only in precursor form, as plasminogen. Therefore, the critical step in fibrinolysis is the formation of plasmin, and if it is formed, its inactivation becomes the crucial process.

Beside hemostasis, fibrinolysis contributes to several other biological functions as well,[395-400] i.e., it takes part in inflammation, cancer development and metastasis, defense mechanisms against bacterial invasion, ovulation and embryo implantation, major surgery and traumatic injuries, in wound healing, etc. (not discussed in this chapter).

A. Action of Plasmin on Fibrin

The biological significance of the action of plasmin on fibrin is that a water-insoluble molecule is solubilized. In biochemical terms, fibrin dissolution means a limited proteolysis of the fibrin molecule by the proteinase plasmin. The precise sequence of the biochemical reactions is not known at present, although it is clear that first the α-chain, thereafter the β-chain, and finally the γ-chain of fibrin(ogen) are hydrolyzed, resulting in the formation of four major soluble degradation products designated X, Y, D, and E.[401]

The molecular events, however, are more complicated since different types of fibrin can serve as substrate for plasmin, i.e., fibrinogen, noncross-linked fibrin, and partly and totally cross-linked fibrin. The attack of plasmin on noncross-linked fibrin is very similar to that on fibrinogen, as only the lack of fibrinopeptides A and B distinguishes noncross-linked fibrin from fibrinogen. During the action of plasmin, as a first step, Fragment X with M_r of approximately 280,000 daltons is formed from fibrinogen (M_r 340,000 daltons) by the action of plasmin on the C-terminal part of α-chain. By a second attack of plasmin on 1 side of the dimer Fragment X, a Fragment D, with M_r 94,000 daltons, is released resulting also in the formation of Fragment Y, with M_r 150,000 daltons. In the next step of plasmin action, the remaining other Fragment D is released from Fragment Y, resulting in Fragment E, with M_r 50,000 daltons (Figure 18). These fragments, Fragment E and two Fragment D's, are the final main soluble products of plasmin action on noncross-linked fibrin(ogen). Although fibrinogen and noncross-linked fibrin are very similar, there is a discrete structural difference between Fragment Y and Fragment D derived from them.[403]

Due primarily to the γ-chain, and not to α-chain cross-links,[402,404,405] cross-linked fibrin is less susceptible to digestion by plasmin than noncross-linked fibrin. During fibrin for-

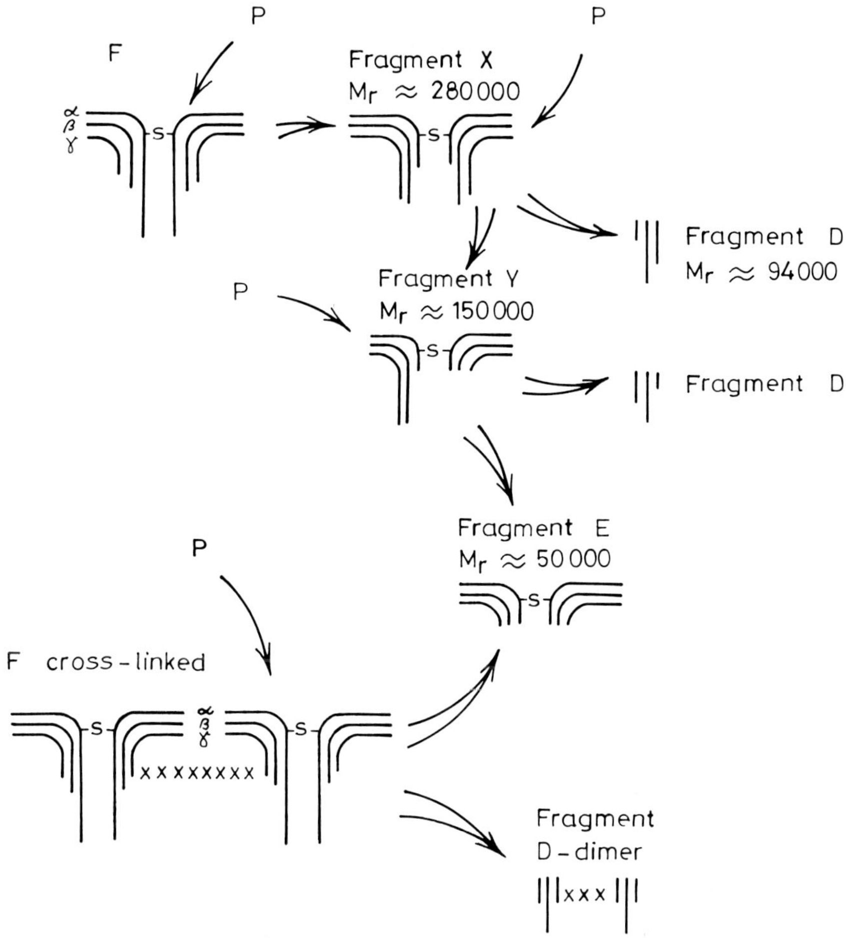

FIGURE 18. Action of plasmin on fibrin. Both fibrin (F) and cross-linked fibrin can be degraded and solubilized by plasmin (P). The cross-links, symbolized by xx, are formed mainly between the γ-chains of two fibrin(ogen)s via glutamine and lysine residues. The fragments formed are soluble (on the basis of References 399, 401, and 402).

mation, as mentioned earlier, the fibrin strands become stabilized by the action of F-XIIIa. F-XIIIa, formed from F-XIII by the action of thrombin and Ca^{2+}, cross-links γ- as well as α-chains of fibrin(ogen) between intermolecular glutamine and lysine residues of the protein.[406] This cross-linking process begins before insoluble fibrin develops and continues after deposition.[407] Cross-links between γ-chains are formed rapidly, whereas between α-chains they are formed more slowly.[408,409] All thrombi developed in artery or vein contain fibrin with both γ-chain dimers and highly cross-linked α-chains.[410] It is probable that α-chain cross-linked fibrin is present mainly in "aged" thrombus and that is the reason why only fresh clots are dissolved easily. Nevertheless, plasmin can digest α-cross-linked fibrin as well, although the degradation products differ from that emerged from fibrinogen or noncross-linked fibrin. Namely, by the action of plasmin, Fragment E and Fragment D dimer appear from cross-linked fibrin[411,412] (Figure 18). The Fragment D dimer is held together by γ-γ-cross-links. The mechanism of dissolution of the α-cross-linked fibrin, however, is rather complicated and is beyond the aim of the present survey (for more details see Reference 401).

B. Control of the Amount and Activity of Plasmin

According to the above discussion, the dissolution of fibrin depends on the plasmin activity, i.e., on the amount of plasmin formed, as well as on the conformation of the active enzyme determined by various conditions and factors present in blood and blood vessel wall. Other crucial questions are how, when, and where is plasmin formed, and also, what happens to the ''unnecessary'' enzyme molecules?

1. Formation of Plasmin from Plasminogen(s)

Plasmin is a serine proteinase with the ability to hydrolyze peptide bonds between Lys and another amino acid residue. Although the specificity of plasmin is not restricted to the fibrinolytic system — plasmin affects different proteins involved in blood coagulation, tumor metastasis, inflammation, wound healing, etc. — the main target of this enzyme is the fibrin. Plasmin is a 2-chain glycoprotein, with M_r 25,000 daltons for light chain and M_r 48,000 daltons for heavy chain, linked by the disulfide bridge. The active site region is located on the light chain.[413,414]

a. Structure of Plasminogen(s)

Plasmin is formed from plasminogen, a single polypeptide chain protein with a M_r of about 90,000 daltons, containing 22 disulfide bridges.[415,416] Its primary structure, the complete amino acid sequence and the carbohydrate content, is known.[417,418] Plasminogen consists of 791 amino acid residues, shaping three domains, relevant to the activation process, i.e.,

1. Activation peptide located in residues 1 to 76.
2. A heavy chain (A-chain region) containing five ''Kringle'' structures at residues 77 to 560
3. Light chain (B-chain domain), at residues 561 to 790, where the active site of the enzyme is settled down[419]

Each ''Kringle'' structure in the A-chain region is made up of approximately 80 amino acid residues and stabilized by three disulfide bridges forming a triple loop structure. This structure is responsible for the binding of plasminogen to fibrin. The ''Kringle'' domains contain also high- and low-affinity lysine binding sites which compete for fibrin and/or α_2-antiplasmin during fibrinolysis.

b. Mechanism of Plasminogen Activation

There are two mechanisms for plasminogen activation. One involves proteolytic events in the parent molecule, resulting in an active center, the ''charge-relay system'' formation. In the other one, without proteolytic cleavage, plasminogen conformation is modified in such a way that serine, hystidine, and asparagic acid are ordered to accomplish the active center. During proteolytic activation, two peptide bonds are hydrolyzed in plasminogen: one is at Lys 78, resulting in the formation of Lys-plasminogen, and another is at Val 561, with the consequence of the formation of a two-chain protein, held together by a disulfide bridge. In the latter, the active serine group on the light chain develops. The exact sequence of reactions, for instance, the proteolysis of the bond at Lys 78 by plasmin itself and/or at Arg 560 by proteinases called plasminogen activators, is not known at present. Two pathways seem to be plausible in vivo (Figure 19). One could occur when the first step is the reaction of the activator at Val 561 residue, resulting in Glu-plasmin formation, and thereafter the release of the activation peptide, containing 77 amino acid residues, by the action of plasmin, leading to the formation of Lys-plasmin. The other way would occur by the first attack of catalytic amount of plasmin on plasminogen resulting in Lys-plasminogen formation, and as a next step, the plasminogen activator acts on Lys-plasminogen more easily at Val 561 residue leading to plasmin formation.[421]

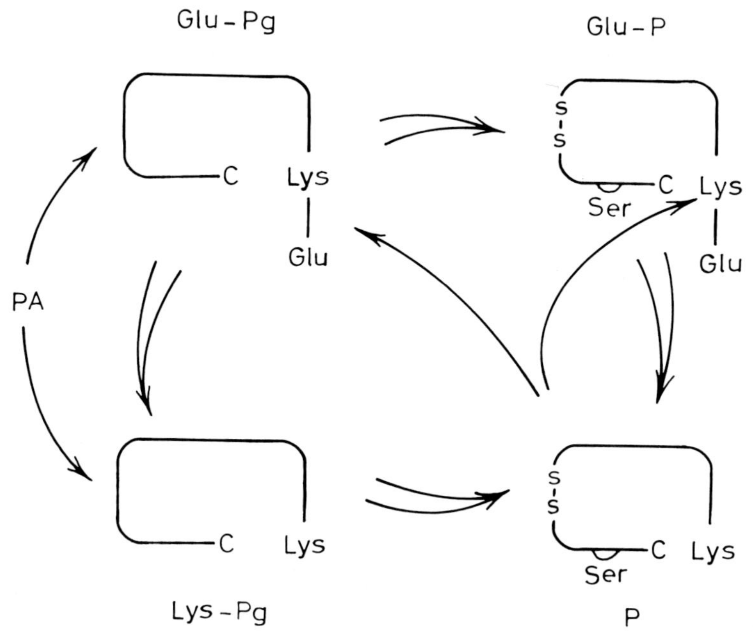

FIGURE 19. Conversion of plasminogen to plasmin. Plasminogen, containing Glu at the N-terminal end of the molecule, designated Glu-plasminogen (Glu-Pg), can be hydrolyzed at two bonds by either plasmin (P) formed or plasminogen activator (PA). Depending on the sequence of events, there are two possible methods for the mechanism of plasminogen activation. First, when plasminogen activator attacks the Arg 560-Val 561 bond, a 2-chain molecule is formed (Glu-P) with the active center serine (Ser) on the light chain. Thereafter, a sequence with approximately 77 amino acid residues is released from the N-terminal end of the molecule by the action of a plasmin resulting in additional plasmin formation. The other way would start with the release of the activation peptide leading to Lys-plasminogen (Lys-Pg) formation; after a second hydrolytic step by plasminogen activator, plasmin develops (on the basis of References 401 and 420).

c. *Factors Influencing the Rate of Plasminogen Activation*

Plasminogen binds preferentially to fibrin during clot formation, i.e., 1 mol of fibrin binds 1 mol of Lys-plasminogen, whereas native Glu-plasminogen shows less affinity to fibrin.[422-425] The interaction between fibrin and plasminogen takes place via the lysine-binding site(s) of the zymogen, and is abolished by 6-aminohexanoic acid.[426,427] On the other hand, at low concentration, 6-aminohexanoic acid changes the conformation of Glu-plasminogen in such a manner that it is easily activated, like Lys-plasminogen. The differences in binding of Glu-plasminogen and Lys-plasminogen to fibrin may be due to the masking of the lysine-binding site in Glu-plasminogen by the activation peptide. Since the lysine binding site of plasminogen mediates the interaction with the inhibitor α_2-antiplasmin as well,[428,429] the mechanism of plasminogen activation in plasma, in the presence of fibrin, α_2-antiplasmin, and additional known (lysine, 6-aminohexanoic acid, etc.) and unknown components, is rather complicated.

Moreover, tissue plasminogen activator, unlike urokinase or streptokinase, also binds strongly to fibrin,[430] and the rate of plasminogen activation is extremely enhanced in this complex, whereas without fibrin, tissue plasminogen activator is a poor effector of the conversion of plasminogen to plasmin. Thus, the exact mechanism of plasminogen activation in vivo is more complicated when the activation involves tissue type plasminogen activator.

In addition, plasminogen also binds to the platelet with a K_d of approximately 2×10^{-6}

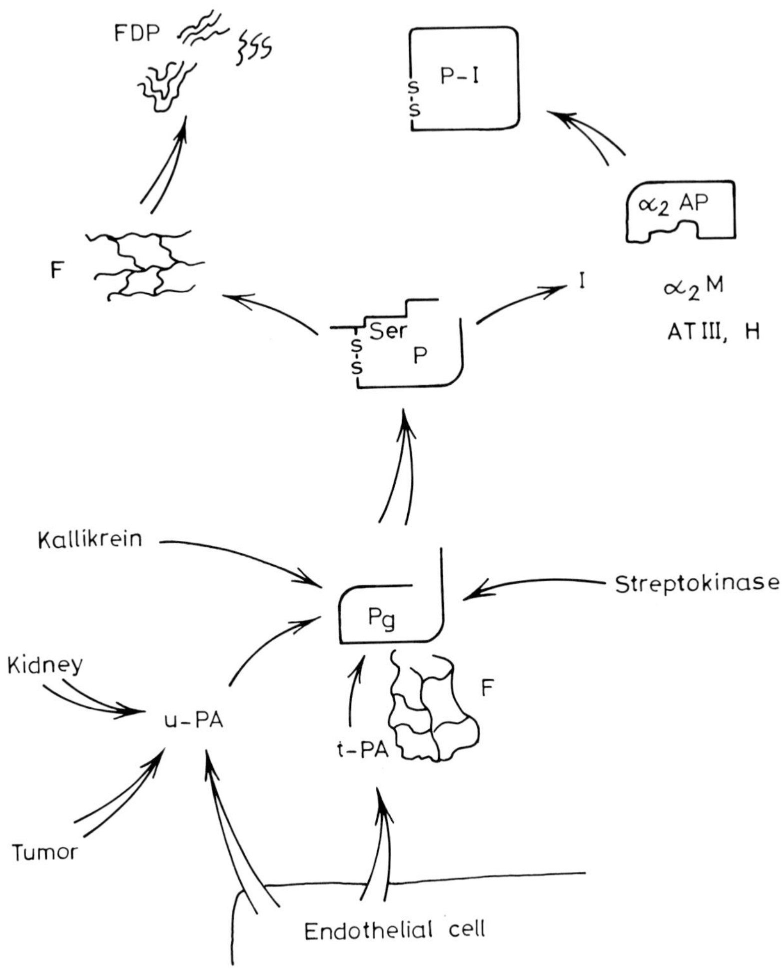

FIGURE 20. Control of the formation and activity of plasmin. Plasminogen (Pg), circulating in blood, can be activated in several ways. One of the most important activators is tissue-type plasminogen activator (t-PA) secreted by endothelial cells and acting on fibrin (F) surface. Urokinase-type plasminogen activator (u-PA), from different tissues, can also be a powerful activator, although its action is not localized to fibrin. Kallikrein is considered to be a proteinase with a rather slow reaction rate in plasminogen proteolysis. The exact control of the trigger(s), and of the rate for activation, are not known, although besides induction of activator release by blood coagulation factor(s), plasma proteinase inhibitor(s) are also assumed to participate in the regulation (not shown in this figure). Plasmin (P), formed by any kind of mechanism, however, may react with fibrin resulting in the formation of fibrin degradation products (FDP) or may be inactivated by plasma proteinase inhibitors (I) like α_2-macroglobulin (α_2-M), antithrombin III (AT III), and heparin (H), but mainly by α_2-antiplasmin (α_2-AP).

M, and the number of receptors increases by fivefold when platelets are activated.[431] This reaction may serve to localize and promote plasminogen activation.

2. *Plasminogen Activators*

A critical step in the determination of fibrinolysis is the conversion of plasminogen to the active enzyme, plasmin. In different tissues there are several plasminogen activators with various functions depending on the normal or pathological conditions (Figure 20).

a. Urokinase-Type Plasminogen Activator(s)

A number of forms of urokinase with different molecular weights can be found. The classical type, synthesized by the kidney and being present in the urine, is a proteolytic enzyme.[432] Its high molecular weight form, M_r 54,000 daltons, can be converted to a low molecular weight form, M_r 31,000 daltons,[433,434] by serine proteinases. Nevertheless, both forms of urokinase are active in vivo, and their different specific activities in vitro depend on the assay conditions.[435] As to the mechanism of plasminogen activation, it has been proposed that as a first step urokinase would split the Arg 560-Val 561 bond resulting in Glu-plasmin formation, and thereafter plasmin formed converts Glu- to Lys-plasmin.[436] Various urokinase-type plasminogen activators (u-PA), with different molecular weights, can also be found in several tumor tissues.[396]

b. Streptokinase

Streptokinase, a protein without proteolytic enzyme activity, is produced by β-hemolytic streptococci. It forms an equimolar complex with plasminogen leading to a conformational change of the proenzyme molecule and the demasking of the active center without proteolytic events.[437] The activated complex formed can directly convert plasminogen to plasmin. The reaction is more complicated in blood plasma.[438] A similar activation process may also be initiated by staphylokinase produced by staphylococci.

c. Factor XIIa and Kallikrein Pathway of Plasminogen Activation

Both F-XIIa and kallikrein can directly activate plasminogen,[439,440] as detailed earlier. The rate of activation of plasminogen on these ways, however, is slow compared with the reaction rate of urokinase or tissue-type plasminogen activator. The biological significance of the plasmin formation initiated by the contact activation phase is not known at present.

d. Tissue-Type Plasminogen Activators; Plasminogen Activator Synthesized by Endothelial Cells

Tissue-type plasminogen activators are widely distributed in various tissues and are different in some properties depending on the origin of the tissue as well as on the species.[441-444] Tissue-type plasminogen activator (t-PA) present in blood vessel perfusate is a single chain polypeptide[445] with M_r 74,000 daltons. In the presence of plasmin, tissue-type kallikrein or F-Xa (but not of F-XIIa, F-XIa, F-VIIa, protein C, and/or thrombin), the 1-chain molecule, is converted to a 2-chain enzyme without a change in the molecular mass.[170]

Endothelial cells synthesize both t-PA and urokinase-type (u-PA) plasminogen activators;[446,447] while bovine aortic endothelial cells secrete u-PA, human umbilical vein endothelial cells produce t-PA. The synthesis and release of plasminogen activators of endothelial cells are stimulated by thrombin, activated protein C, or by vasoactive peptides like bradykinin.[169,370,448]

As mentioned earlier, t-PA activity on plasminogen is enhanced in the presence of fibrin(ogen). Thus, fibrin seems to play a role in localization and acceleration of fibrinolysis at the appropriate place.

This aspect of the possible control of plasminogen activation, however, is not so simple. Not only fibrin, but other factors, such as denatured proteins or the endothelial cell-cofactor (see later) have the ability to enhance the rate of plasminogen activation by t-PA. We have found recently that pronase can activate plasminogen by proteolytic action ($K_m \approx 7\ \mu M$), but also has the capacity (when its active center is blocked) to accelerate plasminogen activation by t-PA.[530] Since pronase has sequence homology with streptokinase, these actions of this proteinase on fibrinolysis may be significant.

3. Plasma Proteinase Inhibitors of Plasmin and Plasminogen Activators

Human plasma contains several proteinase inhibitors and many of them may participate in the control of fibrinolysis, as well.[386] While antithrombin III and heparin cofactor II are believed to play primary role in blood coagulation, α_2-antiplasmin and α_2-macroglobulin are of importance for fibrinolysis.

a. α_2-Antiplasmin

α_2-Antiplasmin, a single-chain glycoprotein with M_r 70,000 daltons, forms a 1:1 stoichiometric complex with plasmin via the active center serine of the enzyme.[449,450] The reaction takes place in two steps, i.e., the first one is very rapid and reversible, with a K_d of 2×10^{-10} *M*, followed by a slower irreversible reaction.[428,429] The reaction between plasmin and α_2-antiplasmin is highly influenced by lysine or 6-aminohexanoic acid, which may be important in regulation of fibrinolysis.[386] The plasma level of α_2-antiplasmin is approximately 1 μM and it may decrease in liver diseases or intravascular coagulation.[451,452]

b. α_2-Macroglobulin

α_2-Macroglobulin is a nonspecific plasma proteinase inhibitor with a wide range of activity on proteinases of the blood coagulation-fibrinolytic system.[453] Regarding the mechanism of its action, α_2-macroglobulin forms a complex with proteinases at a site distinct from the active center, as described earlier. Accordingly, plasmin activity in a complex with α_2-macroglobulin is inhibited against fibrin(ogen), whereas other, small molecular weight substrates are henceforth available for proteolytic action.

Since the possible concentration of plasmin in plasma is approximately 1,5 μM, whereas the level of its primary inhibitor, α_2-antiplasmin, is only 1 μM,[454] it is believed that α_2-macroglobulin is necessary for the neutralization of the excess amount of plasmin. Moreover, α_2-macroglobulin can influence plasminogen activation as well.[455] The relative importance of α_2-macroglobulin compared with other plasma proteinase inhibitors in fibrinolysis, is not known at present.

c. Antithrombin III and Heparin

Beside α_2-antiplasmin and α_2-macroglobulin, at least three additional plasma proteinase inhibitors exist, namely, α_1-proteinase inhibitor, C1-inactivator, and antithrombin III.[456] Purified antithrombin III is an inhibitor of purified plasmin,[457] and heparin accelerates this reaction by a mechanism similar to the thrombin inactivation.[458] Other data in the literature, however, suggest that antithrombin III still does not play a role in fibrinolysis in vivo, since only a small amount of plasmin, formed in plasma, binds to antithrombin III.[459] Nevertheless, the possible role of heparin and antithrombin III in fibrinolysis, especially under some pathological conditions, needs further consideration.

d. Inhibitors of Plasminogen Activators

Our knowledge of the inhibition of plasminogen activators is still very preliminary, although this field is extensively studied nowadays. As to the urokinase inhibition in blood, all α_2-macroglobulin, α_1-proteinase inhibitor, α_2-antiplasmin, as well as antithrombin III, have been described to act as urokinase inhibitors.[449,460-462] Several inhibitors of intrinsic plasminogen activation exist also in human plasma: C1-inactivator, antithrombin III, and α_2-macroglobulin.[385,463,464]

Recently, a plasminogen activator inhibitor has been isolated from both aortic endothelial cells and umbilical vein endothelial cells, with an M_r of approximately 50,000 daltons.[465,466] This protein is a rapid inhibitor of tissue-type plasminogen activator as well as of urokinase-type plasminogen activator synthesized by endothelial cells.[467] This inhibitor also differs from other fibrinolytic inhibitors, like protease nexin, a cellular proteinase inhibitor, or plasma proteinase inhibitors.[468]

C. Role of Endothelial Cells and Polymorphonuclear Neutrophils in Fibrinolysis

Endothelial cells play a crucial role in fibrinolysis, either by the production of plasminogen activators or by the synthesis of their inhibitors. In addition, polymorphonuclear cells bound to endothelial cells may also contribute to the control of fibrinolysis.

1. Regulation of Plasminogen Activator Synthesis in Endothelial Cells

Endothelial cells are the main site of t-PA synthesis. These cells, as mentioned earlier, produce both u-PA and t-PA, and t-PA also contains two subpopulations of this enzyme — a proteinase with M_r of 74,000 daltons, which is comparable to that of t-PA originated from blood plasma, and one with an M_r of 100,000 daltons.[446,466] The latter form very probably represents an enzyme-inhibitor complex.

The factors influencing PA release from endothelial cells are different. Bradykinin, epinephrine, vasopressin, proteinases, and electroshock, as well as physical exercise, have been described to induce the release of PA either directly or indirectly acting on endothelial cells, although the exact mechanism of action is not known.[448,469-473] The effect of these vasoactive agents, however, is of very short duration. On the other hand, anabolic steroids produce long-term stimulation of endogenous fibrinolysis by increasing the synthesis as well as the release of PA.[474] On the basis of these and additional data, it is suggested that the release of PA is under neurohumoral control.[475]

Another very interesting regulation of fibrinolysis is the key enzyme of the blood coagulation system, thrombin. For example, thrombin, besides producing the substrate fibrin for plasmin, can also stimulate the release of PA from the coronary arteries of perfused dog hearts as well as the release of t-PA from cultured human endothelial cells.[169,441] Since venous thrombosis is frequently associated with a decreased fibrinolytic activity,[386] the understanding of the mechanisms resulting in PA release may contribute to the prevention of thromboembolic diseases.

2. Fibrin(ogen) Envelope of Endothelium

Fibrin formation and deposition, as well as fibrinolysis, can occur simultaneously under normal conditions on the endothelium. As a consequence of an equilibrium between blood coagulation and fibrinolysis, an endothelial fibrin lining is supposed.[476] Endothelial cells, at least those that are capillary, are covered by fibrin at the basement membrane, in the interendothelial space, and on the luminal surface of the cells. This fibrin lining may contribute to the rigidity and elasticity of the blood capillary wall, to microcircular hemorrheology, and to the maintenance of the antithrombotic nature of the blood vessel wall. It may also participate, as a porous Ca^{2+}-fibrin cement substance, in transport processes between blood plasma and tissues.

The exact mechanism of the formation of the fibrin lining is not known at present. A possible explanation would be the association of fibrinogen with endothelial cells and the high affinity of plasmin to endothelial cells. Fibrinogen, bound to endothelial cells with a K_d of approximately 2×10^{-7} *M*, may cause cell migration,[477] and it may serve as a substrate for plasmin, since plasmin also binds to endothelial cells very rapidly (and with high affinity) with a K_d of approximately 10^{-9} *M*.[171] Furthermore, Lys-plasminogen, but not Glu-plasminogen, shows high affinity to endothelial cells, and Lys-plasminogen is easily converted to plasmin on the endothelial cell surface.[478] Thus, it is possible that the endothelium is a "subtle" place for the fibrinolytic system. For instance, endothelial cells synthesize and release plasminogen activators, and activate plasminogen, preferentially Lys-plasminogen, bound to endothelial cell. The plasmin formed also binds to the cells and commences to dissolve fibrin, formed from fibrinogen on the endothelial cell surface. Accordingly, plasmin(ogen), fibrin(ogen), and plasminogen activator(s) operate in concert.

3. Endothelial Cell-Cofactor for Tissue-Type Plasminogen Activator

Since plasmin(ogen) binds to endothelial cells, where the reaction rate of plasminogen activation is accelerated, endothelial cells may contribute to the control of fibrinolysis not only by the synthesis of some components of the fibrinolytic system, but also by the regulation of the reaction rate(s) on the surface. Recently, we have found a protein cofactor in the extract of coronary and cultured valve endothelial cells (but not in platelets or red and white blood cells) which can accelerate the plasminogen-t-PA by a rate of at least two orders of magnitude. The mechanism of action of this cofactor differs from that of fibrin(ogen); endothelial cell-cofactor does not influence K_m, but increases V_{max}.[531] The cofactor for t-PA seems to be an endothelial cell membrane component.

4. Polymorphonuclear Neutrophils and Fibrinolysis

Polymorphonuclear cells also participate in fibrinolysis, i.e., they have components of alternative fibrinolysis.[479] Neutrophil granules have the capacity to degrade both fibrinogen and fibrin.[480] Since these cells secrete lytic agents,[481] and are able to adhere directly to endothelial cells, approximately four to five blood cells per single endothelial cell,[165] it has been suggested that granulocytes, and not plasmin, play the primary role in spontaneous fibrinolysis.[482] Moreover, polymorphonuclear leukocytes activated by chemoattractants can also trigger the PGI_2 production of endothelial cells.[483] Although investigation of the roles of granulocytes in hemostasis is one of the most rapidly developing aspects in the field discussed above, the exact actions of polymorphonuclear cells in fibrinolysis, especially in inflammation, however, are not known at present.

VI. ROLE OF LIVER IN HEMOSTASIS

Of the proteins present in circulating blood, large amounts originate from the liver. Among them, almost all proenzymes and inhibitors of the blood coagulation-fibrinolytic system are synthesized and secreted by the liver.[485] It synthesizes proteins intensively, i.e., approximately 1 to 2 mg/g of tissue per hour.[484] The liver takes part, however, not only in the production, but also in the elimination of the components of hemostasis.

This function of the liver in hemostasis is a consequence of a well-controlled mutual action of various types of cells. Thus, whereas hepatocytes are considered as part of the biosynthetic process, the macrophage system, the Kupffer cells are mainly responsible for the degradation of several molecules and the liver endothelial cells would play a role in the transport and barrier processes.

Although many aspects of the protein synthesis as well as the modification of the proenzymes are clear at present, the regulation of the biosynthetic process, the modification of amino acid residues of the proteins, and the fate of the components of blood coagulation-fibrinolytic system taken up by the liver are rather unknown.

A. Synthesis of the Molecular Components of the Blood Coagulation-Fibrinolytic System

The liver participates in hemostasis directly and indirectly through synthetic processes, namely liver cells synthesize proenzymes and proteinase inhibitors as well as modify the proteins to be suitable for functions.

1. Biosynthesis of Proteins Involved in the Blood Coagulation-Fibrinolytic System

Most secretory proteins, like proenzymes of the blood coagulation system, are synthesized in a precursor form with an N-terminal leader sequence. This sequence, which is highly hydrophobic, containing 15 to 30 amino acid residues, binds to specific membrane sites. The precursor form of prothrombin, called preprothrombin, for example, is cleaved by the signal peptidase leading to the emergence and secretion of prothrombin. The proteolysis of the bond between the signal peptide and prothrombin part of the preprothrombin molecule, as well as the initial glycosylation of the polypeptide chain, occur as cotranslational events prior to the release of the completed protein from ribosomes.[486]

The liver, however, synthesizes and secretes not only prothrombin, but other vitamin K-dependent factors, components of the fibrinolysis as well as inhibitors of proteinases of the blood coagulation-fibrinolytic system. Thus, synthesis of the vitamin K-dependent proteins, like F-X, F-IX, F-VII, protein C and protein S, is liver dependent,[487] although macrophages are also able to produce these proteins.[488] The production of F-XI and F-XII by liver is supported only by indirect proof.[489] A F-X activating component, inducible by lipopolysaccharides,[490] has also been found in hepatic macrophages. Fibrinogen is also synthesized and secreted by hepatocytes.[491-493]

Among the plasma proteinase inhibitors, α_2-macroglobulin,[494,495] antithrombin III,[496,497] α_1-proteinase inhibitor,[498] and α_2-antiplasmin[499,500] are known at present to by synthesized and secreted by hepatocytes. Hepatocytes also produce heparan sulfate.[501] VLD-lipoprotein,[502] and plasminogen.[503,504]

The main question at present is, how is the plasma level of these proteins controlled? There are several possibilities for the regulation of the synthesis and secretion of these proteins, although only few experimental data exist which mainly concern prothrombin synthesis. Accordingly, a prothrombin degradation product, residues 1 to 42 at the N-terminal region of prothrombin also containing the γ-carboxyglutamyl acids, induces prothrombin synthesis.[505] Indirect evidence for endocrine control of prothrombin synthesis has also been published.[506] Furthermore, a humoral factor, coagulopoietin-III, that regulates prothrombin level in the circulating blood has also been found.[507] Its chemical nature, however, has not yet been determined and the question of whether this factor is identical with any degradation product of the clotting factors cannot be answered at present.

Endocrine control for fibrinogen synthesis has been suggested, since its relatively selective increase by dexamethasone was found.[493,508] Furthermore, estrogens seem to decrease the synthesis of antithrombin III.[509]

2. *Modification of Proteins Synthesized by Liver Cells; Role of Vitamin K*

As mentioned earlier, a critical step in blood coagulation is the surface formation in blood plasma, mainly phospholipid surface of platelet or damaged tissues, for the acceleration of the cascade reaction. This surface, if formed, is available for the binding of proteins containing γ-carboxyglutamic acids (Gla) via Ca^{2+} bridges between Gla residues of protein and phospholipids of blood vessel wall and/or platelets. The Gla moieties of proteins are formed by the modification of some glutamic acid residues of the polypeptide chain during protein biosynthesis in the liver.

Three enzyme actions seem to be involved in Gla formation. A carboxylase catalyzes CO_2 incorporation into the carbon atom at γ-position in glutamic acid. This reaction also requires the labilization of the hydrogen atom. The exact mechanism of the carboxyl group incorporation, however, is not known at present.[484] Superoxide anion formation via semiquinone, as well as peroxy radical production, are supposed as probable mechanisms.[510,511] Whichever is the mechanism, the reactions are coupled to the vitamin K cycle, i.e., to hydroquinone, quinone, epoxide, and hydroquinone conversions. The cycle involves two additional enzyme reactions catalyzed by an epoxide reductase and a dehydrogenase* with NADPH as the hydrogen donor. The energy required for the carboxylation reaction is supplied by the oxido-reduction cycle. Under pathological conditions, in certain liver diseases,[485] or in the absence of viatmin K_1, hemorrhage may develop.

* Coumarins, e.g., warfarin, used for the prevention of thrombus development are assumed to inhibit this dehydrogenase reaction.

397. **Hawiger, J., Hammond, D. K., and Timmons, S.,** Human fibrinogen possesses binding sites for staphylococci on Aα and Bβ polypeptide chains, *Nature (London),* 258, 643, 1975.
398. **Verstraete, M. and Vermylen, J.,** Fibrinolysis, in *Thrombosis,* Verstraete, M. and Vermylen, J., Eds., Pergamon Press, Oxford, 1984, 40.
399. **Murano, G. and Bick, R. L.,** Fibrino(geno)lysis, in *Basic Concepts of Hemostasis and Thrombosis,* Murano, G. and Bick, R. L., Eds., CRC Press, Boca Raton, Fla., 1980, 61.
400. **Duckert, F. and Beck, E. A.,** Clinical disorders due to the deficiency of Factor XIII (fibrin stabilizing factor, fibrinase), *Semin. Hematol.,* 5, 83, 1968.
401. **Gaffney, P. J.,** The fibrinolytic system, in *Hemostasis and Thrombosis,* Bloom, A. L. and Thomas, D. P., Eds., Churchill Livingstone, Edinburgh, 1981, 198.
402. **Marder, V. J. and Francis, C. W.,** Plasmin degradation of cross-linked fibrin, *Ann. N.Y. Acad. Sci.,* 408, 397, 1983.
403. **Edgington, T. W. and Plow, E.,** Differentiation between fibrinogen and fibrin cleavage fragments based on immunochemical correlates of structure and clinical implications, in *Haemostasis and Thrombosis,* Neri-Serneri, G. G. and Prentice, C. R. M., Eds., Academic Press, London, 1979, 27.
404. **Gormsen, J., Fletcher, A. P., Alkjaersig, N., and Sherry, S.,** Enzymic lysis of plasma clots. The influence of fibrin stabilization on lysis rates, *Arch. Biochem. Biophys.,* 120, 654, 1967.
405. **Schwartz, M. L., Pizzo, S. V., Hill, R. C., and McKee, P. A.,** Human factor XIII from plasma and platelets. Molecular weights subunit structures, proteolytic activation and cross-linking of fibrinogen and fibrin, *J. Biol. Chem.,* 248, 1395, 1973.
406. **Lorand, L. and Konishi, K.,** Activation of the fibrin stabilizing factor of plasma by thrombin, *Arch. Biochem. Biophys.,* 105, 58, 1964.
407. **Gaffney, P. J.,** Fibrinolysis by plasmin and brinase: in vitro and in vivo observations, in *Progress in Chemical Fibrinolysis and Thrombosis,* Vol. 3, Davidson, J. F., Cepelak, V. M., Samama, M. M., and Desnoyers, P. C., Eds., Raven Press, New York, 1978, 349.
408. **Pisano, J. J., Finlayson, J. S., and Peyton, M. P.,** Crosslink in fibrin polymerized by factor XIII; ε-(γ-glutamyl)lysine, *Science,* 160, 892, 1968.
409. **McKee, P. A., Mattock, P., and Hill, R. L.,** Subunit structure of human fibrinogen, soluble fibrin and crosslinked insoluble fibrin, *Proc. Natl. Acad. Sci. U.S.A.,* 66, 738, 1970.
410. **Gaffney, P. J., Brasher, M., Lord, K., Strachan, C. J. L., Wilkinson, A. R., Kakkar, V. V., and Scully, M. F.,** Fibrin subunits in venous and arterial thromboembolism, *Cardiovasc. Res.,* 10, 421, 1976.
411. **Kopec, M., Teisseyre, E., Dudek-Wojciechowska, G., Klocewiak, M., Pankiewicz, A., and Latallo, Z. S.,** Studies on the "double D" fragment from stabilized bovine fibrin, *Thromb. Res.,* 2, 283, 1973.
412. **Gaffney, P. J.,** Subunit relationships between fibrinogen and fibrin degradation products, *Thromb. Res.,* 2, 201, 1973.
413. **Wallen, P. and Wiman, B.,** On the generation of intermediate plasminogen and its significance for activation, in *Proteases and Biological Control,* Reich, E., Rifkin, D. B., and Shaw, E., Eds., Cold Spring Harbor Laboratory, Cold Spring Harbor, N.Y., 1975, 291.
414. **Robbins, K. C., Summaria, L., and Barlow, G. H.,** Activation of Plasminogen, in *Proteases and Biological Control,* Reich, E., Rifkin, D. B., and Shaw, E., Eds., Cold Spring Harbor Laboratory, Cold Spring Harbor, N.Y., 1975, 305.
415. **Wiman, B. and Collen, D.,** Molecular mechanism of physiological fibrinolysis, *Nature (London),* 272, 549, 1978.
416. **Sjöholm, I., Wiman, B., and Wallen, P.,** Studies on the conformational changes of plasminogen induced during activation to plasmin and by 6-aminohexanoic acid, *Eur. J. Biochem.,* 39, 471, 1973.
417. **Wiman, B. and Wallen, P.,** Structural relationships between "glutamic acid" and "lysine" forms of human plasminogen and their interaction with the amino terminal activator peptide as studied by affinity chromatography, *Eur. J. Biochem.,* 50, 489, 1975.
418. **Sottrup-Jensen, L., Claeys, H., Zajdel, M., Petersen, T. E., and Magnussen, S.,** The primary structure of human plasminogen: isolation of two lysine-binding fragments and one "mini"-plasminogen (MW 38,000) by elastase-catalysed-specific limited proteolysis, in *Progress in Chemical Fibrinolysis and Thrombosis,* Vol. 3, Davidson, J. F., Rowan, R. M., Samama, M. M., Desnoyers, P. C., Eds., Raven Press, New York, 1978, 191.
419. **Collen, D.,** On the regulation and control of fibrinolysis, *Thromb. Haemost.,* 43, 77, 1980.
420. **Saksela, O.,** Plasminogen activation and regulation of pericellular proteolysis, *Biochim. Biophys. Acta,* 823, 35, 1985.
421. **Walther, P. J., Hill, R. L., and McKee, P. A.,** The importance of the preactivation peptide in the two-stage mechanism of human plasminogen activation, *J. Biol. Chem.,* 250, 5926, 1975.
422. **Blix, S.,** Studies on the fibrinolytic systems in the euglobulin fraction of human plasma. A: Methodological study. B: Application of the methods, *Scand. J. Clin. Lab. Invest.,* 13, 3, 1961.
423. **Cederholm-Williams, S.,** The binding of plasminogen (MW 84,000) and plasmin to fibrin, *Thromb. Res.,* 11, 421, 1977.

424. **Thorsen, S.,** Differences in the binding to fibrin of native plasminogen and plasminogen modified by proteolytic degradation. Influence of omega-amino-carboxylic acids, *Biochim. Biophys. Acta,* 393, 55, 1975.
425. **Moroi, M. and Aoki, N.,** Inhibition of plasminogen binding to fibrin by α_2-plasmin inhibitor, *Thromb. Res.,* 10, 851, 1977.
426. **Markus, G., De Pasquale, J. L., and Wissler, F. C.,** Quantitative determination of the binding of epsilon-aminocaproic acid to native plasminogen, *J. Biol. Chem.,* 253, 727, 1978.
427. **Rakoczi, I., Wiman, B., and Collen, D.,** On the biological significance of the specific interaction between fibrin, plasminogen and antiplasmin, *Biochim. Biophys. Acta,* 540, 295, 1978.
428. **Christensen, U. and Clemmensen, I.,** Kinetic properties of the primary inhibitor of plasmin from human plasma, *Biochem. J.,* 163, 389, 1977.
429. **Wiman, B. and Collen, D.,** On the kinetics of the reaction between human antiplasmin and plasmin, *Eur. J. Biochem.,* 84, 573, 1978.
430. **Camiolo, S. M., Thorsen, S., and Astrup, T.,** Fibrinogenolysis and fibrinolysis with tissue plasminogen activator, urokinase, streptokinase-activated human globulin and plasmin, *Proc. Soc. Exp. Biol. Med.,* 38, 277, 1971.
431. **Miles, L. A. and Plow, E. F.,** Binding and activation of plasminogen on the platelet surface, *J. Biol. Chem.,* 260, 4303, 1985.
432. **MacFarlane, R. G. and Pilling, J.,** Fibrinolytic activity of normal urine, *Nature (London),* 159, 779, 1947.
433. **White, F. W., Barlow, G. H., and Mozen, M. M.,** The isolation and characterization of plasminogen activators (urokinase) from human urine, *Biochemistry,* 5, 2160, 1966.
434. **Lesuk, A., Terminiello, L., and Traver, J. H.,** Crystalline human urokinase: some properties, *Science,* 147, 880, 1965.
435. **Philo, R. D. and Gaffney, P. J.,** Assay methodology for urokinase: its use in assessing the composition of mixtures of high- and low-molecular weight urokinase, *Thromb. Res.,* 21, 81, 1981.
436. **Thorsen, S., Suenson, E., Mullertz, S., and Kok, P.,** Transformation of plasminogen (PLG) and the selective degradation of fibrin (FN) in human blood plasma, Proc. 5th Int. Conf. Synth. Fibr. Thromb. Agents, (Abstr.) 23, 1980.
437. **Castellino, F. J.,** A unique enzyme-protein substrate modifier reaction: plasmin/streptokinase interaction, *Trends Biochem. Sci.,* 4, 1, 1979.
438. **Robbins, K. C. and Markus, G.,** The interaction of human plasminogen with streptokinase, in *Fibrinolysis: Current Clinical and Fundamental Concepts,* Gaffney, P. J. and Balkuv-Ulutin, S., Eds., Academic Press, London, 1978, 61.
439. **Goldsmith, G. H., Saito, H., and Ratnoff, O. D.,** The activation of plasminogen by Hageman Factor (Factor XII) and Hageman Factor fragments, *J. Clin. Invest.,* 21, 54, 1978.
440. **Vennerod, A. M. and Laake, K.,** Prekallikrein and plasminogen proactivator. Absence of plasminogen proactivator in Fletcher factor deficient plasma, *Thromb. Res.,* 8, 519, 1976.
441. **Matsubara, F., Sueishi, K., Ishii, Y., and Tanaka, K.,** Release of plasminogen activator from isolated perfused dog heart, *Thromb. Haemost.,* 53, 126, 1985.
442. **Holemans, R., Johnston, J. G., and Reddick, R. L.,** Release of plasminogen activator by the isolated perfused dog kidney, *Nature (London),* 208, 291, 1965.
443. **Onoyama, K. and Tanaka, K.,** Fibrinolytic activity of the arterial wall, *Thromb. Diath. Haemorrh.,* 21, 1, 1969.
444. **Auerswald, W., Binder, B., and Doleschel, W.,** "Angiokinase" — molecular weights of proteins representing a perivascular plasminogen activator, *Thromb. Diath. Haemorrh.,* 26, 411, 1971.
445. **Binder, B. A., Spragg, J., and Austin, K. F.,** Purification and characterization of human vascular plasminogen activator derived from blood vessel perfusates, *J. Biol. Chem.,* 254, 1998, 1979.
446. **Levin, E. G. and Loskutoff, D. J.,** Cultured bovine endothelial cells produce both urokinase and tissue-type plasminogen activators, *J. Cell Biol.,* 94, 631, 1982.
447. **Bykowska, K., Levin, E. G., Rijker, D. C., Loskutoff, D. J., and Collen, D.,** Characterization of a plasminogen activator secreted by cultured bovine aortic endothelial cells, *Biochim. Biophys. Acta,* 703, 113, 1982.
448. **Smith, D., Gilbert, M., and Owen, W. G.,** Tissue plasminogen activator release in vivo in response to vasoactive agents, *Blood,* 66, 835, 1985.
449. **Moroi, M. and Aoki, N.,** Isolation and characterization of alpha-2-plasmin inhibitor from human plasma. A novel proteinase inhibitor which inhibits activator-induced clot lysis, *J. Biol. Chem.,* 251, 5956, 1976.
450. **Wiman, B. and Collen, D.,** Purification and characterization of human antiplasmin, the fast-acting plasmin inhibitor in plasma, *Eur. J. Biochem.,* 78, 19, 1977.
451. **Edy, J., Collen, D., and Verstraete, M.,** Quantitation of the plasma protease inhibitor antiplasmin with the chromogenic substrate S-2251, in *Progress in Chemical Fibrinolysis and Thrombosis,* Vol. 3, Davidson, J. F., Rowan, R. M., Samama, M. M., and Desnoyers, P. C., Eds., Raven Press, New York, 1978, 315.

452. **Teger-Nilsson, A. C., Friberg, P., and Gyzander, E.,** Determination of a new rapid plasmin inhibitor in human blood by means of a plasmin specific tripeptide substrate, *Scand. J. Clin. Lab. Invest.*, 37, 403, 1977.
453. **Feldman, S. R., Gonias, S. L., and Pizzo, S. V.,** Model of α_2-macroglobulin structure and function, *Proc. Natl. Acad. Sci. U.S.A.*, 82, 5700, 1985.
454. **Müllertz, S. and Clemmensen, I.,** The primary inhibitor of plasmin in human plasma, *Biochem. J.*, 159, 545, 1976.
455. **McConnell, D. J.,** Inhibitors of kallikrein in human plasma, *J. Clin. Invest.*, 51, 1611, 1972.
456. **Steinbuch, M.,** Les antiprotéases du plasma, *Rev. Fr. Trans.*, 14, 61, 1971.
457. **Highsmith, R. and Rosenberg, R. D.,** The inhibition of human plasmin by human-antithrombin-heparin cofactor, *J. Biol. Chem.*, 249, 4335, 1974.
458. **Machovich, R., Bauer, P. I., Arányi, P., Kecskés, E., Büki, K., and Horváth, I.,** Kinetic analysis of the heparin-enhanced plasmin/antithrombin III reaction. Apparent catalytic role of heparin, *Biochem. J.*, 199, 521, 1981.
459. **Collen, D., Semerano, N., Telesforo, P., and Verstraete, M.,** The inhibition of plasmin by antithrombin III-heparin complex during thrombolytic therapy in man, *Br. J. Haematol.*, 39, 101, 1978.
460. **Ogston, D., Bennett, B., Herbert, R. J., and Douglas, A. S.,** The inhibition of urokinase by α_2-macroglobulin, *Clin. Sci.*, 44, 73, 1973.
461. **Clemmensen, I. and Christensen, U.,** Inhibition of urokinase by complex formation with human α_1-antitrypsin, *Biochim. Biophys. Acta,* 249, 591, 1976.
462. **Clemmensen, I.,** Inhibition of urokinase by complex formation with human antithrombin III in absence and presence of heparin, *Thromb. Haemost.*, 39, 616, 1978.
463. **Cluft, C.,** Elimination of inhibition in euglobulin fibrinolysis by use of flutenamate: involvement of C1-inactivator, *Haemostasis,* 6, 351, 1977.
464. **Cluft, C., Jie, A. F. H., Sprengers, E. D., and Verheijen, J. H.,** Identification of a reversible inhibitor of plasminogen activators in blood plasma, *FEBS Lett.*, 190, 315, 1985.
465. **van Mourik, J. A., Lawrence, D. A., and Loskutoff, D. J.,** Purification of an inhibitor of plasminogen activator (antiactivator) synthesized by endothelial cells, *J. Biol. Chem.*, 259, 14,914, 1984.
466. **Philips, M., Juul, A.-G., and Thorsen, S.,** Human endothelial cells produce a plasminogen activator inhibitor and a tissue-type plasminogen activator-inhibitor complex, *Biochim. Biophys. Acta,* 802, 99, 1984.
467. **Loskutoff, D. J. and Edgington, T. S.,** An inhibitor of plasminogen activator in rabbit endothelial cells, *J. Biol. Chem.*, 256, 4142, 1981.
468. **Hekman, C. M. and Loskutoff, D. J.,** Endothelial cells produce a latent inhibitor of plasminogen activators that can be activated by denaturants, *J. Biol. Chem.*, 260, 11,581, 1985.
469. **Markwardt, F. and Klocking, H. P.,** Studies on the release of plasminogen activator, *Thromb. Res.*, 8, 217, 1976.
470. **Marsh, N. A. and Gaffney, P. J.,** Some observations on the release of extrinsic and intrinsic plasminogen activators during exercise in man, *Haemostasis,* 9, 238, 1980.
471. **Hijikata, A., Hirata, M., and Kitaguchi, H.,** Effect of proteases on plasminogen activator release from isolated perfused dog leg, *Thromb. Res.*, 20, 521, 1980.
472. **Pina-Cabral, J. M. and Rodrigues, C.,** Blood catecholamine levels, factor VIII and fibrinolysis after therapeutic electroshock, *Br. J. Haematol.*, 28, 371, 1974.
473. **Hawkey, C. M., Britton, B. J., Wood, W. G., Peele, M., and Irving, M. H.,** Changes in blood catecholamine levels and blood coagulation and fibrinolytic activity in response to graded exercise in man, *Br. J. Haematol.*, 29, 377, 1975.
474. **Nilsson, I. M.,** Effect of drugs on plasminogen activator synthesis and release, in *Progress in Chemical Fibrinolysis and Thrombolysis,* Vol. 3, Davidson, J. F., Rowan, R. M., Samama, M. M., and Desnoyers, P., Eds., Raven Press, New York, 1978, 77.
475. **Cash, J. D.,** Control mechanisms of activator release, in *Progress in Chemical Fibrinolysis and Thrombolysis,* Vol. 3, Davidson, J. F., Rowan, R. M., Samama, M. M., and Desnoyers, P. C., Eds., Raven Press, New York, 1978, 65.
476. **Copley, A. L.,** The physiological significance of the endothelial fibrin lining as the critical interface in the "vessel-blood organ" and the importance of in vivo "fibrinogenin" formation in health and disease, *Thromb. Res.*, Suppl. 5, 105, 1983.
477. **Dejana, E., Langulno, L. R., Polentarutti, N., Balconi, G., Ryckewaert, J. J., Larrieu, M., Donatti, M. B., Mantovani, A., and Marguerie, G.,** Interaction between fibrinogen and cultured endothelial cells; induction of migration and specific binding, *J. Clin. Invest.*, 75, 1, 1985.
478. **Machovich, R.,** The role of the blood coagulation-fibrinolytic system and endothelial cell in malignancy, in *Hemostasis and Cancer,* Vol. 1, Muszbek, L., Ed., CRC Press, Boca Raton, Fla., 1987, 1.
479. **Plow, E. and Edgington, T. S.,** An alternative pathway for fibrinolysis. I. The cleavage of fibrinogen by leucocyte protease at physiological pH, *J. Clin. Invest.*, 56, 30, 1975.

480. **Kopéc, M., Wegrzynowicz, Z., Ardelt, W., Teisseyre, E., and Latallo, Z. S.,** Effect of elastolytic enzymes from human leukocyte granules and from pig pancreas on plasminogen, fibrinogen and fibrin, in *Progress in Chemical Fibrinolysis and Thrombolysis,* Vol. 3, Davidson, J. F., Rowan, R. M., Samama, M. M., and Desnoyers, P. C., Eds., Raven Press, New York, 1978, 417.
481. **Kwaan, H. C. and Hatem, A. A.,** The lysis of early fibrin by eosinophils, in *Progress in Chemical Fibrinolysis and Thrombolysis,* Vol. 3, Davidson, J. F., Rowan, R. M., Samama, M. M., and Desnoyers, P. C., Eds., Raven Press, New York, 1978, 413.
482. **Moroz, L. A. and Gilmore, N. J.,** Fibrinolysis in normal plasma and blood: evidence for significant mechanisms independent of the plasminogen-plasmin system, *Blood,* 48, 531, 1976.
483. **Miller, D. K., Sadowski, S., Soderman, D. D., and Kuehl, F. A.,** Endothelial cell prostacyclin production induced by activated neutrophils, *J. Biol. Chem.,* 260, 1006, 1985.
484. **Machovich, R.,** Biosynthesis of prothrombin, in *The Thrombin,* Vol. 2, Machovich, R., Ed., CRC Press, Boca Raton, Fla., 1984, 43.
485. **Flute, P. T.,** Clotting abnormalities in liver disease, in *Progress in Liver Diseases,* Vol. 6, Popper, M. and Schaffner, F., Eds., Grune and Stratton, New York, 1979, chap. 16.
486. **Chung, D. W., MacGillivray, R. T. A., and Davie, E. W.,** The biosynthesis of bovine fibrinogen, prothrombin and albumin in a cell-free system, *Ann. N.Y. Acad. Sci.,* 343, 210, 1980.
487. **Suttie, J. W., McTigue, J., Larson, A. E., and Wallin, R.,** Biosynthesis of prothrombin complex proteins, *Ann. N.Y. Acad. Sci.,* 344, 271, 1981.
488. **Østerud, B., Lindahl, U., and Seljelid, R.,** Macrophages produce blood coagulation factors, *FEBS Lett.,* 120, 41, 1980.
489. **Walker, I. R., Milner, R. A., Johnston, M. A., Rand, A. C. A., Neame, P. B., and Hirsh, J.,** Factors XI and XII are low in subjects with liver disease, *Digest. Dis. Sci.,* 28, 967, 1983.
490. **Maier, R. V. and Ulevitch, R. J.,** The induction of a unique procoagulant activity in rabbit hepatic macrophages by bacterial lipopolysaccharides, *J. Immunol.,* 127, 1596, 1981.
491. **Grieninger, G., Hertzberg, K. M., and Pindyck, J.,** Fibrinogen synthesis in serum-free hepatocyte cultures: stimulation by glucocorticoids, *Proc. Natl. Acad. Sci. U.S.A.,* 75, 5506, 1978.
492. **Amrani, D. L., Plant, P. W., Pindyck, J., Mosesson, M. W., and Grieninger, G.,** Structural analysis of fibrinogen synthesized by cultured chicken hepatocytes in the presence or absence of dexametasone, *Biochim. Biophys. Acta,* 743, 394, 1983.
493. **Grieninger, G., Plant, P. W., Liang, T. J., Kalb, R. G., Amrani, D., Mosesson, M. W., Hertzberg, K. M., and Pindyck, J.,** Hormonal regulation of fibrinogen synthesis in cultured hepatocytes, *Ann. N.Y. Acad. Sci.,* 408, 469, 1983.
494. **Andus, T., Gross, V., Tran-Thi, T.-A., and Heinrich, P. C.,** Synthesis of α_2-macroglobulin in rat hepatocytes and in a cell-free system, *FEBS Lett.,* 151, 10, 1983.
495. **Northemann, W., Andus, T., Gross, V., and Heinrich, P. C.,** Cell-free synthesis of rat α_2-macroglobulin and induction of its mRNA during experimental inflammation, *Eur. J. Biochem.,* 217, 258, 1983.
496. **Watada, M., Nagakawa, M., Kitani, T., Okajima, Y., Maeda, Y., Urano, S., and Ijichi, N.,** Identification of the AT III synthesizing hepatocytes by immunofluorescent technique, *Thromb. Haemost.,* 46, 284, 1981.
497. **Leon, M., Aiach, M., Guennec, J. Y., Yarnet, J., Girot, R., Fiessinger, J. N., and Jaubert, F.,** Antithrombin III in rat hepatocytes, *Thromb. Res.,* 28, 115, 1982.
498. **Eriksson, S., Alm, R., and Astedt, B.,** Organ cultures of human fetal hepatocytes in the study of extra- and intracellular α_1-antitrypsin, *Biochim. Biophys. Acta,* 542, 496, 1978.
499. **Saito, H., Goodnough, L. T., Aden, D. P., and Knowles, B. B.,** Synthesis and secretion of α_2-antiplasmin by human liver cell lines, *Blood,* 58, 225a, 1981.
500. **Högstorp, H. and Saldeen, T.,** Synthesis of α_2-antiplasmin by rat liver cells, *Thromb. Res.,* 28, 19, 1982.
501. **Sinn, W., Sudhakaran, P. R., and von Figura, K.,** Stimulation of heparan sulphate synthesis in cultured rat hepatocytes by (+)-catechin, *Biochem. J.,* 200, 51, 1981.
502. **Haagsman, H. P. and van Golde, L. M. G.,** Synthesis and secretion of very low density lipoproteins by isolated rat hepatocytes in suspension: role of diacylglycerol acyltransferase, *Arch. Biochem. Biophys.,* 208, 395, 1981.
503. **Raum, D., Marcus, D., Alper, C. A., Levey, R., Taylor, P. D., and Starzl, T. E.,** Synthesis of human plasminogen by the liver, *Science,* 208, 1036, 1980.
504. **Bohmfalk, J. F. and Fuller, G. M.,** Plasminogen is synthesized by primary cultures of rat hepatocytes, *Science,* 209, 408, 1980.
505. **Graves, C. B., Munns, T. W., Carlisle, T. L., Grant, G. A., and Strauss, A. W.,** Induction of prothrombin synthesis by prothrombin fragments, *Proc. Natl. Acad. Sci. U.S.A.,* 78, 4772, 1981.
506. **Siegfried, C. M., Knauer, G. R., and Matschiner, J. T.,** Evidence for increased formation of preprothrombin and the noninvolvement of vitamin K-dependent reactions in sex-linked hyperprothrombinemia in the rat, *Arch. Biochim. Biophys.,* 194, 486, 1979.

507. **Karpatkin, M. and Karpatkin, S.,** Humoral factor that specifically regulates prothrombin levels, *Proc. Natl. Acad. Sci. U.S.A.,* 76, 491, 1979.
508. **Amrani, D. L., Mosesson, M. W., and Coide, T.,** Evidence that chicken antithrombin III is a developmentally regulated glycoprotein synthesized by hepatocytes, *Biochim. Biophys. Acta,* 847, 324, 1985.
509. **Verstraete, M. and Vermylen, J.,** Thrombosis in association with oral contraceptives and other drugs, in *Thrombosis,* Verstraete, M. and Vermylen, J., Eds., Pergamon Press, Oxford, 1984, 67.
510. **Esnouf, M. P., Green, M. R., Hill, H. A. O., and Walter, S. J.,** The inhibition of the vitamin K-dependent carboxylation of glutamyl residues in prothrombin by copper complexes, *FEBS Lett.,* 107, 146, 1979.
511. **Larson, A. E., McTigue, J. J., and Suttie, J. W.,** Investigation of the role of oxygen in the vitamin K-dependent carboxylase reaction, in *Vitamin K Metabolism and Vitamin K-Dependent Proteins,* Suttie, J. W., Ed., University Park Press, Baltimore, 1979, 413.
512. **Spolarics, Z., Mandl, J., Machovich, R., Lambin, P., Garzó, T., Antoni, F., and Horváth, I.,** Association of α_2-macroglobulin-thrombin and α_2-macroglobulin-plasmin complexes with isolated hepatocytes, *Biochim. Biophys. Acta,* 845, 389, 1985.
513. **Fuchs, H. E., Shifman, M. A., and Pizzo, S. V.,** In vivo catabolism of α_1-proteinase inhibitor-trypsin, antithrombin III-thrombin and α_2-macroglobulin-methylamine, *Biochim. Biophys. Acta,* 716, 151, 1982.
514. **Vogel, C. N., Kingdon, H. S., and Lundblad, R. L.,** Correlation of in vivo and in vitro inhibition of thrombin by plasma inhibitor, *J. Lab. Clin. Med.,* 93, 661, 1979.
515. **Lam, L. S. L., Regoeczi, E., and Hatton, M. W. C.,** In vivo behaviour of some antithrombin III-protease complexes, *Br. J. Exp. Pathol.,* 60, 151, 1979.
516. **Shifman, M. A. and Pizzo, S. V.,** The in vivo metabolism of antithrombin III and antithrombin III complexes, *J. Biol. Chem.,* 257, 3243, 1982.
517. **Bauer, P. I., Mandl, J., Machovich, R., Antoni, F., Garzó, T., and Horváth, I.,** Specific binding of thrombin-antithrombin III complex to hepatocytes, *Thromb. Res.,* 28, 595, 1982.
518. **Collen, D. and Wiman, B.,** Turnover of antiplasmin, the fast-acting plasmin inhibitor of plasma, *Blood,* 53, 313, 1979.
519. **Gliemann, J., Larsen, T. R., and Sottrup-Jensen, L.,** Cell association and degradation of α_2-macroglobulin-trypsin complexes in hepatocytes and adipocytes, *Biochim. Biophys. Acta,* 756, 230, 1983.
520. **Owen, W. G.,** Hemostasis. Role of endothelium in the regulation of inhibitory and catabolic pathways, *Arch. Pathol. Lab. Med.,* 106, 209, 1982.
521. **Comp, P. C. and Esmon, C. T.,** Evidence for multiple roles for activated protein C in fibrinolysis, in *The Regulation of Coagulation,* Mann, K. G. and Taylor, F. B., Eds., Elsevier/North-Holland, Amsterdam, 1980, 583.
522. **Machovich, R. and Arányi, P.,** Effect of heparin on thrombin inactivation by antithrombin III, *Biochem. J.,* 173, 869, 1978.
523. **Pomerantz, M. W. and Owen, W. G.,** A catalytic role for heparin. Evidence for a ternary complex of heparin cofactor, thrombin and heparin, *Biochim. Biophys. Acta,* 535, 66, 1978.
524. **Sim, R. B. and Reboul, A.,** Preparation and properties of human C1 inhibitor, *Methods Enzymol.,* 80, 43, 1981.
525. **Machovich, R.,** Choices among the possible reaction routes catalyzed by thrombin, *Ann. N.Y. Acad. Sci.,* 485, 170, 1986.
526. **Mandl, J., Spolarics, Z., and Machovich, R.,** unpublished.
527. **Papp, B., Kovacs, T., Lerant, I., Nagy, Zs., and Machovich, R.,** Conditions of formation of the heparin-fibronectin-collagen complex and the effect of plasmin, *Biochim. Biophys. Acta,* in press.
528. **Gebremedhin, D., Ballagi-Pordany, G., Hadhazi, P., Magyar, K., and Machovich, R.,** Species specificity of thrombin-induced changes in vascular tone, *Eur. J. Pharmacol.,* 132, 71, 1986.
529. **Nichols, W., Gerrard, J., and Didisheim, P.,** Platelet structure, biochemistry, and physiology, in *Recent Advances in Blood Coagulation,* Poller, L., Ed., Churchill Livingstone, Edinburgh, 1981, 1.
530. **Machovich, R. and Owen, G.,** unpublished.
531. **Machovich, R. and Owen, G.,** unpublished.

Chapter 2

GLYCOSAMINOGLYCANS OF THE BLOOD VESSEL WALL

J. Dawes and D. S. Pepper

TABLE OF CONTENTS

I. INTRODUCTION

Glycosaminoglycans are negatively charged polysaccharides which occur in the tissues mainly as proteoglycans, in which one or more polysaccharide chains are attached to a core protein. They are found in almost all mammalian tissues and serve many diverse structural and organizational functions. This chapter reviews the structure and occurrence of the glycosaminoglycans of the blood vessel wall and discuss current views of their functions, including maintenance of the integrity of the vessel wall and interaction with circulating components of the blood. Glycosaminoglycans have been implicated in the evolution of the atherosclerotic plaque, in angiogenesis, in regulation of lipid metabolism, and in control of coagulation and fibrinolysis. We believe that they are of central relevance to the development of thrombosis.

II. GLYCOSAMINOGLYCANS: CHEMICAL STRUCTURE

Glycosaminoglycans consist of unbranched chains of repeating disaccharide units in which one of the monosaccharides is an amino sugar and the other is usually a hexuronic acid; all except hyaluronic acid are sulfated. Their classification is based on the structure of the disaccharide units and is summarized in Table 1. Thus, keratan sulfate contains galactose instead of a hexuronic acid and the chondroitin sulfates are distinguished from heparan sulfate and heparin by the presence of galactosamine rather than glucosamine, as well as the absence of *N*-sulfate groups. However, within each type of glycosaminoglycan there remains considerable heterogeneity with respect to the length of the polysaccharide chains, the ratio of glucuronic acid to iduronic acid, and the amount and distribution of sulfate groups along the carbohydrate backbone. Unlike proteins, carbohydrate molecules are not directly genetically defined and are therefore variable. The variable factors can have a major effect on their properties and functions, probably the most important being charge density. The presence of sulfate and/or carboxyl groups on each of the disaccharide units means that glycosaminoglycans are strong polyanions, and this dominates their physical characteristics and to a large extent mediates their interaction with other molecules.[1]

With the possible exception of hyaluronic acid, glycosaminoglycan chains do not seem to occur in tissues in the free state. They are bound to core proteins in high molecular weight complexes in which 5 to 10% of the mass is a single protein chain. This may carry a single type of glycosaminoglycan or, as in cartilage, a range of different side chains, further increasing the potential for variation in the proteoglycan. The major type of carbohydrate-protein linkage is an *O*-glycosidic bond between D-xylose on the polysaccharide and the hydroxyl group of serine. This bond appears to be unique to connective tissue proteoglycans; it provides the attachment for chondroitin sulfate, heparan sulfate, and heparin chains[2] and is found in the linkage region of most proteoglycans in the blood vessel wall. Keratan sulfate does not contain xylose at its linkage region, but is attached to the protein core in connective tissue proteoglycan by an *O*-glycosidic bond between *N*-acetylgalactosamine and serine or threonine residues on the protein chain.[3,4] Little is known about the structures and functions of the core proteins, though it is clear that different ones exist. We will therefore concentrate our attention on the glycosaminoglycan side chains. For recent reviews covering proteoglycan structure in more detail, the reader is referred to Hascall and Hascall[5] and Hook et al.[6]

The most important blood vessel glycosaminoglycans are the chondroitin sulfates and heparan sulfate. The chondroitin sulfates contain galactosamine with an ester sulfate attached to C-4 (chondroitin 4-sulfate) or C-6 (chondroitin 6-sulfate). This is usually the only sulfate group per disaccharide, but oversulfated[7,8] and undersulfated[9] chondroitin sulfate chains have been reported. The proportion of glucuronic acid and iduronic acid residues varies, and traditionally those molecules with a high proportion of glucuronate have been termed chon-

Table 1
GLYCOSAMINOGLYCAN STRUCTURE

Glycosaminoglycan	Uronic acid	Substituent	Amino sugar	Substituent
	Repeating disaccharide			
Hyaluronate	β-D-Glucuronic acid	—	β-D-Glucosamine	*N*-acetyl
Chondroitin and dermatan sulfates	β-D-Glucuronic acid α-L-Iduronic acid	— 2-*O*-sulfate	β-D-Galactosamine	4- and 6-*O*-sulfate *N*-acetyl
Heparan sulfate and heparin	β-D-Glucuronic acid α-L-Iduronic acid	— 2-*O*-sulfate	α-D-Glucosamine	3- and 6-*O*-sulfate *N*-acetyl or -sulfate
Keratan sulfate	β-D-Galactose[a]	—	β-D-Glucosamine	6-*O*-sulfate *N*-acetyl

[a] Keratan sulfate contains galactose rather than a uronic acid.

droitin sulfates, and those in which iduronic acid predominates have been known as dermatan sulfate. However, there is a continuous gradation between the two and this group of glycosaminoglycans is probably best thought of as a family of chondroitin sulfates.

The same is true of heparan sulfate and heparin, which have the common repeating disaccharide unit of glucosamine and glucuronic or iduronic acid. In heparin many of the glucosamine residues are *N*-sulfated rather than *N*-acetylated and also carry an ester sulfate in the C-6 position. In addition most of the iduronic acid residues, which predominate over glucuronic acid, are sulfated at C-2; heparin is the most highly sulfated of the naturally occurring glycosaminoglycans. Heparan sulfate contains fewer *N*-sulfate residues, is *O*-sulfated to a lower degree, and often carries, on average, only one sulfate group per disaccharide unit. This is not evenly distributed, with the chains composed of block structures in which some regions contain no *N*-sulfate and little *O*-sulfate.[10] However, heparan sulfates containing considerably more, or less, sulfate than this characteristic molecule have been isolated.[11] Typically heparan sulfate also contains glucuronic acid as the predominant uronic acid, but again intermediate forms exist and there is no clear demarcation between heparan sulfate and heparin.[1,12,13]

III. OCCURRENCE IN THE VESSEL WALL

Vessel wall proteoglycans occur in the intima, media, and adventitia and are contributed by several cell types, including smooth muscle cells, fibroblasts, and endothelial cells. Until recently, little attempt was made to characterize the intact molecules, and analysis was confined to the glycosaminoglycan content of the large vessels. The major aortic glycosaminoglycans were identified as hyaluronic acid, chondroitin 4- and 6-sulfates, and dermatan sulfate and heparan sulfate, with only trace amounts of heparin and keratan sulfate. The relative amounts of each type of glycosaminoglycan varied according to the species[14-16] and there was no general pattern detectable. Reports of changes in concentration and type of glycosaminoglycan with age are conflicting.[17-19] It has, however, been shown that glycosaminoglycans were more concentrated in the intima than in the other layers of the blood vessel, where they differed in type from those in the media and adventitia. Murata et al.[20] found that although all three layers of the bovine aorta contained chondroitins 4- and 6-sulfate, dermatan sulfate, heparan sulfate, and hyaluronic acid, chondroitin 6-sulfate was predominant in the intima; the highest levels of hyaluronic acid, dermatan sulfate, and heparin sulfate were found in the adventitia. Gamse et al.[21] extended this work by examining the products of cells cultured from the intima and media of the bovine aorta and comparing them with those of endothelial cells. All the glycosaminoglycans except keratan sulfate were found in the extracellular, pericellular, and intracellular fractions of all three cell types, but there was more heparan sulfate in the pericellular and intracellular fractions than in the culture supernatant. Dermatan sulfate formed only a small fraction of the surface-associated glycosaminoglycan, and the chondroitin sulfates were largely extracellular and pericellular. The endothelial cells displayed a unique distribution pattern, with high levels of heparan sulfate and chondroitin 6-sulfate in each pool and a very low content of dermatan sulfate. Moreover, the endothelial heparan sulfate was more highly *N*-sulfated than that synthesized by the other cells, and some of the heparan sulfate associated with the endothelial cell membrane resembled heparin. Winterbourne et al.[22] found that local regions of bovine aortic endothelial cell heparan sulfate were highly sulfated. These molecules may interact in a very specific fashion with the cells which produce them. Waxler et al.[23] have found that bovine aortic endothelial cells in culture orient on the extracellular matrix, which contained heparan sulfate, chondroitin sulfate, and dermatan sulfate in similar amounts. Smooth muscle cells from the same bovine aorta produced chondroitin sulfate and dermatan sulfate, but very little heparan sulfate, and did not display any polarity toward their extracellular matrix.

Intact proteoglycans have now been isolated from porcine,[24] bovine,[25,26] and human[27,28] aorta. One class of molecules contained principally chondroitin and dermatan sulfates and formed aggregates with hyaluronic acid in the same way as cartilage proteoglycans;[26,29] the other class was present in smaller amounts and contained mainly heparan sulfate and heparin.[26,30]

Further definition of vessel wall proteoglycans has been possible by analysis of the products of cultured cells. Buonassisi[31] first showed that vascular endothelial cells from rabbit aorta synthesized and secreted glycosaminoglycans, which he tentatively identified as chondroitin 4-sulfate and heparan sulfate. He later confirmed the presence of heparan sulfate in the culture medium and suggested that it was also present on the endothelial cell surface.[32] The proteoglycans from which these glycosaminoglycan chains were derived have now been identified. Proteoglycans containing heparan sulfate[33,34] and others containing chondroitin sulfate with a small amount of dermatan sulfate[35] are secreted into the culture medium; endothelial cells secreted several heparan sulfate proteoglycans carrying two distinct types of heparan sulfate chain, whereas a subendothelial cell line only produced a single heparan sulfate proteoglycan.[34] In addition, heparan sulfate proteoglycans, one of which was lipid associated and probably a component of the plasma membrane, have been found in the cells,[33,35] and different heparan sulfate proteoglycans have been identified in the basement membrane.[33,36]

Another recent development has been the culture of microvascular endothelial cells, which are probably more relevant to the physiology of much vascular disease than those derived from the aorta. Proteoglycan was found in the basement membrane of human microvascular endothelial cells,[37] and Bar et al.[38] compared the glycosaminoglycans synthesized by bovine capillary endothelial cells with those produced by bovine pulmonary artery, pulmonary vein and aorta, and human umbilical vein. All the endothelial cells produced more heparan sulfate than smooth muscle cells, chondrocytes, and fibroblasts, and in this study heparin was also identified. However, all five endothelial cultures displayed their own characteristic pattern of glycosaminoglycan distribution in the cellular, pericellular, and secreted compartments. As these authors point out, glycosaminoglycan metabolism is modulated by many factors including interactions with other cell types,[39] and the in vitro findings may not accurately reflect the in vivo situation. Nevertheless, their studies are strongly indicative of the presence of significantly different glycosaminoglycan contents in the endothelia of different vessel walls. Simionescu et al.[40] used a different approach. They had identified anionic sites on murine visceral capillary endothelium *in situ* by labeling with cationized ferritin. Perfusion

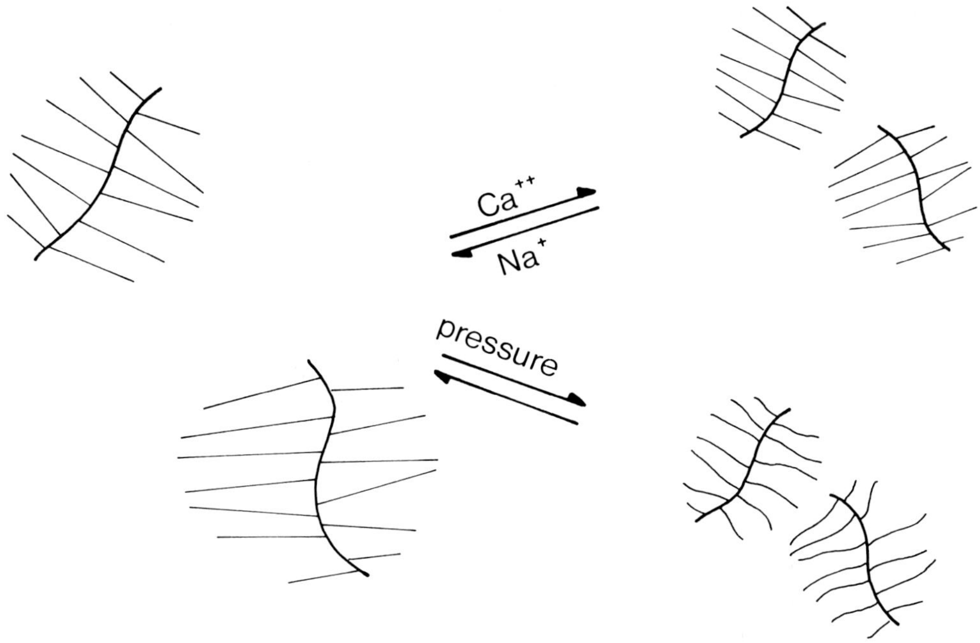

FIGURE 1. Viscoelastic properties of proteoglycans. Proteoglycans have extended structures and occupy large hydrodynamic volumes, which are reduced by pressure or by substituting divalent calcium ions for the sodium counterion.

of the capillaries with different enzymes indicated that the fenestral diaphragms contained locally high concentrations of heparan sulfate, whereas the anionic sites on the rest of the endothelial surface were more diverse.

IV. FUNCTION IN THE VESSEL WALL

A. Contribution to Viscoelasticity and Permeability

The major arteries are highly elastic structures, and their constituent proteoglycans are major contributors to the maintenance of their viscoelasticity. Because of their high negative charge density, proteoglycans have extended structures in solution and occupy very large hydrodynamic volumes in relation to their molecular weight.[41,42] They form a hydrated, viscous gel which confers a degree of spatial order on the intercellular matrix of the vessel wall and is reversibly compressible, absorbing and dissipating stress imposed on the blood vessel. Under normal physiological conditions, monovalent sodium ions provide the counterion to most of the sulfate groups,[43] and the gel is expanded and tissue turgor is maintained. Too high a proteoglycan content can thus further increase turgor, altering vessel viscoelasticity and even reducing the lumen, with an increase in vascular resistance which contributes to hypertension.[43,44] Substitution of the sodium counterion by divalent calcium ions, which is known to occur in arterial walls, has the opposite effect. The glycosaminoglycan chains move closer together, the configuration of the gel changes so that it contracts, and the elasticity of the wall decreases. These effects are illustrated in Figure 1.

The same properties of the proteoglycan molecule allow it to affect the movement of other molecules, both large and small, through the blood vessel wall. The proteoglycan matrix excludes all molecules above a certain size and prevents their passage across the wall; the higher the proteoglycan concentration, the smaller the pore size in the matrix and the smaller the molecules which can pass through. After perfusion of porcine aortas with glycosaminoglycan degrading enzymes, the vessel wall becomes much more permeable to dye markers.[45] In addition, molecules can become trapped in the proteoglycan matrix by ionic interaction with the negatively charged sulfate groups. Thus, that part of the vasculature containing the highest concentration of proteoglycans has the greatest effect on the diffusion of both calcium and water across the arterial wall.[46]

B. Effect on Cell Growth

Cell growth is relatively unimportant in the intact blood vessel, for a characteristic feature of the normal, healthy arterial wall is that the intimal endothelial cells form a continuous quiescent monolayer overlying medial smooth muscle cells which are also quiescent. However, cell growth and division assume major significance both when new vessels are formed — angiogenesis — and when a vessel wall is damaged. Angiogenesis is initiated by the local degradation of the basement membrane of the parent vessel,[47] and this is followed by endothelial cell migration and growth. The vascular endothelial cell seems to express all the information necessary for angiogenesis,[48] and there is some evidence that heparin may be able to modulate, though not initiate, angiogenesis by stimulating both growth and migration of endothelial cells. Vigorous in vitro growth of human vascular endothelial cells was achieved by supplementation of the medium with heparin;[49] this effect may be attributable to the ability of heparin to release endothelial cell-derived mitogens.[50] It has also been reported that heparin derived from mast cells stimulates the migration of capillary endothelial cells in vitro[51] and that angiogenesis can be promoted by heparin in vivo.[52] However, reports that it will also induce tumor regression are conflicting,[53,54] and there is no evidence to indicate whether endogenous glycosaminoglycans display similar effects.

The effect of heparin on intimal smooth muscle cells, however, appears to be quite different from that on endothelial cells. If the endothelium is damaged, smooth muscle cell proliferation occurs until the endothelium regenerates, and this myointimal proliferation is inhibited by heparin. Clowes and Karnofsky[55] first demonstrated this effect of heparin in vivo, after denudation of rat carotid artery endothelium by air-drying injury. It was not mediated by effects on other cells at the level of the arterial wall, and nonanticoagulant heparin fractions were as effective as those with high anticoagulant activity.[56] Growth of vascular smooth muscle cells in vitro is similarly suppressed by heparin, which blocks the stimulatory effect of platelet derived growth factor.[57] Moreover, further work has indicated that the glycosaminoglycans of the vessel wall function in the same way as heparin. Conditioned medium from confluent, but not exponential bovine aortic endothelial cells, specifically inhibited the proliferation of growth-arrested smooth muscle cells, and the inhibitory activity was heparin or heparan sulfate[58] released from the cultured endothelial cells, perhaps by the action of platelet heparitinase.[59] The endothelium also appears to influence glycosaminoglycan synthesis in the inner media. Merrilees and Scott[39] found that cultured endothelial cells produce a factor which stimulates glycosaminoglycan synthesis by smooth muscle cells and confirmed this observation in segments of rat carotid artery maintained in organ culture,[60] where altered glycosaminoglycan synthesis in the inner media was related to the presence and activity of the endothelium, but independent of smooth muscle cell growth. Thus, it seems likely that the vessel wall glycosaminoglycans are crucial to the regulation of cell growth within normal and injured vessels. The high content of glycosaminoglycans in the extracellular matrix of both intima and media will inhibit proliferation of medial smooth muscle cells in the undamaged wall. After injury or removal of endothelial cells and the consequent degranulation of adherent platelets, the suppressing action of the residual glycosaminoglycans may be negated by neutralization with locally high concentrations of platelet factor 4 (PF4) and platelet heparitinase, and the smooth muscle cells, stimulated by platelet derived growth factor, can migrate into the intima and proliferate. However, once the damaged area is reendothelialized, smooth muscle cell growth ceases.[61] There is clearly a complex interplay of factors involved in the regulation of cell growth after vascular wall injury, the balance of which may determine whether healthy vessel wall is restored or the development of atherosclerotic plaque initiated.

C. Regulation of Lipid Metabolism

Vessel wall glycosaminoglycans are also fundamental to the regulation of lipid metabolism at the luminal surface, for they interact with both lipoproteins and the enzyme which degrades them, lipoprotein lipase. Heparin binds to very low-density lipoproteins (VLDL) and low-density lipoproteins (LDL) at physiological ionic strength[62] by interaction of its sulfate groups with positively charged sequences on apolipoproteins B[63] and E[64] which are found in LDL and VLDL, respectively. A small fraction of high-density lipoprotein (HDL) also contains apolipoprotein E and binds to heparin.[65] The affinity of this interaction depends upon the type of glycosaminoglycan and is strongest with iduronic acid-containing molecules, i.e., heparin, dermatan sulfate, and heparan sulfate. Moreover, subfractions of heparan sulfate containing highly *N*-sulfated sequences display higher affinity for LDL than does heparin.[66] The relevance of these interactions is indicated by the close correlation between the presence of glycosaminoglycans and lipid observed in developing atherosclerotic plaques[67] and the isolation of lipoprotein-glycosaminoglycan complexes from fatty streaks of human aorta.[68]

The second mechanism by which proteoglycans influence the lipid content of the vascular wall is by their affinity for the catabolic enzymes, lipoprotein lipase, and possibly also hepatic triglyceride lipase. Hahn, in 1943,[69] first noticed that the injection of heparin resulted in the clearing of alimentary lipemia, and the active principle was identified as a lipolytic enzyme by Korn in 1955.[70] The interaction between heparin and lipoprotein lipase is ionic and is not related to the ability of heparin to bind antithrombin III.[71] Moreover, heparin has little or no effect on the ability of lipoprotein lipase to hydrolyze acylglycerols either in the presence or absence of apolipoprotein CII, which stimulates lipoprotein lipase.[72] However, under normal physiological conditions, lipoprotein lipase is not present in the plasma in high concentrations as it is after administration of heparin, but located on the vascular endothelium, where the degradation of chylomicra and VLDL has been shown to occur.[73] Nevertheless, cultured endothelial cells do not contain lipoprotein lipase,[74] and it appears that the enzyme is synthesized and secreted by adipocytes and other parenchymal cells and then taken up by the endothelial cell surface; its receptor is probably a heparan sulfate-containing glycosaminoglycan. Bengtsson et al.[75] showed that glycosaminoglycans other than heparin will bind lipoprotein lipase, though with lower affinity; heparan and dermatan sulfates bound more strongly than chondroitin sulfates. Direct evidence for lipoprotein lipase attachment to cultured bovine aortic endothelial cells through heparan sulfate on the cell surface was then supplied by the studies of Shimada et al.[76] These workers found that treatment of the cells with purified heparinase totally inhibited the binding of lipoprotein lipase, but the enzymic removal of chondroitin and dermatan sulfates had no effect. Heparin, with its higher affinity for the enzyme, released it from its receptor. The function of hepatic triglyceride lipase is less clear than that of lipoprotein lipase. It, too, binds to heparin[77] and other glycosaminoglycans,[75] though with lower affinity than lipoprotein lipase. It has not been demonstrated on the vascular endothelium and may be associated with the plasma membrane of the hepatocyte or hepatic sinusoidal endothelium where it could metabolize the chylomicron remnants produced by lipoprotein lipase.

Thus, it seems probable that vessel wall glycosaminoglycans bind both lipoprotein lipase and its substrate, LDL and VLDL. The complexes are then subjected to lipolysis and cholesterol-rich β-lipoprotein or chylomicron remnants are formed. These have a lower affinity for glycosaminoglycans than the large complexes and most of them are probably released into the bloodstream to be degraded by the liver. However, some may remain attached to the intimal surface long enough to be incorporated. The significance of this sequence is underlined by a recent report of a strong negative correlation between the severity of coronary artery disease and postheparin lipoprotein lipase activity,[78] implying an association between impaired availability of lipoprotein lipase and coronary artery disease, though whether of cause or effect has yet to be established.

D. Involvement in Coagulation and Fibrinolysis

The healthy vascular endothelium maintains the fluidity of blood by presenting a nonthrombogenic surface to circulating plasma proteins, as long as the turbulent, pulsatile flow of blood is presented to the vessel wall — if flow is stagnant then the bulk of the blood is no longer anticoagulated. No other equally anticoagulant surface is known. When endothelial injury and denudation occur, the subendothelium is exposed to the circulating blood, and platelets and surface-active procoagulants are activated, initiating a sequence which should theoretically lead to thrombus formation. However, extensive thrombi rarely form as a consequence of endothelial denudation alone; platelets adhere to the damaged sites,[79] but there is little deposition of fibrin and the platelet layer disappears with the regrowth of the endothelium. The vessel wall proteoglycans are fundamental to its nonthrombogenic properties, affecting coagulation factors, platelets and fibrinolysis. Heparin is a long-established antithrombotic drug, and both heparan sulfate[80] and dermatan sulfate[81] are now known to be effective in preventing thrombosis in animal models and clotting in vitro. Bovine aortic proteoglycans containing dermatan sulfate[82] and heparan sulfate proteoglycans from cultured endothelial cells but not those from the subendothelium[83] have similarly been shown to inhibit clotting.

Heparin itself is believed to exert its anticoagulant action largely by potentiating the inactivation of the coagulation factors, particularly thrombin and Factor Xa, by antithrombin III (ATIII).[84,85] However, it is rapidly becoming clear that the interactions involved are much more complex than this. Only glycosaminoglycans containing a specific pentasaccharide sequence — about 30% of heparin molecules — bind with high affinity to ATIII,[86] and this sequence apparently occurs only at low frequency in heparan sulfate and not at all in dermatan sulfate. It is likely that the antithrombotic action of dermatan sulfate is mediated through interaction with heparin cofactor II,[87,88] which neutralizes thrombin, but not the other clotting factors. In addition, glycosaminoglycans can inhibit formation of the "tenase" and "prothrombinase" complexes independently of both ATIII and heparin cofactor II,[89,90] and this may contribute significantly to their antithrombotic properties. However, experimental studies of the anticoagulant properties of the vessel wall glycosaminoglycans at a molecular level have been largely confined to their interaction with ATIII and thrombin. Stern et al.[91] have convincingly demonstrated that the bovine aortic endothelium binds ATIII and that the binding is mediated by heparan sulfate on the endothelial cell surface. Rabbit aortic segments also bind ATIII,[92] but although proteoglycans were shown to be involved in the interaction with subendothelium after damage by ballooning, they were not implicated in binding by intact endothelium. Inactivation of Factors IXa and Xa was facilitated by bovine aortic segments[91] and by glycosaminoglycans released by cultured human endothelial cells;[93] at the present state of knowledge, this implies binding of the glycosaminoglycans to ATIII. It is also reported that the vascular endothelium mediates the interaction between ATIII and thrombin;[94] unlike the neutralization of Factor Xa, however, that of thrombin requires binding of glycosaminoglycan to both ATIII and thrombin for optimal catalytic effect.[95] There are several reports of thrombin binding to the vascular endothelium[92,96-98] as well as to the subendothelium,[99] and an interesting comparison of thrombin binding to aortic endothelium and neointima developing on vascular grafts.[100] It is clear that thrombin does bind to endothelial cells with high affinity,[96] but the role of vessel proteoglycans in binding thrombin is disputed. Their major contribution to inactivation of the coagulation factors may well be through the binding of ATIII.

There are numbers of reports that heparin can both enhance and inhibit platelet aggregation, depending on the heparin concentration and the stimulus for aggregation, but the few studies of the effect of vessel wall proteoglycans on platelets indicate that they act as inhibitors of aggregation. Ts'ao et al.[82] found that a highly purified bovine aortic proteoglycan containing chondroitin and dermatan sulfates inhibited thrombin-induced platelet aggregation in the presence of plasma, but had no effect on aggregation induced by ADP, adrenaline, or human collagen. A later report[101] indicated that proteoglycans will inhibit collagen-induced platelet aggregation when both collagen and platelets are from the same species. Of particular interest, however, is the work of Colburn and Buonassisi,[83] who found that the addition of rabbit plasma to rabbit subendothelial cell cultures caused the rapid formation of large platelet aggregates followed by the deposition of fibrin strands. No aggregates were formed in endothelial cell cultures unless the cells were pretreated with antiserum against endothelial cell heparan sulfate proteoglycan, when platelet aggregates and fibrin strands were formed. This is a clear demonstration of the importance of specific vascular proteoglycans in maintaining the antithrombotic properties of the intact vessel wall.

There is, however, another aspect to platelet-proteoglycan interactions, which is the effect of platelet release proteins on glycosaminoglycans. Several of the proteins released from activated platelets bind to heparin and other glycosaminoglycans, and one of these, PF4 has a higher affinity for heparin than any other known protein.[102] PF4 binds to cultured human endothelial cells.[103] apparently through cell surface glycosaminoglycans, and the formation of this complex will mask the glycosaminoglycan, favoring hemostasis by interfering with its ability to inhibit platelet aggregation and coagulation. Platelets also release platelet-derived growth factor, which has some affinity for glycosaminoglycans and stimulates the growth of arterial smooth muscle cells,[57] and a lysosomal heparitinase.[104] This has recently been shown to degrade heparan sulfate in the extracellular matrix of cultured vascular endothelial cells[105] and on the surface of the cells themselves.[106] Thus, platelet release products can reduce both the concentration and the availability of vessel wall glycosaminoglycans.

In recent years, heparin has also been reported to enhance fibrinolysis by increasing the release of plasminogen activator into the blood.[107,108] There are as yet no studies of the effect of vessel wall glycosaminoglycans on fibrinolysis, but as plasminogen activator is synthesized by the vascular endothelium, it is possible that changes in its content resulting from injury could alter plasminogen activator release.

E. Contribution to Atherosclerosis

The weight of evidence presented so far indicates that vessel wall glycosaminoglycans are intimately involved in maintaining the health and integrity of the vascular system. It comes as something of a surprise, therefore, to find that they have also been implicated in the pathogenesis of atherosclerosis for many years. During naturally occurring human atherosclerosis, glycosaminoglycans increase preferentially in the intima during early intimal fibrosis and fatty streak formation, but decrease in the fibrous plaque and complicated lesion state.[109-111] Attempts have been made to define changes in specific types of glycosaminoglycan, but some reports indicate an increase in dermatan sulfate;[112,113] others indicate an increase in chondroitin sulfate during formation of the fatty streak.[114,115] These differences may have technical causes, or they could be related to dietary differences, which have been shown to influence the composition of aortic glycosaminoglycans in rhesus monkeys.[116] Certain species, such as pigeon and rabbit, are susceptible to atherosclerosis, and they have a higher content of aortic glycosaminoglycan than the rat and mouse, which are resistant.[117] A similar pattern is found in different strains of pigeon with different susceptibilities to atherosclerosis,[118] and arterial cells cultured from the susceptible strain synthesized and secreted three- to fourfold the amount of chondroitin sulfate-containing glycosaminoglycans produced by the resistant strain.[119] Glycosaminoglycans also increase in early proliferative lesions induced by balloon catheter injury[120] or chronic hyperlipidemia,[121] as well as in other conditions that result in atherogenesis such as hypoxia[122] and diabetes.[123] Following injury, both lipid and glycosaminoglycans accumulated preferentially in the region covered by regenerated endothelium, and this increase was largely contributed by heparan sulfate.[124]

Little is known of the control of glycosaminoglycan synthesis in the vessel wall. PDGF, which also stimulates smooth muscle cell proliferation, is probably the factor reported by Castor et al.[125] to increase glycosaminoglycan synthesis. Similarly, LDL will stimulate arterial smooth muscle cells in culture to divide[126] and to synthesize glycosaminoglycans at an increased rate.[127] In these instances glycosaminoglycan synthesis may simply reflect the rate of cell growth and division. However, Leung et al.[128] have reported that the rates of glycosaminoglycan and collagen synthesis increased when the subculture of rabbit aorta underwent cyclic stretching; DNA synthesis was not affected.

V. SUMMARY

Glycosaminoglycans fulfill a range of complex functions in the blood vessel wall. They are intrinsic to the maintenance of its considerable viscoelasticity and play a major part in the transport of molecules across the wall, the exchange process fundamental to the basic function of the blood in distributing nutrients and removing waste products from the tissues. They stimulate angiogenesis and inhibit smooth muscle cell growth in the healthy vessel wall. They interact with both lipoprotein and the lipoprotein-degrading enzymes so that the luminal surface of the blood vessel is a major site for lipoprotein catabolism. Finally, they are essential to the nonthrombogenicity of the surface presented to circulating blood. Most of these functions result from the high negative charge of the glycosaminoglycans, but it is becoming increasingly apparent that within the wide range of naturally occurring proteoglycans, particular functions are related to specific structures. The distribution and control of synthesis of different proteoglycans at a particular site will determine the extent to which that site functions in the various ways described. Thus, if a vessel is damaged and stripped of its endothelium, it loses its nonthrombogenic properties, although the subendothelial layers are well supplied with glycosaminoglycans — not, it seems, the specific ones suited to this purpose. Similarly, atherosclerotic plaques contain high levels of glycosaminoglycan, but are thrombogenic. Many of the answers are indicated by the current state of our knowledge, but further detailed analysis is necessary before we can define the exact role of glycosaminoglycans in the complex balance which determines whether atherosclerosis will develop or thrombosis occur.

REFERENCES

1. **Lindahl, U. and Hook, M.,** Glycosaminoglycans and their binding to biological macromolecules, *Annu. Rev. Biochem.,* 47, 385, 1978.
2. **Lindahl, U. and Roden, L.,** Carbohydrate-peptide linkages in proteoglycans of animal, plant and bacterial origin, in *Glycoproteins,* Gottschalk, A., Ed., Elsevier, Amsterdam, 1972, 491.
3. **Bray, B. A., Lieberman, R., and Meyer, K.,** Structure of human skeletal keratosulfate: the linkage region, *J. Biol. Chem.,* 242, 3373, 1967.
4. **De Luca, S., Lohmander, L. S., Nilsson, B., Hascall, V. C., and Caplan, A. I.,** Proteoglycans from chick limb bud chondrocyte cultures: keratan sulfate and oligosaccharides which contain mannose and sialic acid, *J. Biol. Chem.,* 255, 6077, 1980.
5. **Hascall, V. C. and Hascall, C. K.,** Proteoglycans, in *Cell Biology of the Extracellular Matrix,* Hay, E., Ed., Plenum Press, New York, 1981, 39.
6. **Hook, M., Kjellen, L., Johansson, S., and Robinson, J.,** Cell surface glycosaminoglycans, *Annu. Rev. Biochem.,* 53, 847, 1984.

7. **Razin, E., Stevens, R. L., Akiyama, F., Schmid, K., and Austen, K. F.,** Culture from mouse bone marrow of a subclass of mast cells possessing a distinct chondroitin sulfate proteoglycan with glycosaminoglycans rich in *N*-acetylgalactosamine-4,6-disulfate, *J. Biol. Chem.*, 257, 7229, 1982.
8. **Kolset, S. O., Kjellen, L., Seljelid, R., and Lindahl, U.,** Changes in glycosaminoglycan biosynthesis during differentiation in vitro of human monocytes, *Biochem. J.*, 210, 661, 1983.
9. **Ito, K., Kimata, K., Sobue, M., and Suzuki, S.,** Altered proteoglycan synthesis by epiphyseal cartilages in culture at low SO_4^{2-} concentrations, *J. Biol. Chem.*, 257, 917, 1982.
10. **Muir, H. and Hardingham, T.,** Structure of proteoglycans, in *Biochemistry of Carbohydrates,* Whelan, W. J., Ed., Butterworths, London, 1975, 153.
11. **Johnson, E. A.,** Heparan sulphates from porcine intestinal mucosa. Preparation and physicochemical properties, *Thromb. Res.*, 35, 583, 1984.
12. **Jacques, L. B.,** Simplified and rational nomenclature for heparins, glycosaminoglycans and sulfated mucopolysaccharides, *Artery,* 4, 144, 1978.
13. **Busch, C. and Owen, W. G.,** Identification in vitro of an endothelial cell surface cofactor for antithrombin III: parallel studies with isolated perfused rat hearts and microcarrier cultures of bovine endothelium, *J. Clin. Invest.*, 69, 726, 1982.
14. **Engel, U. R.,** Glycosaminoglycans in the aorta of six animal species, *Atherosclerosis,* 13, 45, 1971.
15. **Stefanovich, V. and Akiyama, K.,** Comparative studies of aortic acid mucopolysaccharides in fifteen species, *Comp. Biochem. Physiol.*, 34, 125, 1970.
16. **Gardais, A., Picard, J., and Hermelin, B.,** Glycosaminoglycan (GAG) distribution in aortic wall from five species, *Comp. Biochem. Physiol. B,* 44, 507, 1973.
17. **Kaplan, D. and Meyer, K.,** Mucopolysaccharides of aorta at various ages, *Proc. Soc. Exp. Biol. Med.*, 105, 78, 1960.
18. **Gore, I., Tanaka, Y., and Kimoto, E.,** Changes in the acid mucopolysaccharides of human aorta with age and atherosclerosis, *Circulation,* 30(Suppl. 3), 10, 1964.
19. **Kumar, V., Berenson, G. S., Ruiz, H., Dalferes, E. R., and Strong, J. P.,** Acid mucopolysaccharides of human aorta. I. Variations with maturation, *J. Atheroscler. Res.*, 7, 573, 1967.
20. **Murata, K., Nakazawa, K., and Hamai, A.,** Distribution of acidic glycosaminoglycans in the intima, media and adventitia of bovine aorta and their anticoagulant properties, *Atherosclerosis,* 21, 93, 1975.
21. **Gamse, G., Fromme, H. G., and Kresse, H.,** Metabolism of sulfated glycosaminoglycans in cultured endothelial cells and smooth muscle cells from bovine aorta, *Biochim. Biophys. Acta,* 544, 514, 1978.
22. **Winterbourne, D. J., Schor, A. M., and Gallagher, J. T.,** Synthesis of glycosaminoglycans by cloned bovine endothelial cells cultured on collagen gels, *Eur. J. Biochem.*, 135, 271, 1983.
23. **Waxler, B., Schumacher, B., and Eisenstein, R.,** Cell stroma interactions in aortic endothelial cell cultures, *Lab. Invest.*, 41, 128, 1979.
24. **Dunstone, J. and Cleland, S.,** Some further observations on the proteoglycans from ox nasal cartilage and pig aorta, *Connect. Tissue Res.*, 3, 105, 1975.
25. **Radhakrishnamurthy, B., Ruiz, H. A., and Berenson, G. S.,** Isolation and characterisation of proteoglycans from bovine aorta, *J. Biol. Chem.*, 252, 4831, 1977.
26. **Oegema, T. R., Hascall, V. C., and Eisenstein, R.,** Characterisation of bovine aorta proteoglycan extracted with guanidine hydrochloride in the presence of protease inhibitors, *J. Biol. Chem.*, 254, 1312, 1979.
27. **Muthiah, P. L.,** Proteoglycans and atherosclerosis, *Artery,* 4, 183, 1978.
28. **Tomaszewski, J. J., Hanzlik, J. A., and Donica, H.,** Isolation of proteoglycans from human aorta, *Artery,* 4, 408, 1978.
29. **McMurtrey, J., Radhakrishnamurthy, B., and Dalferes, E. R.,** Isolation of proteoglycan-hyaluronate complexes from bovine aorta, *J. Biol. Chem.*, 254, 1621, 1979.
30. **Jacobs, S. and Muir, H.,** A heparan sulphate-peptide from human aorta, *Biochem. J.*, 87, 38P, 1963.
31. **Buonassisi, V.,** Sulfated mucopolysaccharide synthesis and secretion in endothelial cell cultures, *Exp. Cell Res.*, 76, 363, 1973.
32. **Buonassisi, V. and Root, M.,** Enzymatic degradation of heparin-related mucopolysaccharides from the surface of endothelial cell cultures, *Biochim. Biophys. Acta,* 385, 1, 1975.
33. **Oohira, A., Wight, T. N., and Bornstein, P.,** Sulfated proteoglycans synthesised by vascular endothelial cells in culture, *J. Biol. Chem.*, 258, 2014, 1983.
34. **Buonassisi, V. and Colburn, P.,** Antibodies to the heparan sulfate proteoglycans synthesized by endothelial cell cultures, *Biochim. Biophys. Acta,* 760, 1, 1983.
35. **Buonassisi, V. and Colburn, P.,** Biological significance of heparan sulfate proteoglycans, *Ann. N.Y. Acad. Sci.*, 401, 76, 1982.
36. **Norling, B., Glimelius, B., and Wasteson, A.,** Heparan sulfate proteoglycan of cultured cells: demonstration of a lipid- and a matrix-associated form, *Biochem. Biophys. Res. Commun.*, 103, 1265, 1981.
37. **Kramer, R., Davison, P., and Karasek, M.,** Characterisation of a basement membrane matrix synthesised by cultured human microvascular endothelial cells, *Clin. Res.*, 31, A580, 1983.

38. **Bar, R. S., Dake, B. L., and Spanheimer, R. S.,** Sulfated glycosaminoglycans in cultured endothelial cells from capillaries and large vessels of human and bovine origin, *Atherosclerosis,* 56, 11, 1985.
39. **Merrilees, M. J. and Scott, L.,** Interaction of aortic endothelial and smooth muscle cells in culture — effect on glycosaminoglycan levels, *Atherosclerosis,* 39, 147, 1981.
40. **Simionescu, M., Simionescu, N., Silbert, J. E., and Palade, G. E.,** Differentiated microdomains on the luminal surface of the capillary endothelium. II. Partial characterization of their anionic sites, *J. Cell Biol.,* 90, 614, 1981.
41. **Pasternak, S. G., Veis, A., and Breen, M.,** Solvent-dependent changes in proteoglycan subunit conformation in aqueous guanidine hydrochloride solutions, *J. Biol. Chem.,* 249, 2206, 1974.
42. **Reihanian, H., Jamieson, A. M., Tang, H. L., and Rosenberg, L.,** Hydrodynamic properties of proteoglycan subunit from bovine nasal cartilage. Self-association behaviour and interaction with hyaluronate studied by laser light scattering, *Biopolymers,* 18, 1727, 1979.
43. **Palaty, V., Gustafson, B. K., and Friedman, S. M.,** The role of protein polysaccharides in the hydration of the arterial wall, *Can. J. Physiol. Pharmacol.,* 48, 54, 1970.
44. **Feigl, E. O., Peterson, L. H., and Jones, A. W.,** Mechanical and chemical properties of arteries in experimental hypertension, *J. Clin. Invest.,* 42, 1640, 1963.
45. **Klynstra, F. B.,** On the passage-restricting role of acid mucopolysaccharides in the endothelium of pig aortas, *Atherosclerosis,* 19, 215, 1974.
46. **Glatz, C. E. and Massaro, T. A.,** Influence of glycosaminoglycan content on mass transfer behaviour of porcine artery wall. II. Differences in mass transfer rates related to variations in glycosaminoglycan content, *Atherosclerosis,* 25, 165, 1976.
47. **Burger, P. C., Chandler, D. B., and Klintworth, G. K.,** Corneal neovascularization as studied by scanning electron microscopy of vascular casts, *Lab. Invest.,* 48, 169, 1983.
48. **Folkman, J.,** What is the role of endothelial cells in angiogenesis?, *Lab. Invest.,* 51, 601, 1984.
49. **Thornton, S. C., Mueller, S. N., and Levine, E. M.,** Human endothelial cells: use of heparin in cloning and long-term serial cultivation, *Science,* 222, 623, 1983.
50. **Gajdusek, C. M. and Reidy, M. A.,** Heparin release of endothelial cell-derived mitogens, *Fed. Proc.,* 44, 1655, 1985.
51. **Azizkhan, R. G., Azizkhan, J. C., Zetter, B. R., and Folkman, J.,** Mast cell heparin stimulates migration of capillary endothelial cells in vitro, *J. Exp. Med.,* 152, 931, 1980.
52. **Taylor, S. and Folkman, J.,** Protamine is an inhibitor of angiogenesis, *Nature (London),* 297, 307, 1982.
53. **Folkman, J., Langer, R., Linhardt, R. J., Haudenschild, C., and Taylor, S.,** Angiogenesis inhibition and tumor regression caused by heparin or a heparin fragment in the presence of cortisone, *Science,* 221, 719, 1983.
54. **Penhaligon, M. and Camplejohn, R. S.,** Treatment of two transplantable tumors with the putative anti-angiogenic combination of heparin plus cortisone, *Br. J. Cancer,* 51, 601, 1985.
55. **Clowes, A. W. and Karnofsky, M. J.,** Suppression by heparin of smooth muscle cell proliferation in injured arteries, *Nature (London),* 265, 625, 1977.
56. **Guyton, J. R., Rosenberg, R. D., Clowes, A. W., and Karnofsky, M. J.,** Inhibition of rat arterial smooth muscle cell proliferation by heparin. In vivo studies with anticoagulant and nonanticoagulant heparin, *Circ. Res.,* 46, 625, 1980.
57. **Hoover, R. L., Rosenberg, R., Haering, W., and Karnofsky, M. J.,** Inhibition of rat arterial smooth muscle cell proliferation by heparin. II. In vitro studies, *Circ. Res.,* 47, 578, 1980.
58. **Castellot, J. J., Addonizio, M. L., Rosenberg, R., and Karnofsky, M. J.,** Cultured endothelial cells produce a heparinlike inhibitor of smooth muscle cell growth, *J. Cell Biol.,* 90, 372, 1981.
59. **Castellot, J. J., Favreau, L. V., Karnofsky, M. J., and Rosenberg, R.,** Inhibition of vascular smooth muscle cell growth by endothelial cell-derived heparin. Possible role of a platelet endoglycosidase, *J. Biol. Chem.,* 259, 11256, 1982.
60. **Merrilees, M. J. and Scott, L. J.,** Effects of endothelial removal and regeneration on smooth muscle glycosaminoglycan synthesis and growth in rat carotid artery in organ culture, *Lab. Invest.,* 52, 409, 1985.
61. **Wight, T. N., Curwen, K. D., Litrenta, M. M., Alonso, D. R., and Minick, C. R.,** Effect of endothelium on glycosaminoglycan accumulation in injured rabbit aorta, *Am. J. Pathol.,* 113, 156, 1983.
62. **Iverius, P. H.,** The interaction between human plasma lipoproteins and connective tissue glycosaminoglycans, *J. Biol. Chem.,* 247, 2607, 1972.
63. **Shaefer, E., Eisenberg, S., and Levy, R. I.,** Lipoprotein apoprotein metabolism, *J. Lipid Res.,* 19, 667, 1978.
64. **Shelburne, F. A. and Quarfordt, S. H.,** Interaction of heparin with an apoprotein of human very low-density lipoprotein, *J. Clin. Invest.,* 60, 944, 1977.
65. **Quarfordt, S. H., Jain, R. S., Jakoi, L., Robinson, S., and Shelburne, F. A.,** The heterogeneity of rat high density lipoproteins, *Biochem. Biophys. Res. Commun.,* 83, 786, 1978.
66. **Fransson, L. A. and Havsmark, B.,** Glycosaminoglycan-lipoprotein interactions. II. Structure of heparin-related variants with high affinity for low density lipoprotein, *Int. J. Biol. Macromol.,* 3, 361, 1981.

67. **Robinson, R. W., Likar, I. N., and Likar, L. J.,** Glycosaminoglycans and arterial disease, in *Monographs of Atherosclerosis,* Vol. 5, Kirk, J. E., Kritchevsky, D., Pollack, O. J., and Simms, H., Eds., S. Karger, New York, 1975, 1.
68. **Srinivasan, S. R., Dolan, P., Radhakrishnamurthy, B., and Berenson, G. S.,** Isolation of lipoprotein-acid mucopolysaccharide complexes from fatty streaks of human aortas, *Atherosclerosis,* 16, 95, 1972.
69. **Hahn, P. F.,** Abolishment of alimentary lipemia following injection of heparin, *Science,* 98, 19, 1943.
70. **Korn, E. D.,** Clearing factor, a heparin-activated lipoprotein lipase. I. Isolation and characterization of the enzyme from normal rat heart, *J. Biol. Chem.,* 215, 1, 1955.
71. **Bengtsson, G. and Olivecrona, T.,** Interaction of heparin with proteins. Demonstration of different binding sites for antithrombin and lipoprotein lipase, *FEBS Lett.,* 79, 59, 1977.
72. **Bengtsson, G. and Olivecrona, T.,** Heparin-bound lipoprotein lipase is catalytically active and can be stimulated by apolipoprotein CII, *FEBS Lett.,* 128, 9, 1981.
73. **Scow, R. O., Blanchette-Mackie, E. J., and Smith, L. C.,** Role of capillary endothelium in the clearance of chylomicrons. A model for lipid transport from blood by lateral diffusion in cell membranes, *Circ. Res.,* 39, 149, 1976.
74. **Howard, B. V.,** Uptake of very low density lipoprotein triglyceride by bovine aortic endothelial cells in cultures, *J. Lipid Res.,* 18, 561, 1977.
75. **Bengtsson, G., Olivecrona, T., Hook, M., Riesenfeld, J., and Lindahl, U.,** Interaction of lipoprotein lipase with native and modified heparin-like polysaccharides, *Biochem. J.,* 189, 625, 1980.
76. **Shimada, K., Gill, P. J., Silbert, J. E., Douglas, W. H. J., and Fanburg, B. L.,** Involvement of cell surface heparin sulfate in the binding of lipoprotein lipase to cultured bovine endothelial cells, *J. Clin. Invest.,* 68, 995, 1981.
77. **Assman, G., Krauss, R. M., Fredrickson, D. S., and Levy, R. I.,** Characterization, subcellular localization and partial purification of a heparin-released triglyceride lipase from rat liver, *J. Biol. Chem.,* 248, 1992, 1973.
78. **Breier, C., Muhlberger, V., Drexel, H., Herold, M., Lisch, H.-J., Knapp, E., and Braunsteiner, H.,** Essential role of post-heparin lipoprotein lipase activity and of plasma testosterone in coronary artery disease, *Lancet,* 1, 1242, 1985.
79. **Baumgartner, H. R. and Haudenschild, C.,** Adhesion of platelets to subendothelium, *Ann. N.Y. Acad. Sci.,* 201, 22, 1972.
80. **Thomas, D. P., Johnson, E. A., and Barrowcliffe, T. W.,** The antithrombotic action of heparan sulphate, in *Vascular Occlusion: Epidemiological, Pathophysiological and Therapeutic Aspects,* Tesi, M. and Dormandy, J., Eds., Academic Press, London, 1981, 377.
81. **Teien, A., Abildgaard, U., and Hook, M.,** The anticoagulant effect of heparan sulfate and dermatan sulfate, *Thromb. Res.,* 8, 859, 1976.
82. **Ts'ao, C.-H., Eisenstein, R., and Schumacher, B.,** Effect of an aortic proteoglycan on platelet aggregation and thrombin time: plasma requirement and active moieties, *Proc. Natl. Acad. Sci. U.S.A.,* 156, 162, 1977.
83. **Colburn, P. and Buonassisi, V.,** Anticlotting activity of endothelial cell cultures and heparan sulfate proteoglycans, *Biochem. Biophys. Res. Commun.,* 104, 220, 1982.
84. **Abildgaard, U.,** Inhibition of the thrombin-fibrinogen reaction by heparin and purified cofactor, *Scand. J. Haematol.,* 5, 440, 1968.
85. **Rosenberg, R. D. and Damus, P. S.,** The purification and mechanism of action of human antithrombin-heparin cofactor, *J. Biol. Chem.,* 248, 6490, 1973.
86. **Rosenberg, R. D. and Lam, L.,** Correlation between structure and function of heparin, *Proc. Natl. Acad. Sci. U.S.A.,* 76, 1218, 1979.
87. **Tollefsen, D. M., Pestka, C. A., and Monafo, M. J.,** Activation of heparin cofactor II by dermatan sulfate, *J. Biol. Chem.,* 258, 6713, 1983.
88. **Ofosu, F. A., Modi, G. J., Smith, L. M., Cerskus, A. L., Hirsh, J., and Blajchman, M. A.,** Heparan sulfate and dermatan sulfate inhibit thrombin generation by complementary pathways, *Blood,* 64, 742, 1984.
89. **Ofosu, F. A., Blajchman, M. A., and Hirsh, J.,** The inhibition by heparin of the intrinsic pathway activation of factor X in the absence of antithrombin III, *Thromb. Res.,* 20, 391, 1980.
90. **Walker, F. J. and Esmon, C. T.,** Interactions between heparin and factor Xa. Inhibition of prothrombin activation, *Biochim. Biophys. Acta,* 585, 405, 1979.
91. **Stern, D., Nawroth, P., Marcum, J., Handley, D., Kisiel, W., Rosenberg, R., and Stern, K.,** Interaction of antithrombin III with bovine aortic segments. Role of heparin in binding and enhanced anticoagulant activity, *J. Clin. Invest.,* 75, 272, 1985.
92. **Hatton, M. W. C. and Moar, S. L.,** Comparison of binding properties of thrombin and antithrombin III (ATIII) by rabbit thoracic aorta endothelium and subendothelium in vitro, *Thromb. Haemost.,* 54, 232, 1985.

93. **Shimada, K., Kusumoto, I., and Ozawa, T.**, The potency of heparin-like activity of glycosaminoglycans released by human endothelial cells in culture, *Experientia*, 41, 671, 1985.
94. **Brandt, J. T., Stephens, R. E., Joseph, L. B., and Miller, L.**, Human endothelial cells mediate the interaction between human antithrombin III and thrombin, *Fed. Proc.*, 44, 1847, 1985.
95. **Nesheim, M. E.**, A simple rate law that describes the kinetics of heparin-catalysed reaction between antithrombin III and thrombin, *J. Biol. Chem.*, 258, 14708, 1983.
96. **Aubrey, B. J., Hoak, J. C., and Owen, W. G.**, Binding of human thrombin to cultured human endothelial cells, *J. Biol. Chem.*, 254, 4092, 1979.
97. **Dryjski, M., Olsson, P., and Swedenborg, J.**, Uptake and inhibition of thrombin by the vascular wall, *Thromb. Res.*, 27, 467, 1982.
98. **Lollar, P., Mackintosh, S. C., and Owen, W. G.**, Reaction of antithrombin III with thrombin bound to the vascular endothelium. Analysis in a recirculating perfused rabbit heart preparation, *J. Biol. Chem.*, 259, 4335, 1984.
99. **Hatton, M. W. C. and Moar, S. L.**, A role for pericellular proteoglycan in the binding of thrombin or antithrombin III by the blood vessel endothelium? — The effects of proteoglycan-degrading enzymes and glycosaminoglycan-binding proteins on ^{125}I-thrombin binding by the rabbit thoracic aorta in vivo, *Thromb. Haemostas.*, 53, 228, 1985.
100. **Dryjski, M., Swedenborg, J., and Wasiutynski, A.**, Uptake and inactivation of thrombin on aortic endothelium and neo-intima, *Eur. Surg. Res.*, 17, 1, 1985.
101. **Zucker-Franklin, D. and Rosenberg, L.**, Platelet interaction with modified articular cartilage: its possible relevance to joint repair, *J. Clin. Invest.*, 59, 641, 1977.
102. **Moore, S., Pepper, D. S., and Cash, J. D.**, Platelet antiheparin activity. The isolation and characterization of platelet factor 4 released from thrombin-aggregated washed human platelets and its dissociation into subunits and the isolation of membrane-bound antiheparin activity, *Biochim. Biophys. Acta*, 379, 370, 1975.
103. **Busch, C., Dawes, J., Pepper, D. S., and Wasteson, A.**, Binding of platelet factor 4 to cultured human umbilical vein endothelial cells, *Thromb. Res.*, 19, 129, 1980.
104. **Wasteson, A., Hook, M., and Westermark, B.**, Demonstration of a platelet enzyme, degrading heparan sulphate, *FEBS Lett.*, 64, 218, 1976.
105. **Yahalom, J., Eldor, A., Fuks, Z., and Vlodavsky, I.**, Degradation of sulfated proteoglycans in the subendothelial extracellular matrix by human platelet heparitinase, *J. Clin. Invest.*, 74, 1842, 1984.
106. **Rosenberg, R. D., Fritze, L. M. S., Castellot, J. J., and Karnovsky, M. J.**, Heparin-like molecules as regulators of atherogenesis, *Nouv. Rev. Fr. Hematol.*, 26, 225, 1984.
107. **Vinazzer, H. A., Sternberger, A., Haas, S., and Blumel, E.**, Influence of heparin, of different heparin fractions, and of a low molecular weight heparin-like substance on the mechanism of fibrinolysis, *Thromb. Res.*, 27, 341, 1982.
108. **Vairel, G. E., Brouty-Borge, H., Toulemonde, F., Doutremepuich, C., Marsh, N. A., and Gaffney, P. J.**, Heparin and a low-molecular weight fraction enhance thrombolysis and by this pathway exercise a protective effect against thrombosis, *Thromb. Res.*, 30, 219, 1983.
109. **Bottcher, C. J. F. and Klynstra, F. B.**, Acid mucopolysaccharides in human aortic tissue: their distribution at different stages of atherosclerosis, *Lancet*, 2, 439, 1963.
110. **Berenson, G. S., Radhakrishnamurthy, B., Dalferes, E. S., and Srinivasan, S. R.**, Carbohydrate macromolecules and atherosclerosis, *Hum. Pathol.*, 2, 57, 1971.
111. **Smith, E. B.**, Acid glycosaminoglycan, collagen, and elastin content of normal artery, fatty streaks, and plaques, *Adv. Exp. Med. Biol.*, 43, 125, 1974.
112. **Kumar, V., Berenson, G. S., Ruiz, H., Dalferes, E. R., and Strong, J. P.**, Acid mucopolysaccharides of human aorta. III. Variations with atherosclerotic involvement, *J. Atheroscl. Res.*, 7, 583, 1967.
113. **Stevens, R. L., Colombo, M., Gonzales, J. J., Hollander, W., and Schmid, K.**, The glycosaminoglycans of the human artery and their changes in atherosclerosis, *J. Clin. Invest.*, 58, 470, 1976.
114. **Klynstra, F. B., Bottcher, C. J. F., Van Melsen, J. A., and van der Laan, E. J.**, Distribution and composition of acid mucopolysaccharides in normal and atherosclerotic human aortas, *J. Atheroscler. Res.*, 7, 301, 1967.
115. **Toledo, O. M. S. and Mouro, P. A. S.**, Sulfated glycosaminoglycans of human aorta: chondroitin 6-sulfate increase with age, *Biochem. Biophys. Res. Commun.*, 89, 50, 1979.
116. **Radnakrishnamurthy, B., Ruiz, H. A., Dalferes, E. R., Vesselinovitch, D., Wissler, R. W., and Berenson, G. S.**, The effect of various dietary regimens and cholestyramine on aortic glycosaminoglycans during regression of atherosclerotic lesions in rhesus monkeys, *Atherosclerosis*, 33, 17, 1979.
117. **Mullinger, R. N. and Manley, G.**, Glycosaminoglycans and atherosclerosis in animal aortas, *Atheroscler. Res.*, 9, 108, 1969.
118. **Kurwen, K. D. and Smith, S. C.**, Aortic glycosaminoglycans in atherosclerosis-susceptible and resistant pigeons, *Exp. Mol. Pathol.*, 27, 121, 1977.

119. **Wight, T. N.,** Differences in the synthesis and secretion of sulfated glycosaminoglycans by aorta explant monolayers cultured from atherosclerosis-susceptible and -resistant pigeons, *Am. J. Pathol.*, 101, 127, 1980.
120. **Helin, P., Lorenzen, I., and Garbarsch, G.,** Repair in arterial tissue: morphological and biochemical changes in rabbit aorta after a single dilation injury, *Circ. Res.*, 29, 542, 1971.
121. **Saxena, I. D. and Nagchaudhuri, J.,** Effect of high fat diets on acid mucopolysaccharides of the aorta in rabbits, *Indian J. Exp. Biol.*, 8, 15, 1970.
122. **Helin, G., Helin, P., and Lorenzen, I.,** The aortic glycosaminoglycans in arteriosclerosis induced by systemic hypoxia, *Atherosclerosis*, 12, 325, 1970.
123. **Ichida, T. and Kalant, N.,** Aortic glycosaminoglycans in atheroma and alloxan diabetes, *Can. J. Biochem.*, 46, 249, 1968.
124. **Wight, T. N., Curwen, K., Homan, W., and Minick, C. R.,** Effect of regenerated endothelium on glycosaminoglycan accumulation in the arterial wall, *Fed. Proc.*, 38, 1075, 1979.
125. **Castor, C. W., Ritchie, J. C., Scott, M. E., and Whitney, S. L.,** Connective tissue activation. IX. Stimulation of glycosaminoglycan and DNA formation by a platelet factor, *Arthritis Rheum.*, 20, 859, 1977.
126. **Fischer-Dzoga, K., Fraser, R., and Wissler, R. W.,** Stimulation of proliferation in stationary primary cultures of monkey and rabbit aortic smooth muscle cells. I. Effects of lipoprotein fractions of hyperlipemic serum and lymph, *Exp. Mol. Pathol.*, 24, 346, 1976.
127. **Erhlich, K. and Murray, M.,** Effect of low density lipoprotein on proteoglycan synthesis by aorta cells in culture, *Experientia*, 34, 179, 1978.
128. **Leung, D. Y. M., Glagov, S., and Mathews, M. B.,** Cyclic stretching stimulates synthesis of matrix components by arterial smooth muscle cells in vitro, *Science*, 191, 475, 1976.

Chapter 3

EICOSANOIDS

Jozsef Mandl

TABLE OF CONTENTS

I. INTRODUCTION

Eicosanoids are the derivatives of polyunsaturated fatty acids containing 20 carbon atoms; the 3 most common precursors in animals are 8-cis-, 11-cis-, 14-cis-eicosatrienoic acid (dihomo-γ-linolenic acid), 5-cis-, 8-cis-, 11-cis-, 14-cis-eicosatetraenoic acid (arachidonic acid), and 5-cis-, 8-cis-, 11-cis-, 14-cis-, 17-cis-eicosapentaenoic acid. The most important eicosanoid precursor is arachidonic acid, and this chapter covers mainly the derivatives of arachidonic acid.

More than 50 years ago, von Euler and Goldblatt independently discovered a new vasodepressor in genital glands and human semen which exhibited smooth muscle contracting activity; von Euler named it "prostaglandin". In the 1960s Bergstrom's and van Dorp's groups simultaneously demonstrated that prostaglandins were produced from polyunsaturated fatty acids. The rapid expansion of the research in these fields led to the discoveries of new prostanoid derivatives, thromboxanes and prostacyclin, identified in the middle of the 1970s by Samuelsson et al. and Vane and Moncada et al. In 1979 another structure of oxygenated arachidonic acid derivatives was identified, termed leukotriene, a completely new system of biological regulators.

Nearly all mammalian cells (perhaps the most important exception is the erythrocyte) have the enzymes to form these very effective molecules "on demand", but frequently not every kind of them. There are wide qualitative and quantitative differences in the ability of different tissues to synthesize eicosanoids. The profile of oxygenated arachidonic acid derivatives in various cell types is often characteristic for their biological function. In spite of the fact that the ability of the cells to synthesize various eicosanoids represents a universal mechanism, an overall view on their biological significance and role is lacking.

II. ARACHIDONIC ACID METABOLISM

A. Arachidonic Acid Supply

Arachidonic acid is synthesized in the cells mainly from linoleate and linolenate, which are essential fatty acids furnished by the diet. The availability of free arachidonic acid is considered to be rate limiting in the biosynthesis of eicosanoids.[1] Its concentration in the cytosol and plasma is kept low normally;[2,3] the large amount of arachidonate like the other polyunsaturated fatty acids in mammalian cells is esterified almost exclusively in the 2-acyl position of glycerophospholipids.[4] Thus, phospholipids constitute the main intracellular source of arachidonate, while the contribution of the major neutral storage lipids — triacylglycerols — to arachidonate liberation is practically negligible.

It is assumed that the enzymes of arachidonate (re)esterification play a dominant role in keeping free arachidonate level low within the cell. First, arachidonic acid is esterified with CoA by acyl-CoA synthetase (which is very much favored over acyl hydrolase catalyzing the hydrolysis of arachidonoyl CoA) and then it is transferred into the 2-acyl position of phospholipids by acyl transferase (Figure 1). While no pronounced specificity of long chain fatty acid acyl CoA synthetase has been found for arachidonic acid, the affinity of lysophosphoglyceride acyltransferase(s) is high for arachidonoyl CoA.[1,4] The importance of reesterification in the regulation of free arachidonate level in the cell is generally accepted, but this does not influence the concept; free arachidonate supply for eicosanoid synthesis is controlled by phospholipases.[1,5,6]

In stimulated cells the increased liberation of arachidonate derives from the hydrolysis of glycerolipids. Phosphatidylethanolamine and phosphatidylcholine are generally assumed to be hydrolyzed by phospholipase A2 (PLA2). In the case of phosphatidylinositol, it can be hydrolyzed first by phospholipase C (PLC) and then both the formed diacylglycerol or its metabolite, the phosphatidic acid, might be hydrolyzed further to liberate arachidonic

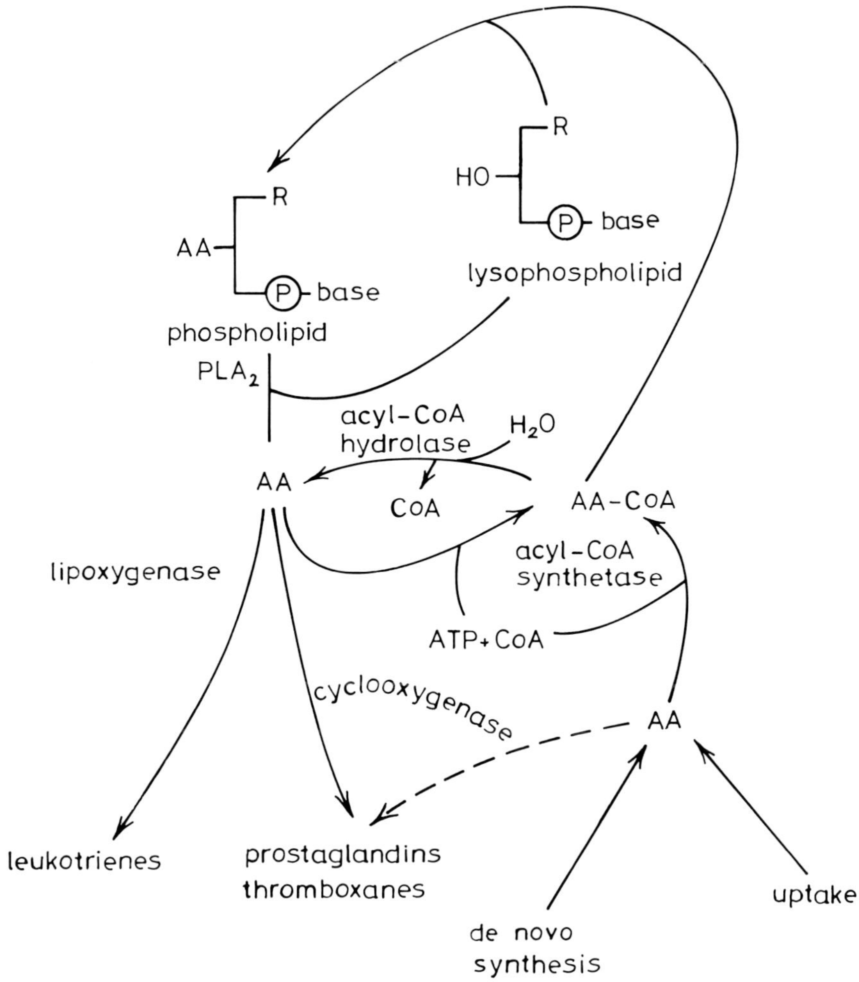

FIGURE 1. Arachidonic acid metabolism in the cell. Abbreviations: AA, arachidonic acid; PLA2, phospholipase A2; R, fatty acid.

acid.[7-9] There are differences among the various phosphatidate esters in their contribution to arachidonate supply depending on cell type examined and the trigger used. The physiological stimulus for arachidonic acid liberation and its further metabolism can be hormonal, e.g., angiotensin II, bradykinin, epinephrine; formation of a protease, e.g., thrombin; immunological, e.g., certain antibody-antigen complexes, etc. A great variety of effectors which cause various kind of membrane perturbation or ischemia may also induce eicosanoid synthesis.

Little is known about the presumably different mechanisms controlling the activity of phospholipases involved, how the (patho)physiological stimuli or other effectors ignite an increase of PLA2 activity. PLA2, diacylglycerol, and phosphatidic acid lipase activities are membrane bound; the bulk of the activities is associated with the microsomal fraction. PLA2 is a Ca^{2+}-calmodulin dependent enzyme, thus its action is related to the changes of intracellular calcium concentration.[1,10] However, it should be noted that at stimulated hydrolysis of phosphatidylinositol by PLC, the activity of diacylglycerol and phosphatidic acid lipase can also be increased at lower level of calcium. There is a view that phosphatidylinositol is the principal source of arachidonate for eicosanoid production induced by "receptor mediated" agonists.[11]

The liberation of arachidonic acid by PLA2 can be reduced by corticosteroids,[12] which induce synthesis of proteins (macrocortin, lipomodulin, renocortin) inhibitory on PLA activity.[13-15] This action of corticosteroids might constitute a long-term regulatory mechanism of arachidonate liberation. This is the mechanism underlying the inhibitory action of anti-inflammatory steroids.

The regulation of arachidonate liberation is further complicated by (1) the cell type specific differences, even within one organ like the kidney[16,17] or the liver[18] (PLA2-s may differ depending upon the cellular origin), and (2) the possibility of various arachidonate pools (even the existence of hormone-linked arachidonate pools is suggested).[19,20] Moreover, it is supposed that exogenous arachidonate first is not converted directly by oxygenases to prostanoids, but occupies a place in the esterified arachidonate pool and the substrates for cyclooxygenase are liberated from the phospholipids.[17] Contrary to this opinion, in certain cell types prostanoids can be synthesized from exogenous arachidonate, demonstrated in endothelial cells,[21,22] macrophages,[23] etc., and termed PLA2 insensitive prostanoid synthesis. There are also cell type differences in the response to the addition of exogenous arachidonate;[18] thus, in these cases a regulatory role of extracellular arachidonate might be supposed. It has been suggested that liver serves to supply other organs with arachidonate in essential fatty acid deficiency.[11] To summarize, arachidonate liberation is a crucial process in eicosanoid synthesis and really may constitute a site for regulation.

B. Prostaglandins and Thromboxanes

1. Synthesis of Prostaglandins and Thromboxanes

The widely accepted nomenclature of prostaglandins (PG) is based on the prostanoic acid skeleton — a monocarboxylic acid with 20 carbon atoms containing a cyclopentane ring. The letters following the abbreviation PG indicate the nature and position of oxygen containing functional groups present at C9, C11 in the cyclopentane ring. The various thromboxane (TX) derivatives are also designated with various letters (TXA, TXB). Prostanoids also contain one, two, or three double bonds in the side chains indicated by numerical subscripts (PGE_1, PGE_2, PGE_3). The greek subscript indicates that the hydroxyl group at C9 lies on the same side of the cyclopentane ring as the carboxyl side chain ($PGF_{2\alpha}$). Prostaglandins of the 1 series (synthesized in general from eicosatrienoic acid) have a trans double bond in the 13 position. The two double bonds in the side chains (a trans one in the Δ-13 and a cis one in the Δ-5 position) are present in all biologically active arachidonic acid derivatives, while prostaglandins of the 3 series (synthesized from eicosapentaenoic acid) have in addition a cis double bond at Δ-17. The presence of the trans double bond in the Δ-13 position and the 15-hydroxy group is characteristic for all natural biologically active prostanoids independent on the precursor polyunsaturated fatty acid.[24-26]

The enzymes of prostanoid and thromboxane synthesis are localized on the cytosolic surface of several membranes mainly in the endoplasmic reticulum and in nuclear membranes and plasma membranes, as well. Except one, all the enzymes involved are integral membrane proteins. The initial step of the prostanoid synthesis is the oxygenative cyclization of arachidonic acid. In the course of a bis-dioxygenation process, two molecules of oxygen are incorporated into arachidonic acid forming a 9,11-15-hydroperoxy derivative, PGG_2. This reaction is catalyzed by the fatty acid cyclooxygenase which requires heme as cofactor. The reduction of the 15-hydroperoxy group of PGG_2 to 15-hydroxy group (PGH_2) is the second step carried out by prostaglandin hydroperoxidase (Figure 2). It is supposed that the natural electron donor is NADPH. The activity of this enzyme is closely associated with the activity of cyclooxygenase. Therefore, the activities of the two enzymes are frequently termed prostaglandin endoperoxide synthetase.[24]

The bis-dioxygenation reaction catalyzed by the cyclooxygenase is the site of action for several nonsteroidal anti-inflammatory agents. They inhibit the cyclooxygenase activity,

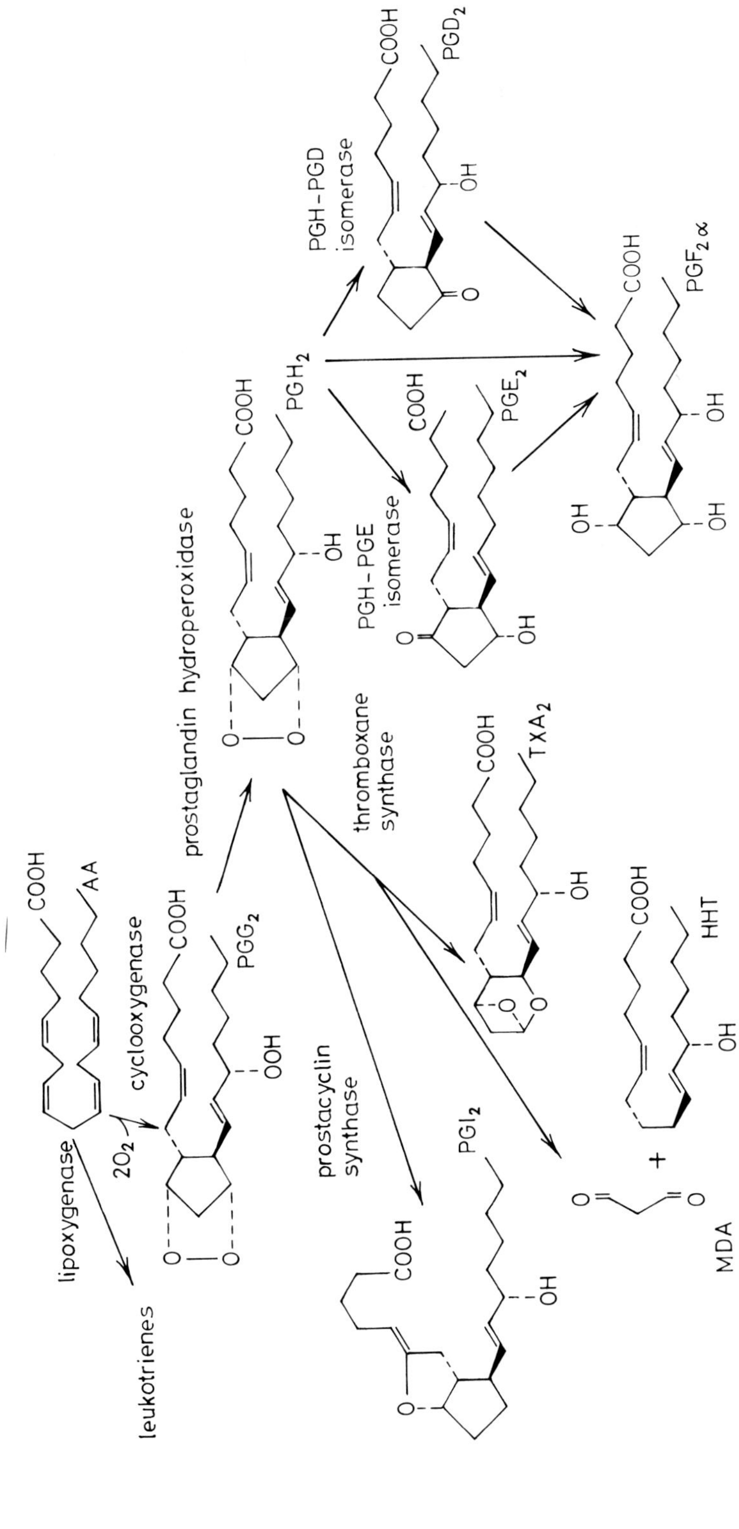

FIGURE 2. Prostaglandin and thromboxane synthesis from arachidonic acid.

however, the activity of peroxidase remains relatively unaffected. The mechanism of inactivation of cyclooxygenase is different. Acetylsalicylic acid causes covalent modification of the enzyme by acetylation of a serine residue, whereas indomethacin irreversibly inactivates it without any covalent modification; several other drugs are only reversible cyclooxygenase inhibitors.[27-30]

PGH_2 is at a central place on the map of various eicosanoid derivatives (Figure 2). The enzymes of different pathways leading to the synthesis of different types of prostanoids utilize PGH_2 as substrate.[31,32] These enzymes attack the 9,11-endoperoxy bridge of PGH_2. It is noted that certain cells (endothelial cells, etc.) might also convert exogenously added PGH_2.[22,33]

Prostaglandin E_2, D_2, and F_2 are subsequently formed from PGH_2 by hydrolytic cleavage combined with oxidoreduction. They have oxygen containing functional groups at carbons 9,11 in the cyclopentane ring. In the course of PGD_2 synthesis an isomerization of the 9,11-endoperoxide of PGH_2 to 9α-hydroxyl and 11-keto groups takes place. This reaction is catalyzed by PGH-PGD isomerases in the cytosol, which are the only nonmembrane-bound enzymes involved in PGH_2 metabolism. The conversion of PGH_2 to PGE_2 is an isomerization of the 9,11-endoperoxide to 9-keto and 11α-hydroxyl groups; glutathione (GSH) as a coenzyme is also required.[31] $PGF_{2\alpha}$ can be produced in three ways: (1) PGH_2 can be reduced in a nonenzymic way, (2) the 9-keto group of PGE_2 can be reduced (3) the 11-keto group of PGD_2 can be reduced, as well. However, it cannot be excluded that $PGF_{2\alpha}$ synthase also exists.[24,26]

In the course of the synthesis of the bicyclic structures of PGI_2 and TXA_2 an intramolecular redox reaction takes place. A hydrogen atom in the side chain of PGH_2 is under attack and displaced. PGI_2 is also a prostanoid, however, in the place of the usual cyclopentane ring TXA_2 contains an oxane-oxetane grouping. The formation of PGI_2 is catalyzed by prostacyclin synthase,[33,34] while the thromboxane synthesis is catalyzed by thromboxane synthase.[25,32,35] These proteins belong to the family of cytochrome P-450 enzymes. However, they do not exhibit monooxygenase activity, NADPH is not effective as a reducing agent, and they do not require electron transport.[36,37] TXA_2 synthase catalyzes cleavages of the endoperoxide bridge between the two oxygen atoms and of the cyclopentane ring between C11 and C12. Ether bridges are formed between C9 and C11 and C11 and C12. Concomitant with TXA_2 formation 12-L-hydroxy-5,8,10-heptadecatrienoic acid (HHT) and malondialdehyde (MDA) are also produced. It is assumed that they are also formed by TXA synthase.[38] TXA synthase inhibitors inhibit HHT formation, as well. In the course of PGI_2 synthesis a transient positive charge appears on the oxygen atom at C9 and a carbon-oxygen bond is formed with concomitant loss of the proton from C6.[39] It is emphasized that PG endoperoxides are unstable in an aqueous medium and under in vitro conditions decompose spontaneously into mixtures containing E-, F-, and D-types of prostaglandins; however, without addition of enzymes, no PGI_2 or TXA_2 formation is observed.[22,35]

The general ability of the cells to synthesize various oxygenated arachidonate derivatives does not mean that each cell is able to produce each kind of eicosanoids. There are cells which synthesize only one or mainly one kind of eicosanoids and this metabolite may determine some of their biological functions. This is especially true for cells playing a pivotal role in the maintenance of hemostasis. On the other hand, certain types of cells (hepatocytes, etc.) produce several types of eicosanoids and synthetic capacities are in the same range. These metabolites may exert opposite effects on the same target; their synthesis can be under different hormonal and other control. Therefore, the selective regulation of various metabolic pathways leading to the synthesis of different prostanoids produced by the same cell but after different stimuli is of special interest. Selective inhibitors of TXA_2 synthase (imidazole derivatives)[35] and PGI synthase (tranylcypromine)[34] have been reported, but the selective regulation of the synthesis of certain eicosanoids is still unknown.

2. Catabolism of Prostaglandins and Thromboxanes

Prostanoids are not stored in the cells, but immediately are secreted. Their catabolism may occur in the blood or in many tissues mainly in the lung, liver, and kidney. In several cases the first step is the uptake of secreted prostanoids into the respective cells. This is followed by intracellular enzymic inactivation.[24] It was emphasized already that the existence of the 15-hydroxyl group is essential for the biological activity of all prostanoid derivatives. The first attack of inactivation transforms the 15-hydroxyl into a keto group catalyzed by 15-hydroxyprostaglandin dehydrogenase (PGDH). PGDH is a cytosolic enzyme; both NAD- and NADP-linked forms have been described. The second step in prostanoid inactivation is the reduction of the 13,14 double bond, also pointed out to be characteristic for all natural prostanoids, by a ketoreductase. After these two reactions the inactive 15-keto 13,14-dihydroprostaglandins are formed. Thus ends the first and functionally most important phase of catabolism, the inactivation. The time is very important; the dehydrogenation of the 15-hydroxy group of prostaglandins in certain parts of the circulation is a very rapid process. A single passage through the pulmonary circulation results in an almost complete inactivation of PGE_2 and $PGF_{2\alpha}$. That is why PGE_2 is much less active in lowering blood pressure when it is given intravenously than when given intraarterially. PGD_2 is inactivated mainly in the blood plasma or in the kidney. Contrary to other prostanoids, the bulk of PGI_2 is not inactivated in the pulmonary circulation, but rather it is decomposed spontaneously, forming its major hydrolysis product 6-keto $PGF_{1\alpha}$, or it is taken up by the liver.[40]

TXA_2 is inactivated mainly by chemical decomposition to TXB_2 inside the "mother" cells or in the blood plasma. TXB_2 is generally considered to be biologically inactive; only some minor effects have been described.[35] The time of inactivation may be belated with the trapping of released TXA_2 by serum proteins (mainly albumin) which protect against hydrolysis. This way a prolonged half-life can be obtained.[41] The formed 15-keto 13,14-dihydroprostanoids subsequently undergo one or more steps of β- or ω-oxidation of the side chain before excretion to the urine.

Arachidonic acid can be also a substrate of monooxygenases in the liver and kidney.[26] Cytochrome P-450 enzymes metabolize arachidonic acid by epoxidation. The epoxides subsequently are hydrolyzed and vicinal diols are formed. This oxidation requires NADPH and it was shown to be inducible by phenobarbital in the liver. The vicinal diols are converted further by ω_1- and ω_2-hydroxylation, as several prostaglandins and leukotrienes. In the liver and renal cortex, ω_1- and ω_2-hydroxylation are also catalyzed by monooxygenases.

C. Leukotrienes

Leukotrienes are also formed from the same polyunsaturated fatty acids as prostanoids and similar to the cyclooxygenase products they are synthesized and released on demand. However, their structure, synthesis, and catabolism are completely different.[42-44] They are noncyclic C20 carboxylic acids with one or two oxygen substituents and three conjugated double bonds. It is assumed that their synthesis, unlike the formation of prostanoids, requires not only the liberation of arachidonic acid, but the activation of lipoxygenases, as well. Lipoxygenases are iron containing proteins, but they do not contain the heme prosthetic group. In several cases 5-lipoxygenase catalyzes the initial step of leukotriene synthesis, which is an insertion of oxygen at C5 of arachidonic acid (Figure 3). Several reports were published on the Ca^{2+} dependence of 5-lipoxygenase.[44] The formed 5(S)-hydroperoxy-6,8,11,14-eicosatetraenoic acid (5 HPETE) (1) is further converted to an epoxy fatty acid 5(S)-trans-oxido-7,9-trans-11,14-cis-eicosatetraenoic acid (leukotriene A_4, LTA_4)[45] (epoxy eicosatetraenoic acid and its derivatives, which already contain the conjugated triene structure are called leukotrienes): (2) can be reduced to the corresponding hydroxy acid, 5(S)-hydroxy-6,8,11,14-eicosatetraenoic acid (5 HETE); (3) can be oxygenated by lipoxygenases at another position in the aliphatic chain and dihydroxy-eicosatetraenoic acids (diHETE-s) produced.

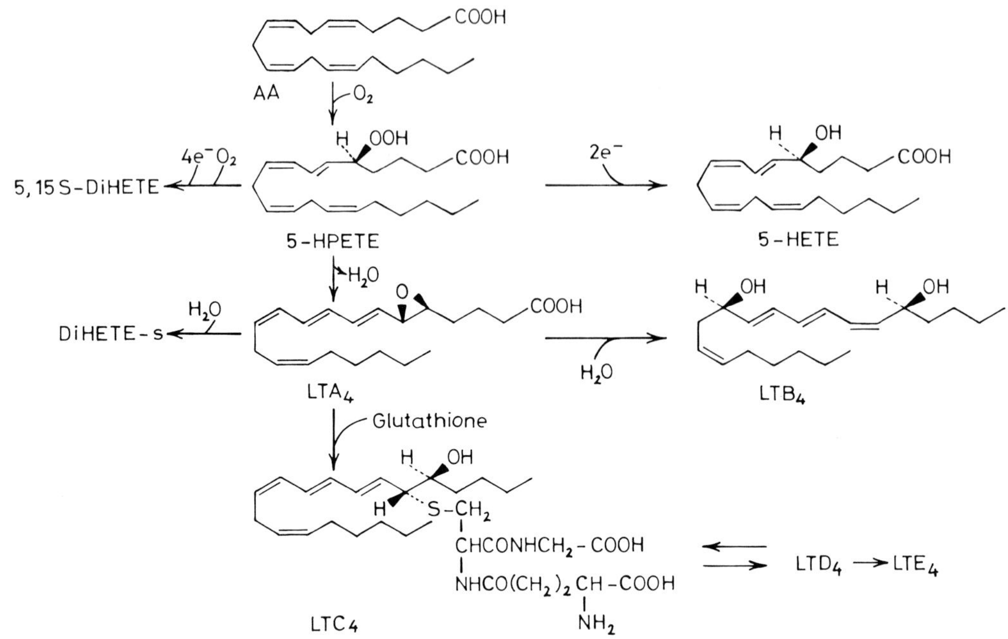

FIGURE 3. Leukotriene synthesis from arachidonic acid.

The first oxygenation of arachidonic acid can occur at C12 and -15, as well resulting in corresponding HPETE-s.

LTA_4 is a common intermediate in the synthesis of both leukotriene B_4 and C_4 (LTB_4, LTC_4). In the formation of LTB_4 (5(S)-12(R)-dihydroxy-6-cis-8,10-trans-14-cis-eicosatetraenoic acid), the dependence of calcium has been observed, while in the study of LTC_4, synthesis investigators have focused their attention on the role of glutathione. In the course of LTC_4 (5(S)-hydroxy-6(R) glutathionyl-7,9-trans-11,14-cis-eicosatetraenoic acid) formation, a nucleophilic opening of the epoxide at C6 of LTA_4 occurs by the sulfhydryl group of glutathione forming a glutathione conjugate of arachidonic acid catalyzed by glutathione -S-transferase, which is a membrane-bound enzyme. Leukotriene D_4, E_4, and F_4 (LTD_4, LTE_4, LTF_4) are formed by a successive elimination of glutamic acid by γ-glutamyl transpeptidase or glycin from the peptide chain of LTC_4. The position (C6) and the free amino and carboxyl groups of the peptide substituent are important for the maximal biological effect of leukotrienes and a partial saturation of the triene also reduces their biological activity.[46,47] The half lives of leukotrienes are very short.[43,44] In their catabolism the role of the liver is dominant; experiments showed a rapid hepatic uptake and biliary excretion of leukotrienes.[39,44,48] Platelets, macrophages, and other cells are able to synthesize both cyclooxygenase and lipoxygenase products. It is supposed that arachidonic acid used by the two enzymes may come from different pools.[39]

III. MECHANISM OF ACTION OF EICOSANOIDS

The expanding research in the field of eicosanoids has produced a huge amount of experimental data on various biological effects of different eicosanoid derivatives, and also several hypotheses on their mechanism of action have been proposed. Most of these actions are ultimately related to (1) their modulating effect on signal transducing processes and (2) their effect on various contractile systems. In this chapter attention has been focused on these two fields.

A. Eicosanoids and Signal Transducing Processes

Both the synthesis and the action of prostanoids are interfering in most cases with the signal transducing mechanisms of the cells. The two best-known signal transducing processes in the cells are linked to adenylate cyclase or to membrane phosphoinositides.

It was previously supposed that plasma membrane prostanoid receptors are connected with adenylate or guanylate cyclases in various types of cells. PGI_2 and PGE_2 receptors have been suggested to be associated with the adenylate cyclase, while $PGF_{2\alpha}$ effects with the changes of guanylate cyclase activity.[25,49] The role of guanylate cyclase in the signal transduction processes is not clear. Much work has been focused on the changes of adenylate cyclase activity induced by eicosanoids. After recent advances on the dual regulation of adenylate cyclase activity mediated by stimulatory (Gs/Ns) or inhibitory (Gi/Ni) guanine-nucleotide-binding regulatory proteins, several previous results in these fields should be reinterpreted. However, the basic concept that cAMP as a second messenger is involved in the action of various prostanoids is not challenged.

The increase or decrease of intracellular cAMP level by prostanoids results in various changes in metabolism of cells and these changes vary depending on the functions of cell types investigated. In the kidney through the decrease of cAMP, PGE_2 modulates the effect of ADH. In this way the changes in cAMP level in the ion transport in brain are connected with the noradrenaline release. The increase of cAMP level in different targets may result in opposite changes in prostanoid synthesis; for example, a Gs guanine-nucleotide-binding regulatory protein mediated stimulation of adenylate cyclase by PGI_2 on platelets causes an increased formation of cAMP,[51] which leads to a decrease of another prostanoid production, like TXA_2. PGI_2 also inhibits its own synthesis in endothelial cells by causing an increase of cAMP concentration.[52-54] In most cases elevation of cAMP level results in a decrease of prostanoid synthesis;[55] this leads to the assumption that cAMP might be involved in a negative feedback control of prostanoid synthesis in various cells.[23] On the other hand, in platelets thrombin and epinephrine causes an Gi guanine nucleotide binding regulatory protein mediated inhibition of adenylate cyclase, cAMP concentration is decreased, and TXA2 is synthesized.

Agonist-receptor interactions connected to the changes of phosphoinositides hydrolysis may represent various types of agonists (hormones, neurotransmitters, other peptides) and various types of receptor classes (α1-adrenergic, H1-histaminergic, V1-vasopressin, muscarinic cholinergic), but their common feature is that they initiate a mechanism which generates several second messengers; this way the whole process is multifunctional. The signal cascade results in a mobilization of calcium, activation of protein kinase C, liberation of arachidonic acid, and stimulation of guanylate cyclase.[56-58]

The crucial first step of this cascade is the hydrolysis of phosphatidylinositol 4,5-bisphosphate (PtdIns 4,5P2) catalyzed by PtdIns 4,5P2 phosphodiesterase (PLC), which is a bifurcation in the signal pathway to yield two second messengers; inositol 1,4,5-trisphosphate (IP3) and diacylglycerol. This cleavage generally occurs at resting levels of calcium. IP3 is a second messenger inducing the mobilization of calcium from intracellular reservoirs and calcium bound to calmodulin acts through phosphorylation of a group of proteins. As it was detailed previously, Ca^{2+}-calmodulin complex also activates PLA2 and thus arachidonate is liberated. Diacylglycerol is also a second messenger, which activates protein kinase C. Protein kinase C also phosphorylates another group of proteins.

In some cells, e.g., in platelets after the stimulation of these receptors, the formed diacylglycerol or phosphatidic acid (after its phosphorylation) may be substrates of specific phospholipases.[7,8] This leads to the liberation of arachidonic acid from phosphoinositides besides the formation of other phosphoinositide derived second messengers. These enzymes require less calcium than those which liberate arachidonic acid by direct stimulation and from other phospholipids.

The mobilization of calcium might stimulate guanylate cyclase, as well, to elevate the intracellular level of cGMP. Several authors have suggested previously that the other second messenger in the action of prostanoids is the cGMP and according to this assumption the controlled release of arachidonic acid or its oxydized metabolites as part of the signal pathway would partly serve as activators (or inhibitors) of guanylate cyclase.

The "cross"-interactions between the various signal transducing processes are of special interest. In platelets the effect of thrombin offers special opportunities to investigate the interrelationship, because its effect is mediated by both the two signal transducing systems. Thrombin exerts a stimulatory action through receptors connected with PLC and PLA2 and an inhibitory action through receptors linked to the adenylate cyclase. The stimulatory effect of thrombin is mediated by a rapid (in 5 sec) formation of IP3 and diacylglycerol by the activation of PLC and it activates PLA2.[59] Via another receptor thrombin may simultaneously decrease the intracellular level of cAMP through a Gi-mediated inhibition of adenylate cyclase. These are synergistic effects and increase TXA_2 synthesis. Alternatively, it has been published recently that in platelets protein kinase C, among others, phosphorylates the characteristic α-subunit of the Gi. Thus, the activation of protein kinase C (as part of the signal cascade) may suppress the inhibitory action of thrombin and epinephrine on adenylate cyclase.[60,61] Activation of adenylate cyclase and thus an increase in intracellular cAMP concentration is known to inhibit the stimulatory action of thrombin; PGI_2, the most powerful antiaggregatory agent, acts through a Gs-mediated activation of adenylate cyclase. A similar regulation exists in endothelial cells as well.[62] Thus, complicated "cross"-reactions between the participants of the two signal transducing processes or within the multifunctional signal cascade initiated by the phosphoinositide hydrolysis constitute a sophisticated regulatory system, where eicosanoids may play several roles. By these methods, prostanoids may have important functions in communication between the various types of cells in different organs or within one organ.

B. Eicosanoids and Contractile Systems

One of the main targets of the different eicosanoids is the various forms of contractile systems. TXA_2 induces the contraction of a cell organelle, the open canalicular system of platelets causing the release of several compounds and resulting in the aggregation of platelets. TXA_2 can also induce smooth muscle cell contraction, similar to leukotrienes or $PGF_{2\alpha}$. It ignites contraction in bronchial smooth muscle as well; thus their role in bronchial asthma is postulated. Alternatively, PGI_2 or PGE_2 causes a relaxation in smooth muscle cells of the blood vessel wall and this way they are vasodilators lowering blood pressure in most species. As Table 1 shows, PGE_2 causes contraction of longitudinal smooth muscle, but a relaxation of the circular smooth muscle of GI tract. Thus, the effect of various eicosanoid derivatives on contractile systems is not a systemic one. They can induce both contraction and relaxation depending on the target or the derivative. The role of calcium in the molecular mechanism of contraction is well established; therefore, it can be supposed that this action of eicosanoids might be linked to their Ca^{2+} ionophoretic properties suggested in several reports.[63-65]

IV. BIOLOGICAL EFFECTS OF EICOSANOIDS

In the course of the last 25 years, a very intensive and exponentially growing research tried to tackle the several problems of eicosanoids. The basic strategy was rather to produce "better" derivatives than to try to influence the synthesis of prostanoids. This is understandable because many drugs of long history, mainly anti-inflammatory drugs, proved to be powerful inhibitors of prostanoid synthesis. It is sometimes more difficult to find one among the anti-inflammatory agents which is not involved in the alteration of arachidonic acid metabolism, than the opposite case. Several analogs of well-known natural prostanoids

Table 1
BIOLOGICAL EFFECTS OF PROSTAGLANDINS AND THROMBOXANE A_2

	PGE_2	PGF_2	PGD_2	PGI_2	TXA_2
Platelet					
Aggregation	+				+
Anti-aggregatory			+	+	
Blood vessel wall					
Vasoconstriction		+			+
Vasodilation	+		+	+	
Smooth muscle cells					
Contraction	Uterus corpus Longitudinal s.m.[a] of GI tract	Uterus cervix Bronchus GI tract	Bronchus GI tract		Bronchus
Relaxation	Uterus cervix Circular s.m.[a] of GI tract Bronchus				
Other	Inhibition of gastric acid secretion Effect on CNS Renal effects	Luteolytic hormone in many species Effects on CNS Renal effects	Effects on kidney function Effects on tumor growth	Effects on CNS Effects on kidney function ''Cytoprotective'' effects	

[a] s.m., smooth muscle.

were synthesized to gain biologically more effective molecules, more effective analogs in time with a longer half-life, and more effective analogs in their biological action. This strategy helped to answer several questions in the structure-effect relation. However, there are several gaps in our knowledge on the regulation of eicosanoid synthesis.

The lack of a general comprehensive view on their general biological significance and function is largely due to those features which confuse and hamper our selective understanding about their unique importance. First, one of the most characteristic features of eicosanoids is their instability. Thus, the time is a fundamental dimension in viewing their function and action, e.g., the half-life for TXA_2 is approximately 30 sec in aqueous solution at 37°C; for PGI_2 it is about 3 min, respectively. Due to their rapid inactivation, they cannot exist as "circulating hormones", and thus, their effect cannot be general. A second point of view is that after the synthesis of eicosanoids they are not stored, but are immediately secreted to the extracellular space. At present no regulation of their release is known to exist. (It is noted that this does not mean that they exert their effect only on other cells; they can also affect the "mother" cell). Being highly unstable and secreted, they usually cause local effects; that is why they are called "local hormones". Third, it is hard to find a single organ in the organism which has not been shown to be influenced directly or indirectly by eicosanoids. The synthesis and effects of various eicosanoids vary depending on the species investigated and the cell type studied or even the age. Table 1 summarizes the most important biological effects of various arachidonic acid derivatives. Having many effects on the vascular system, eicosanoids change the local (micro)circulation and in this way not only directly but indirectly affect several functions, which depend on the local blood flow. Eicosanoids also affect the vascular permeability. It is also shown in Table 1 that the different eicosanoids frequently have opposite effects on the same target. These effects are manifested in several cases through second messenger-mediated processes. Thus, eicosanoids modulate, increase, or decrease the rate of "cell specific" processes: ion transport in kidney tubular cells, acid secretion in gastric mucosa cells, muscle contraction in uterus muscle cells, or proteolytic enzyme secretion in macrophages, etc. Finally, eisosanoids might induce or inhibit prostanoid or leukotriene synthesis as well. Thus, the eicosanoid antagonists are also eicosanoids themselves in several cases. In this chapter I focus attention on the functions of eicosanoids in maintenance of hemostasis and on their role in pathological conditions.

A. Hemostasis and Eicosanoids

The blood vessel wall muscle cells and endothelial cells, the platelets, the coagulation-fibrinolytic system, the liver cells, and the lung cells are considered to be the essential components of the maintenance of hemostasis. All kinds of cells involved in these processes are also dominant sites of eicosanoid synthesis or degradation of general importance for the whole organism, while thrombin is a powerful trigger of prostanoid synthesis in platelets and endothelial cells.

The lung is one of the major sites of eicosanoid synthesis and inactivation. The pathophysiology of bronchial asthma provides a complex and complicated example of interrelationship between the productions of different arachidonic acid derivatives: prostaglandins, thromboxane, and leukotrienes.

The role of the liver in the catabolism of various eicosanoids — prostanoids and leukotrienes — is well known.[39,48,66,67] However, both the parenchymal and the nonparenchymal liver cells are also able to synthesize different eicosanoids.[18,68-70] Major gaps exist in our understanding of the role of eicosanoids in the regulation of various liver functions. Prostanoids are secreted in liver injuries and the various types of liver cells respond to the same injury with the production of different eicosanoids.[69,70] Eicosanoids and even arachidonic acid may take part in the communications between various types of liver cells.[18,71] Phagocytosing Kupffer cells produce and secrete PGE_2.[71] PGE_2 is known (1) to influence the adenylate cyclase activity of parenchymal cells, where the basic regulatory functions of cAMP, as second messenger is established, and (2) to elicit PGI_2 synthesis in liver endothelial cells.[72] In spite of the fact that thrombin and its complexes can bind to hepatocytes[73,74] and also may alter their arachidonic acid metabolism, no change in prostanoid metabolism could have been detected.[75] It is emphasized that hepatocytes can synthesize TXA_2 as well.[18,69,76,77] The TXA_2 synthesis seems to be important in liver regeneration or after various injuries.[46,69]

In this chapter attention was focused on the functions of eicosanoids in the endothelial cell-platelet interaction. One of the basic functions of endothelial cells of the blood vessel wall intima is to prevent the adhesion and aggregation of platelets, while the collagen fibers of the subendothelium trigger the thrombus formation.[78] The main prostanoid product of endothelial cells, PGI_2, plays a pivotal role in these functions and its synthesis is induced by thrombin.[79-81] On the other hand, the most potent inducer of platelet aggregation is also an eicosanoid derivative: TXA_2, produced by platelets themselves (the physiological importance of inductory effects of PGG_2 and PGH_2 on platelet aggregation[30] is dubious). TXA_2 synthesis of platelets is also induced by thrombin. It should be noted that endothelial cells may synthesize TXA_2 as well, but in a smaller amount compared to PGI_2, and also lipoxygenase products.[81-83] There is a view that the primary function of the PGI_2 under "normal" conditions is to prevent platelet aggregation and to protect the vessel wall against deposition of platelets. Platelets are unable to adhere to healthy blood vessel intima. However, the subendothelium does not contain a significant amount of prostacyclin synthase; thus the damage to the blood vessel wall intima results in a limited area where PGI_2 synthesis is markedly reduced and alternatively platelets are exposed to proaggregatory components of the subendothelium, collagen fibers, microfibrils, etc. which induce TXA_2 synthesis in platelets and aggregation. Another possibility is that the role of PGI_2 to bring about a nonthrombogenic surface of endothelial cells is manifested only in the presence of thrombin and not under "normal" conditions. This interpretation would suggest that the primary role of PGI_2 produced by endothelial cells is to prevent and to limit the formation of thrombi in the adjacent area around the damaged internal surface of the blood vessel wall, where the endothelial cells are intact and are able to produce PGI_2, and this continuous production is stimulated by thrombin formed in the coagulation cascade. Thus, the spread of the thrombus either up or down or the entire occlusion of the vessel is prevented. This is supported by the observations that PGI_2 inhibits the cell-cell interactions between thrombocytes (aggregation), but not the thrombocyte-collagen interaction important to adhere thrombocytes to the damaged blood vessel wall, where the endothelial cells are absent.

There is a tempting hypothesis that prostaglandin endoperoxides released from the aggregated adhered thrombocytes are consumed by the intact endothelial cells to produce PGI_2, which limits the growth of the thrombus. The PGI_2 production of vascular endothelial cells can be modified by PGE_2, $PGF_{2\alpha}$, or PGI_2 synthesized by the smooth muscle cells of blood vessel wall media. They also have the capacity to produce prostanoids in significant quantities, and PGE_2 can decrease PGI_2 production of endothelial cells. On the other hand, PGI_2 produced by endothelial cells causes relaxation of smooth muscle through an adenylate cyclase mediated process.[84]

It is well known that circulating polymorphonuclear leukocytes (PMNL) also interact with vascular endothelium; eicosanoids are shown to take part in association of PMNL with endothelial surface. The inhibitory effect of PGI_2 on LTB_4 synthesis of PMNL to vascular endothelium. On the other hand, TXA_2 mediates augmented adhesiveness of PMNL.[85] These interrelationships between endothelial cells, platelets, smooth muscle cells, or PMNL are clear examples of the roles, which eicosanoids play in cell-cell communications.

Nearly every organ contains a blood vessel network; thus, the PGI_2 synthesizing capacity is present everywhere in the organism. Besides thrombin, several other compounds known to play an important role in the regulation of different processes of hemostasis increase the synthesis of PGI_2 in endothelial cells: angiotensin, bradykinin, histamine, LTC_4, LTD_4, and various factors which cause ischemia. PGI_2 production is also increased in essential hypertension. On the other hand, in atherosclerosis and diabetes mellitus — both induce a systemic damage to the blood vessel wall — a deficiency of PGI_2 production[86,87] and at the same time an enhanced TXA_2 synthesis of platelets[34] were observed in an accordance with the increased thrombosis inclination of these patients. It is noteworthy that in atherosclerosis the prostanoid synthesis of smooth muscle cells of the blood vessel wall is also decreased.[86] Conversely, in uremia the TXA_2 formation in platelets is reduced, but the vascular PGI_2 formation is elevated; thus the bleeding tendency is increased. These experimental and clinical observations emphasize the predominant role of eicosanoid derivatives in the maintenance of hemostasis. Furthermore, they suggest a very close interrelationship between TXA_2 and PGI_2 synthesis in different cells. In summary, eicosanoids take part in processes which induce thrombus formation, but they also prevent it.

B. Eicosanoids in Pathological Conditions

It is likely that the importance of eicosanoids increases under various pathological conditions, i.e., the biosynthesis of certain eicosanoids can be enhanced or depressed in several diseases such as inflammations, cardiovascular diseases, renal diseases, ulcerative diseases, asthma bronchiale, diabetes mellitus, schizophrenia, various tumors, etc. Various immunological and pathological stimuli are known to induce the formation of leukotrienes. The sulfidopeptide conjugates are participating mainly in immunological reactions. SRS-A (slow reacting substance of anaphylaxis) — which has long been suggested to be the mediator of bronchoconstriction in asthma bronchiale — consists of a mixture of LTC_4, LTD_4, and LTE_4; all these leukotrienes are able to independently express the activity of SRS-A. Leukotrienes are involved in other allergic responses; they increase vascular permeability in skin and cause vasoconstriction of skin and lung microvessels, transient contraction of arterioles, etc.[43-45,88] LTB_4 takes part mainly in inflammatory reactions. In many systems it displays chemotactic activity; among others it induces adherence of PMNL to endothelial cells and stimulates migration of PMNL into extravascular tissues.[44,89]

Leukotrienes can induce the formation of cyclooxygenase products.[90] In several species, the actions of LTC_4 and LTD_4 are mediated by TXA_2 in bronchial asthma, which is a powerful bronchoconstrictor; similar stimulation has been also shown in macrophages.[91] On the other hand, prostanoids may inhibit leukotriene synthesis, PGI_2 inhibits LTB_4 synthesis in human peripheral PMNL.[90]

The proinflammatory activity of prostanoids has been studied for a long time.[92] At the sites of inflammation, PGE_2, $PGF_{2\alpha}$, or PGI_2 are found in large amounts. Their synthesis and secretion is closely connected with the appearance of the key symptoms of inflammation in general. They participate in the inflammatory response and modify or enhance the effects of locally synthesized inflammatory mediators such as histamine, bradykinin, etc. The inhibitory effect of both steroidal and nonsteroidal antiinflammatory drugs on prostanoid synthesis constitutes an essential part of their action.[25-29,34]

ACKNOWLEDGMENT

The author is grateful to Prof. F. Antoni, T. Garzo, and I. Mucha for their helpful advice and critical reading of the manuscript. This work was supported by a grant of the Hungarian Academy of Sciences (1-3-86-329).

REFERENCES

1. **Irvine, R. F.,** How is the level of free arachidonic acid controlled in mammalian cells?, *Biochem. J.,* 204, 3, 1982.
2. **Bills, T. K., Smith, J. B., and Silver, M. J.,** Selective release of arachidonic acid from the phospholipids of human platelets in response to thrombin, *J. Clin. Invest.,* 60, 1, 1977.
3. **Hagenfeldt, L.,** Turnover of individual free fatty acids in man, *Fed. Proc.,* 34, 2246, 1975.
4. **Normann, P. T., Thomassen, M. S., Christiansen, E. N., and Flatmark, A.,** Acyl CoA synthetase activity of rat liver microsomes. Substrate specificity with special reference to very-long-chain and isomeric fatty acids, *Biochim. Biophys. Acta,* 664, 416, 1981.
5. **Lands, W. E. M. and Samuelsson, B.,** Phospholipid precursor of prostaglandin, *Biochim. Biophys. Acta,* 164, 426, 1968.
6. **Vonkeman, H. and van Dorp, D.,** The action of prostaglandin synthetase on 2-arachidonoyl lecithin, *Biochim. Biophys. Acta,* 164, 430, 1968.
7. **Bell, R. L., Kennerley, D. A., Stanford, N., and Majerus, P. W.,** Diglyceryde lipase: a pathway for arachidonate release from human platelets, *Proc. Natl. Acad. Sci. U.S.A.,* 76, 3238, 1979.
8. **Billah, M. M., Lapetina, E. G., and Cuatrecasas, P. J.,** Phospholipase A2 activity specific for phosphatidic acid, *J. Biol. Chem.,* 256, 5399, 1981.
9. **van den Bosch, H.,** Intracellular phospholipases A, *Biochim. Biophys. Acta,* 604, 191, 1980.
10. **Knapp, H. R., Oelz, O., Roberts, L. J., II, Sweetman, B. J., Oates, J. A., and Reed, P. W.,** Ionophores stimulate prostaglandin and thromboxane biosynthesis, *Proc. Natl. Acad. Sci. U.S.A.,* 74, 4251, 1977.
11. **Lefkowith, J. B., Flippo, V., Sprecher, H., and Needleman, P.,** Paradoxical conversion of cardiac and renal arachidonate content in essential fatty acid deficiency, *J. Biol. Chem.,* 260, 15736, 1985.
12. **Hong, S. and Levine, L.,** Inhibition of arachidonic acid release from cells as the biochemical action of antiinflammatory corticosteroids, *Proc. Natl. Acad. Sci. U.S.A.,* 73, 1730, 1976.
13. **Flower, R. J. and Blackwell, G. J.,** Anti-inflammatory steroids induce biosynthesis of a phospholipase A2 inhibitor which prevents prostaglandin generation, *Nature (London),* 278, 456, 1979.
14. **Hirata, F., Schiffmann, E., Venkatasubramanian, K., Salomon, D., and Axelrod, J.,** A phospholipase A2 inhibitory protein in rabbit neutrophils induced by glucocorticoids, *Proc. Natl. Acad. Sci. U.S.A.,* 77, 2533, 1980.
15. **Blackwell, G. J., Carnuccio, R., Di Rosa, M., Flower, R. J., and Persico, P.,** Macrocortin: a polypeptide causing the antiphospholipase effect of glucocorticoids, *Nature (London),* 287, 147, 1980.
16. **Whorton, A. R., Smigel, P., Oates, J. A., and Frolich, J. C.,** Regional differences in prostacyclin formation by the kidney. Prostacyclin is a major prostaglandin of renal cortex, *Biochim. Biophys. Acta,* 529, 176, 1978.
17. **Schwartzman, M. and Raz, A.,** Selective induction of *de novo* prostaglandin synthesis in rabbit kidney cortex, *Biochim. Biophys. Acta,* 664, 469, 1981.
18. **Spolarics, Z., Mucha, I., Mandl, J., Machovich, R., Banhegyi, G., Tanacs, B., Antoni, F., Horvath, I., and Garzo, T.,** Prostanoid synthesis in isolated parenchymal and nonparenchymal mouse liver cells in the presence of arachidonic acid, *Prostaglandins Leukotrienes Med.,* in press.
19. **Schwartzman, M., Liberman, E., and Raz, A.,** Bradykinin and angiotensin II activation of arachidonic acid deacylation and prostaglandin E_2 formation in rabbit kidney, *J. Biol. Chem.,* 256, 2329, 1981.
20. **Hsueh, W., Isakson, P. K., and Needleman, P.,** Hormone selective lipase activation in isolated rabbit heart, *Prostaglandins,* 13, 1073, 1978.
21. **Hong, S. L. and Levine, L.,** Stimulation of prostaglandin synthesis by bradykinin and thrombin and their mechanism of action on MC5-5 fibroblasts, *J. Biol. Chem.,* 251, 5814, 1976.
22. **Marcus, A. J., Weksler, B. B., and Jaffe, E. A.,** Enzymic conversion of prostaglandin endoperoxide H2 and arachidonic acid to prostacyclin by cultured human endothelial cells, *J. Biol. Chem.,* 253, 7138, 1978.
23. **Lim, K. H., Hunt, N. N., Eichner, R. D., and Weidemann, M. J.,** Cyclic AMP and the regulation of prostaglandin production by macrophages, *Biochem. Biophys. Res. Commun.,* 114, 248, 1983.
24. **Yamamoto, S.,** Enzymes in arachidonic acid cascade, in *Prostaglandins and Related Substances,* Pace-Asciak, C. and Granstrom, E., Eds., Elsevier, Amsterdam, 1983, 171.
25. **Samuelsson, B., Goldyne, M., Granstrom, E., Hamberg, M., Hammarstrom, S., and Malmsten, C.,** Prostaglandins and thromboxanes, *Annu. Rev. Biochem.,* 47, 992, 1978.
26. **Oliw, E., Granstrom, E., and Anggard, E.,** The prostaglandins and essential fatty acids, in *Prostaglandins and Related Substances,* Pace-Asciak, C. and Granstrom, E., Eds., Elsevier, Amsterdam, 1983, 1.
27. **Vane, J. R.,** Inhibition of prostaglandin synthesis as a mechanism of action for aspirin-like drugs, *Nature (London) New Biol.,* 231, 232, 1971.
28. **Smith, J. B. and Willis, A. L.,** Aspirin selectively inhibits prostaglandin production in human platelets, *Nature (London) New Biol.,* 231, 235, 1971.

29. **Ferreira, S. H. and Vane, J. R.,** New aspects of the mode of action of nonsteroid anti-inflammatory drugs, *Annu. Rev. Pharmacol.*, 14, 57, 1974.
30. **van Der Ouderaa, F. J., Buytenhek, M., Nugteren, D. H., and van Dorp, D. A.,** Purification and characterisation of prostaglandin endoperoxide synthetase from sheep vesicular glands, *Biochim. Biophys. Acta*, 487, 315, 1977.
31. **Hamberg, M. and Samuelsson, B.,** Detection and isolation of an endoperoxide intermediate in prostaglandin synthesis, *Proc. Natl. Acad. Sci. U.S.A.*, 70, 899, 1973.
32. **Hamberg, M., Svensson, J., and Samuelsson, B.,** Thromboxanes: a new group of biologically active compounds derived from prostaglandin endoperoxides, *Proc. Natl. Acad. Sci. U.S.A.*, 72, 2994, 1975.
33. **Moncada, S., Gryglewski, R., Bunting, S., and Vane, J. R.,** An enzyme from arteries transforms prostaglandin endoperoxides to an unstable substance that inhibits platelet aggregation, *Nature (London)*, 263, 663, 1976.
34. **Pace-Asciak, C. and Gryglewski, R.,** The prostacyclins, in *Prostaglandins and Related Substances*, Pace-Asciak, C. and Granstrom, E., Eds., Elsevier, Elsevier, Amsterdam, 1983, 95.
35. **Granstrom, E., Diczfalusy, U., and Hamberg, M.,** The thromboxanes, in *Prostaglandins and Related Substances*, Pace-Asciak, C. and Granstrom, E., Eds., Elsevier, Amsterdam, 1983, 45.
36. **Ullrich, V. and Graf, H.,** Prostacyclin and thromboxane synthase as P-450 enzymes, *TIPS*, 352, 1984.
37. **Ullrich, V. and Haurand, M.,** Thromboxane synthase as a cytochrome P450 enzyme, *Adv. Prostaglandins Thromboxanes Leukotriene Res.*, 11, 105, 1983.
38. **Ditzfalusy, U., Falardeau, P., and Hammarstrom, S.,** Conversion of prostaglandin endoperoxides to C17-hydroxy acids catalyzed by human platelet thromboxane synthase, *FEBS Lett.*, 84, 271, 1977.
39. **Smith, W. L. and Borgeat, P.,** The eicosanoids: prostaglandins, thromboxanes, leukotrienes and hydroxyeicosaenoic acids, in *Biochemistry of Lipids and Membranes*, Vance, D. E. and Vance, J. E., Eds., Benjamin/Cummings, Menlo Park, Calif., 1985, 325.
40. **Wong, P. Y-K., Malik, K. U., Desiderio, D. M., McGiff, J. C., and Sun, F. F.,** Hepatic metabolism of prostacyclin (PGI2) in the rabbit: formation of a potent novel inhibitor of platelet aggregation, *Biochem. Biophys. Res. Commun.*, 93, 486, 1980.
41. **Maclouf, J., Kindahl, H., Granstrom, E., and Samuelsson, B.,** Interactions of prostaglandin H2 and thromboxane A2 with human serum albumin, *Eur. J. Biochem.*, 109, 561, 1980.
42. **Samuelsson, B., Borgeat, P., Hammarstrom, S., and Murphy, R. C.,** in *Advances in Prostaglandin and Thromboxane Research*, Vol. 6, Samuelsson, B., Ramwell, P., and Paoletti, R., Eds., Raven Press, New York, 1980, 1.
43. **Hammarstrom, S.,** Leukotrienes, *Annu. Rev. Biochem.*, 52, 355, 1983.
44. **Hansson, G., Malmstein, C., and Radmark, O.,** The leukotrienes and other lipoxygenase products, in *Prostaglandins and Related Substances*, Pace-Asciak, C. and Granstrom, E., Eds., Elsevier, Amsterdam, 1983, 127.
45. **Borgeat, P. and Samuelsson, B.,** Arachidonic acid metabolism in polymorphonuclear leukocytes: effects of ionophore A 23187, *Proc. Natl. Acad. Sci. U.S.A.*, 76, 2148, 1979.
46. **Drazen, J. M., Lewis, R. A., Austen, K. F., Toda, M., Brion, F., Marfat, A., and Corey, E. J.,** Contractile activities of structural analogs of leukotrienes C and D: necessity of a hydrophobic region, *Proc. Natl. Acad. Sci. U.S.A.*, 78, 3195, 1981.
47. **Lewis, R. A., Drazen, J. M., Austen, K. F., Toda, M., Brion, F., Marfat, A., and Corey, E. J.,** Contractile activities of structural analogs of leukotrienes C and D: role of polar substituents, *Proc. Natl. Acad. Sci. U.S.A.*, 78, 4579, 1981.
48. **Appelgren, L. A. and Hammarstrom, S.,** Distribution and metabolism of ^{3}H-labeled leukotriene C3 in the mouse, *J. Biol. Chem.*, 257, 531, 1982.
49. **Mahmud, I., Fukui, N., and Miura, Y.,** Arachidonic acid metabolism in normal and regenerating liver and hepatoma, *Adv. Enzyme Regul.*, 18, 27, 1980.
50. **Hammarstrom, S.,** Biosynthesis and biological actions of prostaglandins and thromboxanes, *Arch. Biochem. Biophys.*, 214, 431, 1982.
51. **Mills, D. C. B.,** in *Cyclic Nucleotides*, Part II, *Physiology and Pharmacology, Handbook of Experimental Pharmacology*, Vol. 58/II, Kebabian, J. W. and Nathanson, J. A., Eds., Springer-Verlag, Berlin, 1982, 723.
52. **Gorman, R. R., Bunting, S., and Miller, O. V.,** Modulation of human platelet adenylate cyclase by prostacyclin (PGX), *Prostaglandins*, 13, 377, 1977.
53. **Hopkins, N. K. and Gorman, R. R.,** Regulation of endothelial cell cyclic nucleotide metabolism by prostacyclin, *J. Clin. Invest.*, 67, 540, 1981.
54. **Adler, B., Gimbrone, M. A., Jr., Schaffer, A. I., and Handin, R. I.,** Prostacyclin and beta-adrenergic catecholamines inhibit arachidonate release and PGI2 synthesis by vascular endothelium, *Blood*, 58, 514, 1981.
55. **Hassid, A.,** Regulation of prostanoid biosynthesis in cultured cells, *Am. J. Physiol.*, 243, C205, 1982.

56. **Berridge, M.,** Inositol triphosphate and diacylglycerol as second messengers, *Biochem. J.*, 220, 345, 1984.
57. **Berridge, M. and Irvine, R. F.,** Inositol triphosphate, a novel second messenger in cellular signal transduction, *Nature (London)*, 312, 315, 1984.
58. **Nishizuka, Y.,** The role of protein kinase C in cell surface signal transduction and tumour promotion, *Nature (London)*, 308, 693, 1984.
59. **Watson, S. P., McConell, R. T., and Lapetina, E. G.,** The rapid formation of inositol phosphates in human platelets by thrombin is inhibited by prostacyclin, *J. Biol. Chem.*, 259, 13199, 1984.
60. **Jakobs, K. H., Bauer, S., and Watanabe, Y.,** Modulation of adenylate cyclase of human platelets by phorbol ester, *Eur. J. Biochem.*, 151, 425, 1985.
61. **Katada, T., Gilman, A. G., Watanabe, Y., Bauer, S., and Jakobs, K. H.,** Protein kinase C phosphorylates the inhibitory guanine-nucleotide-binding regulatory component and apparently suppresses its function in hormonal inhibition of adenylate cyclase, *Eur. J. Biochem.*, 151, 431, 1985.
62. **Adams Brotherton, A. F. and Hoak, J. C.,** Role of Ca^{2+} and cyclic AMP in the regulation of the production of prostacyclin by the vascular endothelium, *Proc. Natl. Acad. Sci. U.S.A.*, 79, 495, 1982.
63. **Malmstrom, K. and Carafoli, E.,** Effects of prostaglandins on the interaction of Ca^{2+} with mitochondria, *Arch. Biochem. Biophys.*, 171, 418, 1975.
64. **Carsten, M. E. and Miller, J. D.,** Comparison of calcium association constants and ionophoretic properties of some prostaglandins and ionophores, *Arch. Biochem. Biophys.*, 185, 282, 1978.
65. **Deelers, M., Grognet, P., and Brasseur, R.,** Structural considerations for calcium ionophoresis by prostaglandins, *Biochem. Pharmacol.*, 34, 3831, 1985.
66. **Garrity, M. J., Brass, E. P., and Robertson, R. P.,** Kinetics of prostaglandin E metabolism in isolated hepatocytes, *Biochim. Biophys. Acta*, 796, 136, 1984.
67. **Okumura, T., Nakayama, R., Sago, T., and Saito, K.,** Identification of prostaglandin E metabolites from primary cultures of rat hepatocytes, *Biochim. Biophys. Acta*, 837, 197, 1985.
68. **Rigas, A. and Levine, L.,** Arachidonic acid metabolism by rat liver cells (the C-9 cell line), *J. Pharmacol. Exp. Ther.*, 231, 230, 1984.
69. **Spolarics, Z., Tanacs, B., Garzo, T., Mandl, J., Mucha, I., Antoni, F., Machovich, R., and Horvath, I.,** Prostaglandin and thromboxane synthesizing activity in isolated murine hepatocytes and nonparenchymal liver cells, *Prostaglandins Leukotrienes Med.*, 16, 379, 1984.
70. **Mucha, I., Spolarics, Z., Mandl, J., Tanacs, B., Banhegyi, G., and Garzo, T.,** Investigation of prostanoid metabolism in mouse liver, *Acta Biochem. Biophys. Acad. Sci. Hung.*, 19, 40, 1984.
71. **Birmelin, M. and Decker, K.,** Synthesis of prostanoids and cyclic nucleotides by phagocytosing rat Kupffer cells, *Eur. J. Biochem.*, 142, 219, 1984.
72. **Tomasi, V., Meringolo, C., Bartolini, G., and Orlandi, M.,** Biosynthesis of prostacyclin in rat liver endothelial cells and its control by prostaglandin E2, *Nature (London)*, 273, 670, 1978.
73. **Bauer, P. I., Mandl, J., Machovich, R., Antoni, F., Garzo, T., and Horvath, I.,** Specific binding of thrombin-antithrombin III complex to hepatocytes, *Thromb. Res.*, 28, 595, 1982.
74. **Spolarics, Z., Mandl, J., Machovich, R., Lambin, P., Garzo, T., Antoni, F., and Horvath, I.,** Association of α2-macroglobulin-thrombin and α2-macroglobulin-plasmin complexes with isolated hepatocytes, *Biochim. Biophys. Acta*, 845, 389, 1985.
75. **Mandl, J., Tanacs, B., Spolarics, Z., Garzo, T., Mucha, I., Antoni, F., Machovich, R., and Horvath, I.,** Uptake of arachidonic acid, arachidic acid, oleic acid and their incorporation into phospholipids and triacylglycerols of isolated murine hepatocytes, *Thromb. Res.*, 35, 407, 1984.
76. **Mahmud, I., Fukui, N., Miura, Y., and Brandenberger, H.,** Thromboxane synthesizing system in rat liver, *Prostaglandins Leukotrienes Med.*, 16, 371, 1984.
77. **Chong, K. P., Burch, R. M., Black, M., Maloney, E., Jollow, D. J., and Halushka, P. V.,** Vasopressin stimulates thromboxane synthesis in isolated hamster hepatocytes: relation to hepatocyte calcium content, *Prostaglandins*, 26, 398, 1983.
78. **Moncada, S. and Vane, J. R.,** The role of prostacyclin in vascular tissue, *Fed. Proc.*, 38, 66, 1979.
79. **Weksler, B. B., Marcus, A. J., and Jaffe, E. A.,** Synthesis of prostaglandin I2 (prostacyclin) by cultured human and bovine endothelial cells, *Proc. Natl. Acad. Sci. U.S.A.*, 74, 3922, 1977.
80. **Weksler, B. B., Ley, C. W., and Jaffe, E. A.,** Stimulation of endothelial cell prostacyclin production by thrombin, trypsin and the ionophore A 23187, *J. Clin. Invest.*, 62, 923, 1978.
81. **Crutchley, D. J., Ryan, J. W., Ryan, U. S., and Fisher, G. H.,** Bradykinin induced release of prostacyclin and thromboxanes from bovine pulmonary artery endothelial cells, *Biochim. Biophys. Acta*, 751, 99, 1983.
82. **Ingerman-Wojenski, C., Silver, M. J., Smith, J. B., and Macarak, E.,** Bovine endothelial cells in culture produce thromboxane as well as prostacyclin, *J. Clin. Invest.*, 67, 1292, 1981.
83. **Hopkins, N. K., Oglesby, T. D., Bundy, G. L., and Gorman, R. R.,** Biosynthesis and metabolism of 15-hydroperoxy-5,8,11,13-eicosatetraenoic acid by human umbilical vein endothelial cells, *J. Biol. Chem.*, 259, 14,048, 1984.
84. **Peach, M. J., Singer, H. A., and Loeb, A. L.,** Mechanism of endothelium dependent vascular smooth muscle relaxation, *Biochem. Pharmacol.*, 34, 1867, 1985.

85. **Spagnuolo, P. J., Ellner, J. J., Hassid, A., and Dunn, M. J.,** Thromboxane A_2 mediates augmented polymorphonuclear leukocyte adhesiveness, *J. Clin. Invest.*, 66, 406, 1980.
86. **Larrue, J., Leroux, C., Daret, D., and Bricaud, H.,** Decreased prostaglandin production in cultured smooth muscle cells from atherosclerotic aorta, *Biochim. Biophys. Acta,* 710, 257, 1982.
87. **Gryglewski, R. J., Dembinska-Kiec, A., Zmuda, A., and Gryglewska, T.,** Prostacyclin and thromboxane A_2 biosynthesis capacities of heart, arteries and platelets at various stages of experimental atherosclerosis in rabbits, *Atherosclerosis,* 31, 385, 1978.
88. **Corey, E. J.,** Chemical studies on slow reacting substances, leukotrienes, *Experientia,* 38, 1259, 1982.
89. **Ford-Hutchinson, A. W., Bray, M. A., Doig, M. V., Shipley, M. E., and Smith, M. J. H.,** Leukotriene B, a potent chemokinetic and aggregating substance released from polymorphonuclear leukocytes, *Nature (London),* 286, 264, 1980.
90. **Kuehl, F. A., Jr., Dougherty, H. W., and Ham, E. A.,** Interactions between prostaglandins and leukotrienes, *Biochem. Pharmacol.*, 33, 1, 1984.
91. **Feuerstein, N., Bash, J. A., Woody, J. N., and Ramwell, P.,** Leukotriene C stimulates prostaglandin release from rat peritoneal macrophages, *Biochem. Biophys. Res. Commun.*, 100, 1085, 1981.
92. **Vane, J. R.,** Prostaglandins as mediators of inflammation, in *Advances in Prostaglandin and Thromboxane Research,* Vol. 2, Samuelsson, B. and Paoletti, R., Eds., Raven Press, New York, 1976, 791.

Chapter 4

BIOLOGY OF ENDOTHELIAL CELLS

Raymund Machovich

TABLE OF CONTENTS

I. INTRODUCTION

Most eukaryotic cells have lost direct contact with the external environment, and their conditions are assured by the blood. The communication between the cells of various organs and the circulating blood, however, is mainly indirect; for example, exchange of metabolites, energy, information, etc., occurs via endothelial cells. Endothelial cells cover the inner surface of the blood vessel walls; they occupy an area of higher than 1000 m^2, which represents approximately 10^{12} endothelial cells per human body.[1] Because of their position, endothelial cells can control several functions of the various eukaryotic cells and also modulate the consistence of the circulating blood, including its cellular and molecular components.

Endothelial cells are highly specialized according to their functions, i.e., every tissue has its own characteristic endothelium. Both the cells and the basement membranes are adapted to the environment. For instance, they are different in the micro- and the macrovasculature. While the main function of microvascular endothelium (arterioles, capillaries, venules) is to fulfill the transport and barrier processes, the exchange between blood and tissues, the macrovascular endothelium (arteries and veins) ought to ensure blood circulation with the highest degree of thromboresistant surface.

Additional differentiations can be recognized in the fine structure of the endothelium at various levels.[2] Endothelium may be continuous (large vessels, arterioles, venules, and capillaries of somatic tissues, nervous system, and lung), fenestrated (visceral capillaries, some pericytic venules, kidney glomeruli), and discontinuous (sinusoids of liver, spleen, bone marrow).[3] There is also a tissue differentiation, namely, vesicle frequency of the endothelial cells may change from organ to organ, or even from segment to segment of arterioles, capillaries, and venules; e.g., in myocardium the cells contain approximately 1000 vesicles per cubic micrometer, whereas in lung or brain capillaries only about 130 vesicles per cubic micrometer or less exist.[4] Another level of differentiation is the different microdomains of the endothelial cell surface formed locally on certain segments of vessel wall depending on the metabolic activities of the cells.[2]

To discuss the morphology and function of various kinds of endothelial cells from a systematic point of view is not possible at present, since the data in the literature are not sufficient. Thus, the aim of this review is to survey the functions and the morphological characteristics of the endothelial cells in general relations.

II. MORPHOLOGY OF ENDOTHELIAL CELLS

Endothelial cells form a monolayer on the inner surface of vessel wall, joined by intercellular junctions. The cells are polygonal, approximately 25 to 40 μm long and 15 μm wide, containing elongated nuclei oriented in the long axis of the vessel. Morphologically several zones of the cell can be described, although their distinction from a functional aspect is rather arbitrary.

A. Membrane Surfaces of Endothelium

There are three kinds of surface on a single endothelial cell: a nonthrombogenic surface, exposed directly to the circulating blood, called luminal surface; a cohesive surface, in the opposite face attached to the basement membrane or to pericytes, called abluminal surface; and the third surface (junctional surface) is an adhesive part of the cell membrane forming cell to cell contact with other endothelial cells.

1. Luminal Surface of Endothelial Cells

The luminal surface of endothelial cells carries an overall negative charge.[5] The distribution of anionic sites, however, is not uniform. The highest concentration of the anionic sites appears on fenestral diaphragms.[6] The fenestral diaphragms consist of proteins in complexes with glycosaminoglycans, mainly with heparan sulfate.[7] Additional components, as acidic glycoproteins and acidic glycolipids, also contribute to the overall negative charge of the anionic sites.[2,8] On the other hand, vesicle and channel diaphragms are neutral, although their polysaccharide components are rich in β-D-galactose, β-*N*-acetyl-D-glucosamine, and neuraminic acids.[2,6]

The most important nature of the endothelial cell in contact with the circulating blood is its ability to prevent thrombus formation, which is maintained by various mechanisms. There are several membrane components, contributing to the nonthrombogenic character of the luminal surface of endothelial cell.[2,9] Thus, thrombomodulin, a specific membrane receptor for thrombin and protein C[10,11] as well as heparan sulfate, as an accelerator of thrombin inactivation, may serve this essential function of the endothelial cell. Other binding sites, involved in arachidonate metabolism, adenosine formation, fibrinolysis initiation, etc., and participating in thromboresistance, are discussed later.

On the luminal surface of the endothelial cell additional receptors can also be found, i.e., receptors for hormones (estrogen, glycocorticoids), lipoproteins, lipoprotein lipase, angiotensin I, insulin, epinephrine, norepinephrine, acetylcholine, serotonin, histamine, kinins, and growth factors have been described.[9,12-28] The possible role(s) of receptors for blood coagulation factors, like fibrinogen, prothrombin, Factor V(F-V), F-VII, F-IX, F-X, proteinase inhibitors (antithrombin III, α_2-macroglobulin), heparin, etc.,[29-37] are discussed in relation to the physiological functions and the pathology of endothelial cells.

2. Intercellular Junctions: Endothelial Cell to Cell Surface

Endothelial cells form a strictly controlled monolayer on the inner side of the blood vessel wall. Thus, these cells are always in direct and close contact with each other. The membrane responsible for the endothelial cell to cell interaction forms intercellular junctions. There are two types of interactions, "gap-junction" and "tight-junction".[2] Gap-junction, also called communicating junction, having a size of 6 nm in diameter,[38] represents the structural element of the intercellular exchange of ions and metabolites with low molecular weight. The tight junctions can be characterized as a close contact, or even as a membrane fusion, of two neighboring cells, with the function of preventing unnecessary transport processes.

Each microvascular segment has characteristic endothelial junctions. In arterioles these are continuous and elaborate, tight (also called occluding junctions) junctions with interpolated large communicating junctions. In capillaries as well as in pericytic venules, communicating junctions are absent.[3o]

3. Subendothelial Matrix: the Abluminal Surface of the Endothelial Cell; Pericytes

Endothelial cells lie on the basement membrane, which is built up from a 40- to 80-nm thick network of collagens, mainly type IV, glycosaminoglycans, fibronectin, laminin, and

F-VIII$_{vW}$. The basement membrane is continuous in the continuous and fenestrated endothelium and discontinuous in sinusoids. The extracellular matrix is important in the maintenance of the shape of the endothelial cell and the vessel wall and also contributes to the transport processes. The components of the subendothelium are synthesized mainly by the endothelial cells.[40-46] The matrix extends into the intercellular space as well.[2]

Endothelial cells also have direct contact with cellular elements of the blood vessel wall, i.e., besides basement membrane, endothelial cells communicate with pericytes. Pericytes, the 150 to 200 μm long and 10 to 25 μm wide cells,[47,48] having numerous cytoplasmic microfilaments, form a discontinuous layer around capillaries and postcapillary venules.[49] They show a phagocytic function in the periendothelial compartment of the blood-brain barrier.[50-52] Besides their phagocytic activity, pericytes provide mechanical support for endothelial cells as well as a contraction system for vasculature.[53]

B. Cytoskeleton and Organelles of the Endothelial Cell

Although endothelial cells show morphological variations according to the function of vasculature, both organelles and contractile proteins are common constituents of the vascular endothelium.

1. Contractile System of Endothelial Cell

The cytoskeleton, in general, is more developed in arteriolar and venular endothelial cells than in capillaries. There are at least four kinds of filaments, located mainly around the nucleus and close to the abluminal membrane or at the parajunctional zone.

1. Thin filaments, approximately 6 nm long, are described as actin-like filaments, found in brain capillaries and postcapillary venules.[24]
2. The intermediate filaments, approximately 10 nm long, form a perinuclear ring playing role in mitosis.[54]
3. Thick filaments, with a 15-nm average size, have been identified as myosin, found in the endothelial cells of arterioles.[55]
4. Microtubules and other fibrils have also been described.[2]

Their functions seem to be controlled by histamine, primarily in venules,[56] where contraction of endothelial cells is triggered via histamine receptors.[57]

2. Organelle Region of the Endothelial Cell

One of the most characteristic granules of endothelial cell is the Weibel-Palade body.[58] They are rod-shaped organelles, 3 μm long and 100 nm thick, having a dense matrix.[2] Weibel-Palade bodies are abundant in the aortic and arteriolar endothelial cells, are less numerous in venules, and are absent in the capillary endothelium. It is interesting that these rod-shaped granules are developed in fish, composing about 70% of the cell volume.[59] Although they contain F-VIII$_{vW}$ and are generally used for identification of endothelial cells, their physiological and pathological roles are hardly known.

Endothelial cells can also be considered as secretory cells, although they have no highly developed rough endoplasmic reticulum, smooth endoplasmic reticulum, Golgi apparatus, mitochondria, and glycogen particles.[2] An increase in the amount of rough endoplasmic reticulum occurs during pathological conditions, such as inflammation, tumor angiogenesis, tissue injury, thyroid hyperplasia, estrogen administration, etc.[60-62] Lysosomes with various sizes are also present in endothelial cells playing a role in endocytosis.[2]

C. Vesicles and Fenestrae

Endothelial cells are rich in various vesicles. They change in form and number with the functions of the various organs and even change sequentially in the same vascular unit.

1. Plasmalemmal Vesicles

They appear in cytoplasm or bound to surface and are also called pinocytotic or transport vesicles. Their size is rather uniform, with a diameter between 60 and 80 nm. The membrane of surface-bound vesicles is continuous with the plasmalemma.[63] The vesicles open to the cell surface have a flask shape with a short neck and a stomatal opening having a diameter of 20 to 40 nm. Most of the open vesicles are closed by diaphragm[2] with a thickness of 6 to 8 nm. The high number of vesicles increases the surface area of endothelial cells, especially in capillary, although the amount of these vesicles may be different by an order of magnitude in the various organs.[64,65] The plasmalemmal vesicles are stable, not affected essentially by pathological conditions.[2] The plasmalemmal vesicle is able to undergo membrane fusion with plasmalemma or other vesicles and to move through the cytoplasm. Finally, attached to the abluminal surface of the cell, they discharge their content in the adjoining extracellular compartment.[66]

The transitional forms of these vesicles suggests that they are the basic elements of the transendothelial channels.[67] For example, the fused vesicles can be opened simultaneously at both the luminal and abluminal surface of the endothelial cell, forming a transendothelial channel.[68] The size of a channel is approximately 20 to 40 nm in diameter at its fusion points.[2] The diaphragms covering the stomatal opening have no lipid bilayers and their glycoprotein content ensures a neutral surface to the periphery.[2] Under pathological conditions such as ischemia or inflammation, the fused vesicles may form large vacuoles with a size of 100 to 200 nm in diameter.[69]

2. Coated Pits and Coated Vesicles

At the luminal front, the endothelial cell membrane displays a fuzzy coat having a thickness of 10 to 20 nm, and it extends into vesicles at the intercellular junctions. The main structure elements of the fuzzy coats are glycosaminoglycans and they behave as diffusion barrier.[70]

Coated pits and coated vesicles, similarly to other eukaryotic cells, also occur in endothelial cells. They have a diameter of 80 to 120 nm. These organelles are particularly numerous in hepatic endothelial cells and bone marrow sinusoids on the luminal surface of the cell.[71,72] They play a role in receptor-mediated endocytosis of low density lipoproteins.[73,74]

3. Fenestrae

Besides vesicles and channels, endothelial cells, especially visceral capillaries, contain fenestrae. Fenestrae can be found in a thin part of the cell in the form of transcellular openings with a size of 60 to 80 nm in diameter.[2] Fenestrae have a central knob with a size of 10 to 15 nm, and from this center a fine fibrillar structure extends radially to the rim.[75] Generally they are closed by a 6- to 8-nm thin diaphragm, which, unlike vesicle diaphragms, shows high net negative charge ensured by heparin-like substances.[76] At some places, e.g., glomerular capillaries, fenestrae are devoid of diaphragms.

The number of fenestrae varies from organ to organ; one order of magnitude[77] difference can be detected, and they can even disappear in cultured endothelial cells of the adrenal cortex.[78] Since fenestrae are members of the endothelial transport system, these changes in their number and diaphragm structure may correlate with the function of a vascular bed.

III. PHYSIOLOGY OF ENDOTHELIAL CELLS

The main function of endothelial cells is to assure the communication between the various cells of different organs and the circulating blood. To fulfill this function, endothelial cells possess the ability to form a barrier for some molecular and cellular components and also represent a highly controlled permeability. Besides the transport processes, endothelial cells, by their biosynthetic and metabolic functions, contribute actively to the regulation of metabolism of various tissues. Without the anticoagulant and, under some conditions, the procoagulant properties of endothelium, however, the cells of the different organs cannot fulfill their main functions.

A. Transport Processes of the Endothelium

1. Permeability

According to the pore theory,[79] two kinds of pores would exist, i.e., a small one with a diameter of approximately 9 nm and an even smaller one, and a large one with a pore size of 50 to 60 nm in diameter. Recent data, however, indicate that this model is oversimplified. The endothelium is highly differentiated, rendering its participation in transport processes more dynamic and active. Nevertheless, a passive transport for water, small nonpolar solutes, as well as for lipid soluble molecules may exist via cell membrane, cytoplasm, and the opposite plasma membrane, called the transmembranous transport process.[8] This route is relatively constant, with a fractional contribution of approximately 10% of the entire transport, and may occur as diffusion or carrier mediated transport.

Another route for transport can be extramembranous, either through the cells, or between two cells via junctions. Thus, the extramembranous routes are transcellular and intercellular. They represent large variability and account for approximately 90% of the volume flow.[2,80] Diffusion and filtration may occur concomitantly through fenestrae coupling protein flux to volume flow.

2. Transcytosis: Endocytosis-Exocytosis

A critical step in the endothelial transport process is the exchange between, at least, two compartments, i.e., blood plasma and interstitial fluid. In addition, large and small molecules move bidirectionally through several plasma membranes and via the cytosol of endothelial cells. In these complicated routes, transcytosis is a major contribution to endothelial transport processes.

Endothelial cells have an apparatus to take up substances from the environment and also to secrete materials into the surroundings by endocytosis and exocytosis, respectively. These two routes are coupled in these cells resulting in transcytosis.[81] Although endothelial cells may function by true endocytosis, its importance is relatively minor. If it occurs, its form can be phagocytosis, pinocytosis, or receptor-mediated endocytosis.

Phagocytosis can be detected only occasionally.[2,82] During pinocytosis, uncoated plasmalemmal vesicles transfer components to the lysosomes, and this event takes place primarily in the endothelial cells of postcapillary venules of lymph nodes.[83,84] This uptake of substances tends toward macromolecules and favors anionic proteins.[2] Low-density lipoproteins are taken up essentially by receptor-mediated endocytosis.[85] After binding, however, these molecules are transferred to lysosomes by coated pits or transcytosed via the cytosol of endothelial cell and discharged into subendothelial space by plasmalemmal vesicles.[73] The function of endocytosis seems to be the supply of the endothelial cell with components, like iron, vitamin B_{12}, cholesterol, hormones, etc. Transcytosis occurs primarily on continuous microvascular endothelium.[81] Molecules in size up to 30 nm in diameter are taken up by vesicles open on the luminal surface, are then internalized, and finally are discharged at the abluminal front.[86,87] A part of the substances passes through transendothelial channels. While endocytotic routes involve coated pits and coated and some uncoated vesicles reaching lysosomes, the transcytotic routes involve plasmalemmal vesicles.[2]

Since the processes discussed above are very dynamic and there are many adaptations to the changing functions, the regulation of endocytosis and transcytosis is an important mechanism. Nevertheless, our present knowledge is rather limited; only factors influencing these transports are known, like temperature, serotonin, divalent cations, glucose concentration, hypertension, etc.[2,88]

3. Junctional Transport and Lateral Movement

While large molecules are prevented from leaving blood vessels between two endothelial cells with tight junctions,[89] communicating (gap) junctions represent the route for a transport between blood and parenchymal cells.

The intercellular junction is modeled as a nonuniform rectangular slit,[90] which would be a 17-nm wide and 700 nm in the total depth. In the middle, a constricted region exists with a size of 70 nm long and 8 nm in diameter.[91] A fibrous network covering the endothelial cell surface penetrates also the intercellular junction. Albumin occupies space, approximately 50% of the volume of this matrix via its positively charged sites bound to the negatively charged parts of the fibers. Such a structure increases the resistance to water flow and diffusion of solutes.[92]

Another mechanism for transport processes is the lateral movement in the cell membrane. Fatty acids, monoacylglycerol, cholesterol, and phospholipids are transported in blood primarily as components of lipoproteins (VLDL, LDL, HDL, and chylomicrons) or bound to albumin.[93-96] At the surface of endothelium, they are converted to amphipathic lipids by lipoprotein lipase. Since cell membranes are lipid bilayers, the lipolytic products may cross the endothelium by movement within cell membranes.[97] Accordingly, lipids move from the blood plasma via the fusion with external leaflet of the plasma membrane of the endothelial cell to the basement membrane, i.e., the lipolytic products move from the luminal surface of endothelial cells to the abluminal surface within cell membrane. Thereafter, the lipolytic products are transported from endothelial cell to parenchymal cell through extracellular spaces. Finally, they are reesterified in the parenchymal cell and stored.

4. Ion Transports

An additional property of endothelial cell functions originates from the polarity of these cells. The transcellular active transport of Na^+ results from the movement of Na^+ into the cell across the luminal surface and subsequent active removal of Na^+ from the cell across the basal membrane. Chloride is also transported via the cell to maintain electroneutrality, and water follows, as a result of the osmotic shift.[98]

The movement of K^+ from blood to cells is extremely slow, at least in brain. The efflux in the opposite direction, however, is mediated by a transport system with a K_m of approximately 2.5 m*M*.[99] This direction of the K^+ transport is partially supported by the finding that a Na^+,K^+-ATP-ase is localized at the abluminal but not at the luminal surface of the brain capillary endothelial cells.[100] As to the Na^+ entry, two separate mechanisms are suggested.[101] Our knowledge on the ion transport mechanisms of endothelial cells is at an early stage and needs further experimentation.

B. Biosynthetic Processes of Endothelial Cells

As mentioned earlier, endothelial cells, by their biosynthetic ability, participate actively in several functions of the surrounding cells, tissues, and the blood. Endothelial cells synthesize connective tissue components, factors participating in hemostasis as well as molecules influencing other cellular functions.

1. Connective Tissue Synthesis: Basement Membrane Components

The components of basement membrane and other extracellular matrix of the blood vessel wall are synthesized by the cellular elements of the vessels. Among these components, endothelial cells synthesize and secrete the following. Based on data obtained mainly with cultured endothelial cells, several types of collagen are synthesized and secreted either into the underlying extracellular matrix or into the culture medium.[102] Thus, collagen I, III, IV, and V, and also a newly described type of collagen, all have been found to be produced by endothelial cells. Their synthesis changes from organ to organ and depends on the vasculature, whether it is artery, vein, or capillary.[103,104] Their contribution to the basement membrane may be controlled by endothelial cells not only via their synthesis, but via their degradation, since endothelial cells, when stimulated, release collagenases as well.[105,106] Elastin is synthesized in the form of tropoelastin and after secretion it becomes cross-linked.[107-109] A high amount of fibronectin and thrombospondin is also synthesized by endothelial cells; approximately 15% of all the proteins secreted into the medium[44,110,111] are fibronectin and thrombospondin, and both proteins are incorporated into the extracellular matrix.[41,112] Laminin production is primarily restricted to the subconfluent phase of the endothelial cell.[113] Some glycosaminoglycans, present in the basement membrane, as well as in the endothelial cell membrane structure or secreted into the medium via the luminal surface of endothelial cell, are synthesized. Heparan sulfate, dermatan sulfate, and chondroitin sulfate are the main types of these glycosaminoglycans.[114-118]

2. Procoagulant Components of Endothelial Cells

Among the factors mentioned above, collagen types III and V induce platelet aggregation/adhesion[119-122] and also may participate in the contact activation phase of blood coagulation. The latter may be amplified by a factor, possibly present in a membrane-bound form, which activates F-XII by proteolytic cleavage.[123]

Platelet adhesion to subendothelium depends on Factor VIII von Willebrand ($F\text{-}VIII_{vW}$) which is also synthesized and secreted by endothelial cells.[124-126] Since $F\text{-}VIII_{vW}$ binds to collagen types I, III, IV, and V[127] and platelet contains receptor for $F\text{-}VIII_{vW}$,[127,128] platelet adheres, very likely, to subendothelium via $F\text{-}VIII_{vW}$. This suggestion is further supported by the fact that in von Villebrand's disease adhesion of platelets to vessel wall decreases and it can be corrected by the addition of exogeneous $F\text{-}VIII_{vW}$.[129,130] The synthesis and release of $F\text{-}VIII_{vW}$ in endothelial cells may be controlled by thrombin and estrogen via stimulation of $F\text{-}VIII_{vW}$ production.[131,132] The thrombin-induced release of $F\text{-}VIII_{vW}$ from endothelial cells is mediated by phospholipid methylation.[131]

Although one of the main functions of endothelium is to prevent thrombus formation, the damage of endothelial cells may contribute to the initiation and/or acceleration of blood coagulation processes. Among blood coagulation factors, besides the F-XII activating enzyme, endothelial cells are able to synthesize tissue factor[133,134] and F-V.[135] As a consequence, tissue factor accelerates F-VII activation, which leads to increased $F\text{-}X_a$ formation. $F\text{-}X_a$ and F-V, in turn, convert prothrombin to thrombin. These processes, however, do not occur on intact endothelial cell.[133,134] When there is endothelium damage or endothelial cells are exposed to thrombin or platelets, tissue factor activity may increase by 40- or 170-fold, respectively.[136,137] Blood coagulation reactions are further modified on endothelium by factors bound to endothelial cells. Thus, $F\text{-}IX_a$ and $F\text{-}X_a$ bind to endothelial cells, and together with prothrombin they may play a role in the localization of the blood coagulation reactions thereby serving to control the place where thrombus formation is necessary.[30,32,138,139]

3. Inhibitors of Blood Coagulation

Only heparan sulfate has been found to be synthesized and secreted by endothelial cell with the capacity to accelerate thrombin inactivation by antithrombin III.[114] Although the presence of α_2-macroglobulin and antithrombin III on endothelial cells has been reported,[35,140] their direct synthesis by endothelial cells is questionable at present. Thrombin can also be inactivated by protease nexin, a protein with M_r 40,000 daltons, synthesized and secreted by endothelial cells. The thrombin-protease nexin complex formed then, is taken up by endothelial cells and degraded by their lysosomal system.[141,142] The role of protein C, as an inhibitor of blood coagulation, is detailed later, in Section III.C.

4. Fibrinolytic Affectors of the Endothelial Cell

Endothelial cells have the capacity to synthesize and secrete both urokinase- and tissue-type plasminogen activators,[143-145] although they preferentially produce the latter. These cells also synthesize and secrete inhibitors of plasminogen activators.[143,146-148] The amount of the activator and inhibitor secreted depends on the phase of the cell cycle, for instance, in confluent cells the secretion of the plasminogen activator dominates, whereas in nonconfluent population, endothelial cells synthesize primarily plasminogen activator inhibitor.[149] Since proteolytically active thrombin increases the release of tissue-type plasminogen activator from human endothelial cells, the ultimate enzyme of blood coagulation may control fibrinolysis, not only by forming the substrate for plasmin action, but also by initiating plasminogen activation.

5. *Endothelial Cell Components Influencing Platelet Functions*

Prostacyclin (PGI_2), a potent vasodilator and inhibitor of platelet aggregation/adhesion, is synthesized and secreted by endothelial cells.[151-156] Although endothelial cells also have the capacity to produce thromboxane A_2 (TXA_2) from arachidonic acid taken up by these cells, the main product of the arachidonate metabolism is PGI_2.[157] The synthesis and/or the release of PGI_2 are influenced by several components present either under physiological conditions or during pathological changes or at pharmacological treatments. Thus, PGI_2 production is stimulated by thrombin,[158] bradykinin,[159] histamine,[160,161] high density lipoproteins,[162,163] ATP,[164] enkephalins,[165] leukotriene C,[166] platelet-derived growth factor,[163] etc. Nicotine,[167] aspirin,[168] and several nonsteroidal antiinflammatory agents,[155] etc., on the other hand, are inhibitory on PGI_2 synthesis. The exact molecular mechanism of regulation of PGI_2 synthesis and secretion by normal endothelial cells is not known at present.

Adenosine, formed from ATP, AMP, and/or ADP on endothelial cell surface, also contributes to the inhibition of platelet aggregation, via activation of adenylate cyclase of platelets (for details see Chapter 1). Endothelial cells are also able to produce platelet-activating factor (PAF) when stimulated with thrombin.[169] Since PAF is a potent stimulus for platelet aggregation and chemotaxis of polymorphonuclear leukocytes, endothelial cells may also contribute to the maintenance of vascular integrity when vessels are damaged.

6. *Endothelial Cell Components Contributing to Smooth Muscle Cell Functions*

The contraction of vascular smooth muscle requires Ca^{2+}, as a trigger, which may be supplied by entry from extracellular space via channels in the cell membrane and/or by release from storage pools within the cell.[170] The vasculature, however, is under neurohumoral control. At least 12 neurotransmitters and several circulating or locally produced substances contribute to the regulation of blood vessel contractions.[171] Some nerves synthesize, store, and release more than one transmitter involving the "classical" transmitters norepinephrine and acetylcholine, together with peptides and purines.[172] While norepinephrine induces contraction of several vessels, acetylcholine results in the relaxation of the smooth muscle cells of the media of the same vessel wall. The relaxation of arteries precontracted by norepinephrine, however, is strictly dependent on the presence of endothelial cells.[173,174] This phenomenon has already been demonstrated in different blood vessels in various mammalian species and can be elicited by several other agents.[175,176] It is supposed that a factor, called endothelium-derived vascular relaxant factor (EDRF) present in the endothelial cells, is released by various stimuli. The exact nature of this component, however, is not known. It is not a lipoxygenase derivative, but an unstable compound, with a species dependent half-life of 24 to 49 sec, containing carboxyl group at or near its active site.[177,178]

Besides acetylcholine, a number of agents have been found to require endothelial cells for exerting their relaxing effects on arteries. Thus, calcium ionophores, but not Na^+ selective ionophores, substance P, bradykinin, histamine, serotonin, arachidonic acid, ATP, ADP, adenosine, thrombin, etc., initiate release of EDRF from endothelial cells.[176,179-186,205] Moreover, most of these substances may also influence prostaglandin synthesis in the endothelial cell, resulting in vasodilation. In addition, adenosine and AMP dilate blood vessels directly via P_1-purinoreceptors of smooth muscle cells, whereas ATP and ADP act via P_2-purinoreceptors located on endothelial cells.[183,187] Since ATP and adenosine inhibit norepinephrine release from sympathic nerves supplying blood vessels,[188] the exact regulatory mechanism of endothelial cells in blood vessel contraction-relaxation is hardly understood at present. Additional difficulty arises in regard to the source of these compounds. Namely, the transmitters, released by perivascular nerves located at the border of the media and adventitia, diffuse through smooth muscle cells before acting on endothelial cells. Furthermore, acetylcholine, ATP, and ADP, from the circulating blood, are rapidly inactivated by ectoenzymes.

7. Endothelial Cell-Derived Growth Factor(s)

Endothelial cells may contribute to the regulation of the underlying cells by synthesizing and secreting components which stimulate or inhibit growth of the smooth muscle cells as well as of fibroblasts. A platelet-derived growth factor-like protein, secreted by endothelial cells (ECDGF), binds to the same receptor as the platelet-derived growth factor (PDGF), resulting in mitosis of the smooth muscle cells, fibroblasts, monocytes, and neutrophils, but without autocrine action, for instance, endothelial cells do not respond to their own growth factor.[189,190] Nevertheless, endothelial cells are able to secrete a component, which is different from ECDGF, and supports the growth of other endothelial cells.[191] Moreover, endothelial cells also produce a heparin-like molecule which is inhibitory for the growth of smooth muscle cells at a concentration of 10 ng/mℓ.[192]

C. Endothelial Cell Membrane as a Nonthrombogenic Surface

Under normal conditions, there is no thrombus formation on the endothelium. Endothelial cell surface inhibits thrombin action on fibrinogen and platelet as well as prevents prothrombin activation. There are two basic mechanisms responsible for this nature of endothelium.[193]

Thrombin, not bound to endothelial cells, has the ability to clot fibrinogen, to activate platelet, F-XIII, and to accelerate its own formation via activation of F-V and F-VIII.[194-197] This form of enzyme may also react with plasma proteinase inhibitors, primarily with antithrombin III, although these reactions are relatively slow.[198] Thrombin, however, binds to endothelial cell very rapidly and with high affinity,[199,200] and the reactivity of this form of the enzyme with its various substrates is modified. For example, if thrombin binds to endothelial cells via heparin-like structures, its inactivation by antithrombin III is facilitated.[37,201,202] If thrombin binds to the endothelial cells via thrombomodulin, a membrane structure protein with M_r 74,000 daltons,[203,204] its formation from prothrombin may be inhibited by a negative feedback control mechanism — the capacity of thrombin to activate protein C in a complex with thrombomodulin increases.[11] Activated protein C, in turn, inactivates activated F-V and F-VIII in the prothrombinase complex.[206,207] In addition, thrombin activity is highly restricted toward fibrinogen, F-V, and platelet when it is bound to thrombomodulin.[208,209,286] Moreover, thrombin, bound to thrombomodulin and/or a protein with M_r 30,000,[200] can be taken up, internalized, and degraded by endothelial cells.[210-212] All of these features of endothelial cell surface result in a thromboresistance of the endothelium. For more details see Chapter 1, Hemostasis, and Chapter 2, Volume II, Role of the Endothelium in the Regulation of Thrombin and Protein C.

The endothelial cell membrane surface may also participate in the control of fibrinolysis; an endothelial cell-cofactor for t-PA has been found recently which can greatly accelerate the rate of plasminogen activation.[288] Since t-PA is synthesized by and plasmin(ogen) binds to these cells,[287] endothelial cells may contribute to the nonthrombogenic nature of the surface this by method as well.

IV. PROLIFERATION AND DIFFERENTIATION OF ENDOTHELIAL CELLS: ROLE OF ENDOTHELIAL CELLS IN ANGIOGENESIS

The vascular endothelium generally shows low rate of cell turnover in the adult. The life span in areas around aortic branches is 60 to 120 days and in the other parts of the aorta, it is approximately 100 to 180 days.[213] Comprising less than 1% of the total number of endothelial cells of aorta, myocardial capillaries enter DNA synthesis each day.[214,215] The low rate of cell turnover in the aorta and large arteries seems to be critical, since denudation of the endothelium leads to the exposure of the thrombogenic subendothelium to platelets. As a consequence, platelet-derived mitogens stimulate the proliferation of the vascular muscle cells.[216-219] Both thrombosis and smooth muscle cell proliferation are responsible for atherosclerosis lesion formation. Thus, endothelial regeneration is an important process to prevent and/or compensate for the consequences of the damage of the vessel wall.

Although endothelial cell turnover is on the average low, locally, especially at sites in the arterial tree, as high as 10% of the endothelial cells can represent replication.[220] Also a relatively high mitotic index occurs in young tissue or during tissue repair, regeneration, and angiogenesis.[221]

Endothelial cells exhibit a polygonal or oval shape with cytoplasm around the centrally located nucleus. During growth, they tend to form round colonies with a generation time of approximately 48 to 72 hr in culture.[9] At confluence, there is a strong contact inhibition. The morphological characteristics of endothelial cells, however, change during differentiation depending on the functions of the various organs and tissues, i.e., endothelium may be continuous, fenestrated, discontinuous, etc.

The proliferation as well as differentiation of endothelial cells are under humoral control.[9,222] Thus, estrogen administration leads to multiplication of liver endothelial cells.[223] Glucocorticoids, primarily dexamethasone, stimulate cell spread and confluency of cultured human endothelial cells.[224] High level of circulating corticosteroids specifically increases the synthesis of 2 proteins (M_r 43,000 and M_r 28,000 daltons) as well as of the angiotensin-converting enzyme of endothelial cells.[225]

Besides hormones, several growth factors are mitogenic for cultured endothelial cells derived from human umbilical vein, i.e., epidermal growth factor (EGF), high density lipoprotein (HDL), extracts of bovine pituitary, hypothalamus, or of whole brain containing a cationic polypeptide called fibroblast growth factor (FGF) as well as an anionic endothelial cell growth factor (ECGF), and the medium conditioned by differentiated human hepatoma cells.[226] Two forms of ECGF have been isolated: a low molecular weight form, with M_r 17,000 to 25,000 daltons, and a high molecular weight form with an M_r of approximately 70,000 daltons. The high M_r ECGF, however, is convertible into biologically active low M_r ECGF.[227] ECGF, the single-chain polypeptide, M_r 20,000 daltons, binds specifically to membrane receptor present on endothelial cells as well as on fibroblasts and induces mitosis. Its mitogenic activity is potentiated by heparin by the stabilization of the tertiary structure of the polypeptide.[228]

The bovine brain-derived acidic fibroblast growth factor (FGF) is a unique protein having amino acid sequence homology with human interleukin 1.[229] The similarity of bovine FGF and human macrophage interleukin 1 suggests that these growth factor proteins are different from the families of PDGF, EGF, and insulin. FGF is a very potent mitogen for both BALB/c3T3 and vascular endothelial cells, and in the presence of heparin, induces blood vessel growth in vivo as well.[229]

Vascular endothelial cells, as mentioned, form a monolayer of contact inhibited polygonal cells.[230] After this phase, however, a second pattern of growth in focal areas may occur.[231] Such parts consist of elongated cells which tend to form new vessels by sprouting.[61,232] This growth mode may depend on growth factors. When endothelial cells in culture have been kept in the presence of FGF after confluence, multifunction of cells continues resulting in sprout cell formation.[233,234] These and additional data in the literature suggest that serum growth factors have a profound effect not only on endothelial cell proliferation, but also on the differentiation and on the expression of morphological phenotype. Whether such a change in endothelial cells caused by different signals means transformation of a single cell population or there exist several distinct types of vascular endothelial cells with different functional potentials controlled by extracellular factors is not clear at present.

A. Regeneration: Injury and Repair

Since subendothelium is rather thrombogenic, the response of endothelial cells to injury and their potential for repair or regeneration is very important. When endothelial cells are removed, platelets adhere to the subendothelium, but they are dislocated by the advancing edge of regenerating endothelium in 24 hr. In almost all instances, such a wound is completely covered by endothelium in 5 days.[235] Injury, however, may occur without loss of endothelial cells. Under such circumstances, there are changes in the cell glycocalyx charges, tight junctions, and contraction, there may occur vacuolization, nuclei disorientation, etc., and the endothelial cells display thrombogenicity.[236]

When endothelium is denuded, the damaged part of the blood vessel wall is replaced by the migration and replication of the cells from the intact endothelium at the edges of the wounded area.[237] Regeneration of aortic endothelium has characteristic forms and events, the cells at the wound edge begin to spread onto the denuded surface, while the endothelial cells become elongated ellipsoid cells with the long axis parallel to blood flow. After 24 hr, the cells start to synthesize DNA and by 48 hr the cell density is two to three times that of the normal.[221] The regeneration is influenced not only by humoral factors as mentioned, but also by blood flow, since regenerating cells move out six times as rapidly along the vessel axis than at the circumference. The early phase of response, the rapid proliferation along the vessel axis, is followed by a phase where the endothelium grows slowly.[237,238] After a few weeks, however, the endothelium has regenerated totally at the damaged part of the vessel. On the other hand, some other areas of injured vessel wall may remain uncovered for a period of months, enabling the smooth muscle cells to proliferate.[239]

Regarding the control of the cell proliferation and differentiation, data are insufficient in the literature to give an exact description of these processes. The only thing that can be said at present is that endothelial cell growth is influenced not only by various growth factors, but also by basement membrane components, like fibronectin, collagen, laminin, F-VIII_{vW}, etc., synthesized by endothelial cells themselves as well as by the neighboring cellular elements like fibroblasts, smooth muscle cells, pericytes, platelets, etc.[28]

B. Angiogenesis

Angiogenesis, the growth of a new capillary, plays an important role in physiological as well as pathological conditions, i.e., tissue regeneration, wound healing, diabetic retinopathy, psoriasis, arteritis, etc., depend highly on the processes of angiogenesis. Furthermore, most tumor cells have angiogenic capacity, and without the development of new capillaries, they would fail to grow.[240]

New blood vessels develop from the walls of existing small vessels by sprouting, the outgrowth of endothelial cells. Tumor tissues, however, release factor(s), called tumor angiogenesis factor(s), that cause(s) the ingrowth of capillaries into tumor cells, supplying them with nutrients.[241] During capillary sprout, pseudopodia of capillary endothelial cells grow into the surrounding connective tissue, and the endothelial cell starts to divide. In the new cell vacuoles are formed to create the lumen of the new capillary.

When capillary endothelial cells in a culture are confluent, they start to form "tubes" after 3 weeks. These "tubes" resemble capillaries found under in vivo conditions. The long tubes develop from cylindrical vacuoles present within endothelial cells, and they seem to connect one cell to another. Tube formation, however, depends on the age of cell culture; for example, once capillary tubes are formed in the primary culture, they appear earlier in subsequent passages. At a stage when four or five cells become connected by a tube, branches begin to appear.[240] The endothelial cells around a tube may migrate along it into the branches. These cells, although they do migrate, are never seen to divide. Endothelial cells, only outside the monolayer, do both divide and migrate. These data suggest that a single cell type contains the information to build up an entire capillary network.

Tumor components, the tumor angiogenesis factor(s), as well as fibroblast growth factor stimulate both migration and proliferation of capillary endothelial cells.[242,243]

The primary event is the endothelial cell migration followed by the cell proliferation.[61] These events may be induced by various molecules and also infuenced by cellular components. Some factors are responsible for neovascularization via affecting both migration and proliferation, whereas others act either on migration or proliferation.[244] Thus, extracts of carcinoma cells possess all the angiogenic components characteristic for neovascularization.[245-248] On the other hand, although ADP, prostaglandin E, or formyl methionyl leucyl phenylalanine induce neovascularization, they do not directly affect migration or proliferation, whereas heparin or copper ions influence angiogenesis through triggering migration.[244,249-252] The level of ceruloplasmin, the blood plasma copper-carrier protein, increases frequently in humans and animals bearing a variety of tumors.[253] Its action on angiogenesis, however, depends on the copper ions bound to the protein. Accordingly, copper ions are involved primarily in the sequence of the events leading to angiogenesis.[254]

Among the cellular components mast cells and leukocytes are supposed to be involved in angiogenesis.[255-258] The number of mast cells in the presence of tumor extracts increases even 40-fold compared to normal tissue within 24 hr. The elevated number of mast cells precedes the appearance of new blood vessels, although these cells do not initiate angiogenesis themselves. Accordingly, mast cells may amplify the rate of angiogenesis through the stimulation of migration of capillary endothelial cells.[255] Among the products of mast cells, only heparin can be found to stimulate the migration of capillary endothelial cells.[256] The effect of mast cell products is blocked by protamine, indicating that heparin is really the component stimulating endothelial cell migration.[250] As to the mechanism of heparin action, whether it is a direct effect or one in combination with tumor-derived endothelial growth factor, it needs further experimentation.[229,259] Regarding the role of leukocytes in angiogenesis, it is assumed that the response of endothelial cells to copper ions or to tumor cell extracts is mediated by leukocytes.[257,258]

V. CONCLUDING REMARKS

Endothelium, as a "widespread organ" with diverse capabilities, displays individual peculiarities in size, shape, intracellular components, intercellular connections, etc., depending on its functions. The differences are the most apparent between capillary and large vessel endothelial cells.[260] Arterial endothelial cells also differ in structure and function from venular endothelial cells. Moreover, even in the capillaries, there are enormous variations among the endothelial cells. They change in vesicle numbers, fenestrae, organelle amounts, junctions, etc. according to their role in transport, biosynthesis, metabolic processes, or regulation of local circulation. While the main function of the kidney endothelial cells is the participation in excretion of materials from blood in one direction, liver endothelial cells may control both the uptake of components from blood and secretion of products of hepatocytes into the blood. Lung endothelial cells, on the other hand, may contribute to the inactivation of metabolites, whereas brain capillaries control the functions of the nervous system.

The diverse activities of these cells correlate with structural modulations, which are only poorly known at present. The only common features which are characteristic for all endothelial cells are their thromboresistant luminal surface and their ability to form a monolayer on a foreign surface. Thus, the description of endothelial cell as a uniform entity is rather misleading. To survey endothelial cells from a consistent aspect of the diverse biological functions, however, is impossible at present, since data in the literature are not sufficient. Therefore, it seems to be reasonable that future endeavors will be directed primarily to the understanding of the specialized functions of the various types of endothelial cells and of the control of their own metabolism.

VI. APPENDIX: ENDOTHELIAL CELL CULTURE TECHNIQUES

To obtain information on endothelial cell biology, a critical step is studying endothelial cells separated from other types of cells as well as from other molecular components of the blood vessel wall. These criteria became available when endothelial cells could be cultured and identified. First, in 1973, Jaffe et al.[261] and Csonka et al.[273] successfully cultured human umbilical vein and bovine aortic endothelial cells, respectively. Thereafter, several methods on various sources have been published. In the next part of this chapter the culture methods for many accessible sources and types of endothelial cells are collected from the literature, and the various techniques are briefly reviewed.

Methods of isolation and culture of endothelial cell are described for human umbilical vein,[199,224,261-265] human umbilical arteries,[266] bovine aortic cells,[267-269] pig artery,[270,271] mini pig aortic cells,[272] rabbit artery,[273,274] rat aortic cells[275] and rat pulmonary artery,[276,277] rat liver,[278] canine vein,[279] capillaries of rat and rabbit brain,[280,281] bovine adrenal cortex[282] and medulla,[283] as well as for bovine corneal endothelium.[28]

These methods generally use proteinases for isolation of endothelial cells from the blood vessel wall and their separation from other cells, such as smooth muscle cells and fibroblasts. Thereafter they are cultured in various media with different additives under sterile conditions. In some cases, the vessel wall support is mimicked by collagen or fibronectin layers or even by their combination with smooth muscle cells. The media may also contain growth factors, hormones, but generally fetal calf serum is present for supplying the cells with nutrients and presently unknown factors necessary for cell growth. A few techniques are briefly described below.

Preparation of a primary culture of human umbilical vein endothelial cells[199,261] — Umbilical veins, collected in medium M-199 containing 10% fetal calf serum (FCS), are washed with phosphate buffered saline (PBS). After clamping at one end, they are filled with 0.25% collagenase and digested for 6 min. The cell suspension formed is drained into 5 to 10 mℓ of medium M-199 containing 20% FCS and rinsed with an additional 40 mℓ of medium-199. The cell pellet formed after centrifugation is resuspended in fresh medium M-199 again with 20% FCS and seeded in petri dishes at a density of 900,000 cells per dish. Thereafter, the cells are incubated at 37°C in 5% CO_2 atmosphere. After 24 hr, the cell layer is washed with fresh medium and kept in medium M-199 containing 20% FCS until experimentation. Human umbilical endothelial cells may also be cultured in the presence of fibroblast growth factor and heparin.[277] After a 10-min treatment of umbilical veins with 1 mg/mℓ of collagenase in medium M-199, the cells are cultured in medium M-199 supplemented with 20% FCS also containing 25 m*M* Hepes, pH 7.4, 100 U/mℓ penicillin and streptomycin, 90 μg/mℓ heparin, 100 ng/mℓ fibroblast growth factor, in 60-mm dishes coated with gelatin. The cells are grown to confluency at 37°C in 5% CO_2 and 95% humidity.

Preparation of rabbit aortic endothelial cell[285] — Rabbit intercostal arteries are ligated and filled with 0.15% collagenase and 0.05% Viokase in F-12 medium. After 20-min incubation at 37°C, the enzyme solution is withdrawn with a syringe and the cells are plated in petri dishes. Thereafter a cloning ring with 4-mm diameter is placed on a colony which appears to be homogeneous for endothelial cells, and they are selectively removed by incubation with 0.5% Viokase solution at 37°C. Finally, the cells are transferred in a 35-mm tissue culture dish and cultured in F-12 medium supplemented with 10% FCS. The processes can be repeated several times.

Preparation of bovine or mini pig aortic endothelial cells[272,273] — Aorta is cleaned in sterilized PBS and cut to a size of approximately 2 cm. The pieces are placed on and covered by sterilized gauze soaked with VERSIN (0.25% trypsin and 0.01% EDTA) and incubated at 22°C for 10 min. Thereafter, the cells are rubbed off and placed into petri dishes containing Dulbecco's modified Eagle's medium (DMEM), 100 U/mℓ penicillin, 50 μg/mℓ streptomycin, and 30% FCS. After 24 hr at 37°C in 5% CO_2 and 95% humidity, the medium is changed for a fresh one. For passages, the endothelial cells are treated by VERSIN in PBS for 5 to 10 min at 22°C and collected by centrifugation. Trypsin action is stopped by the addition of fetal calf serum containing excess plasma proteinase inhibitors.

Preparation of bovine capillary endothelial cells[282] — Bovine adrenal cortex is submerged for a few minutes in Betadine solution and washed with sterile Ringer's solution. Using sterile technique, the tissue is cut into pieces of about 2 mm in diameter and incubated in 0.75% collagenase with 0.5% bovine serum albumin (BSA) at room temperature for 30 min with occasional shaking. Thereafter, these capillary segments are passed through a nylon mesh of 110-μm pore size and centrifuged. The pellet is suspended in DMEM supplemented with 10% calf serum and washed three times. Finally, the cells are cultured in gelatin-coated plastic culture dishes in tumor-conditioned medium. There are some special criteria for migration and proliferation of capillary endothelial cells. They require tumor-conditioned medium, while aortic or umbilical vein endothelium does not. Capillary endothelial cells have matrix requirement, such as gelatin or fibronectin, for their survival, whereas endothelial cells of large vessels do not need special support for growth. Migration of these cells is also stimulated by heparin, at a concentration as low as 1 μg/mℓ, and maximal migration activity occurs at 50 μg/mℓ.[282]

Cocultures of endothelial and smooth muscle cells[266,270] — Sterilized collagen solution is allowed to form a gel on plastic culture wells of 16-mm diameter. Smooth muscle cells, derived from human umbilical arteries, are seeded in RPMI/M 199 medium supplemented with 20% human whole blood serum. After 24 hr, the culture medium is removed and the smooth muscle cell region is covered by collagen gel. On the second collagen region, endothelial cells, isolated from human umbilical veins, are seeded in RPMI/M 199 medium supplemented with 20% human whole blood serum.

The main problem with these culture techniques is to find the factors necessary for migration, proliferation, differentiation, and growth of the endothelial cells and to avoid contamination by either other cells or bacteria. For identification of the endothelial cell, several criteria and markers are used, since each of them is not absolutely unique to this type of cell. For example, although only the endothelial cell contains Weibel-Palade bodies, endothelial cells derived from bovine capillary or rabbit aorta do not possess these structures.[9,233,282] At present, the most frequently used markers for endothelial cell identifications are the following.

1. General morphological characterization involving shape, junctions, vesicles, etc.
2. Presence of the characteristic rod-shaped Weibel-Palade granules in the cytoplasm
3. Synthesis of F-VIII_{vW}
4. Synthesis of Type IV collagen
5. Presence of angiotensin coverting enzyme on the luminal surface of the cell
6. Fibrinolytic activity via synthesis of plasminogen activators
7. Immunological properties of the glycocalyx, containing ABO blood group and HLA-A,B antigens[261,284]

8. Some characteristic glycosaminoglycans may also be used as marker for endothelial cell[9]

ACKNOWLEDGMENTS

I thank Drs. Eva Csonka and Jozsef Csillag for the helpful criticism of the manuscript. This work was supported in part by the Hungarian Ministry of Health and the Hungarian Academy of Sciences, Grant 20.057/85 and the Mayo Foundation, grant HL17430.

REFERENCES

1. **Jaffe, E. A.,** Physiological functions of normal endothelial cells, *Ann. N.Y. Acad. Sci.,* 454, 279, 1985.
2. **Simionescu, M. and Simionescu, N.,** Ultrastructure of the microvascular wall: functional correlations, in *Handbook of Physiology,* Section 2, *The Cardiovascular System,* Vol. 4, Renkin, E. M., Michel, C. C., and Geiger, S. R., Eds., American Physiological Society, Bethesda, Md., 1984, 41.
3. **Majno, G. and Joris, I.,** Endothelium: a review, in *The Thrombotic Process in Atherogenesis,* Chandler, A. B., Eurenius, K., McMillan, G. C., Nelson, C. B., Schwartz, C. J., and Wessler, S., Eds., Plenum Press, New York, 1978, 169.
4. **Simionescu, M., Simionescu, N., and Palade, G. E.,** Morphometric data on the endothelium of blood capillaries, *J. Cell Biol.,* 60, 128, 1974.
5. **Danon, D. and Skutelsky, E.,** Endothelial surface charge and its possible relationship to thrombogenesis, *Ann. N.Y. Acad. Sci.,* 275, 47, 1976.
6. **Simionescu, M., Simionescu, N., and Pallade, G. E.,** Differentiated microdomains on the luminal surface of the capillary endothelium. I. Partial characterization of their anionic sites, *J. Cell Biol.,* 90, 614, 1981.
7. **Simionescu, N.,** The microvascular endothelium: segmental differentiations, transcytosis, selective distribution of anionic sites, in *Advances in Inflammation Research,* Weissman, G., Samuelson, B., and Paoletti, R., Eds., Raven Press, New York, 1979, 61.
8. **Simionescu, N. and Simionescu, M.,** The hydrophilic pathways of capillary endothelium, a dynamic system, in *Water Transport Across Epithelia, Barriers, Gradients, and Mechanisms,* Ussing, H. H., Bindsler, N. B., Lassen, N. A., and Sten-Knudsen, D., Eds., Munksgaard, Copenhagen, 1981, 228.
9. **Buonassisi, V. and Colburn, P.,** Hormone and surface receptors in vascular endothelium, *Adv. Microcirc.,* 9, 76, 1980.
10. **Owen, W. G. and Esmon, C. T.,** Functional properties of an endothelial cell cofactor for thrombin-catalyzed activation of protein C, *J. Biol. Chem.,* 256, 5532, 1981.
11. **Owen, W. G.,** The control of hemostasis: role of endothelium in the regulation of inhibitory and catabolic pathways, *Arch. Pathol. Lab. Med.,* 106, 209, 1982.
12. **Howard, B. V.,** Uptake of very low density lipoprotein triglyceride by bovine aortic endothelial cells in culture, *J. Lipid Res.,* 18, 561, 1977.
13. **Henriksen, T., Mahoney, E. M., and Steinberg, D.,** Interactions of plasma lipoproteins with endothelial cells, *Ann. N.Y. Acad. Sci.,* 401, 102, 1982.
14. **Blanchette-Mackie, E. J. and Scow, R. O.,** Sites of lipoprotein lipase activity in adipose tissue perfused with chylomicrons: electron microscope cytochemical study, *J. Cell Biol.,* 51, 1, 1971.
15. **Wang-Iverson, P. and Brown, W. V.,** Interaction of lipoprotein lipase with cultured endothelial cells, *Ann. N.Y. Acad. Sci.,* 401, 92, 1982.
16. **Richardson, J. B. and Beaulnes, A.,** The cellular site of action of angiotensin, *J. Cell Biol.,* 51, 419, 1971.
17. **Bar, R. S., Hoak, J. C., and Peacock, M. L.,** Insulin receptors in human endothelial cells: identification and characterization, *J. Clin. Endocrinol. Metab.,* 47, 699, 1978.
18. **Bar, R. S.,** Interactions of insulin and insulin-like growth factors (IGF) with endothelial cells, *Ann. N.Y. Acad. Sci.,* 401, 150, 1982.
19. **Heltianu, C., Simionescu, M., and Simionescu, N.,** Histamine receptors of the microvascular endothelium revealed *in situ* with a histamine-ferritin conjugate: characteristic high affinity binding sites in venules, *J. Cell Biol.,* 93, 357, 1982.
20. **Bevan, J. A. and Duckles, S. P.,** Evidence for alpha-adrenergic receptors on intimal endothelium, *Blood Vessels,* 12, 307, 1975.
21. **Apperley, E., Feniuk, W., Humphrey, P. P. A., and Levy, G. P.,** Evidence for two types of excitatory receptor for 5-hydroxytryptamine in dog isolated vasculature, *Br. J. Pharmacol.,* 68, 215, 1980.

22. **Buonassisi, V. and Venter, J. C.,** Hormone and neurotransmitter receptors in an established vascular endothelial cell line, *Proc. Natl. Acad. Sci. U.S.A.*, 73, 1612, 1976.
23. **Flumerfelt, B. A., Lewis, P. R., and Gwyn, D. G.,** Cholinesterase activity of capillaries in the rat brain. A light and electron microscopic study, *Histochem. J.*, 5, 67, 1973.
24. **Owman, C., Edvinsson, L., and Hardebo, J. E.,** Amine mechanisms and contractile properties of the cerebral microvascular endothelium, in *Vascular Neuroeffector Mechanisms*, Bevan, J. A., Ed., Raven Press, New York, 1980, 277.
25. **Ryan, U. S. and Ryan, J. W.,** Correlations between the fine structure of the alveolar-capillary unit and its metabolic activities, in *Lung Biology in Health and Disease. Metabolic Functions of the Lung*, Vol. 4, Bakhle, Y. S. and Vane, J. R., Eds., Marcel Dekker, New York, 1977, 197.
26. **Shepro, D., Barbouta, J. C., Robblee, L. S., Carson, M. P., and Belamarich, F. A.,** Serotonin transport by cultured bovine aortic endothelium, *Circ. Res.*, 36, 799, 1975.
27. **Karnovsky, M. J., Kleinfeld, A. M., Hoover, R. L., Dawidowicz, E. A., McIntyre, D. E., Salzman, E. A., and Klausner, R. D.,** Lipid domains in membranes, *Ann. N.Y. Acad. Sci.*, 401, 61, 1982.
28. **Gospodarowicz, D., Savion, N., and Giguere, L.,** The control of proliferation and differentiation of endothelial cells, in *Pathobiology of the Endothelial Cell*, Nossel, H.L. and Vogel, H. J., Eds., Academic Press, New York, 1982, 19.
29. **Dejana, E., Longulno, L. R., Polentarutti, N., Balconi, G., Ryckewaert, J. J., Larrieu, M., Donatti, M. B., Mantovani, A., and Marguerie, G.,** Interaction between fibrinogen and cultured endothelial cells; induction of migration and specific binding, *J. Clin. Invest.*, 75, 1, 1985.
30. **Rodgers, G. M. and Shuman, M. A.,** Prothrombin is activated on vascular endothelial cells by factor Xa and calcium, *Proc. Natl. Acad. Sci. U.S.A.*, 80, 7001, 1983.
31. **Rodgers, G. M., Broze, G. J., and Shuman, M. A.,** The number of receptors for factor VII correlates with the ability of cultured cells to initiate coagulation, *Blood*, 63, 434, 1984.
32. **Stern, D. M., Drillings, M., Kisiel, W., Nawroth, P., Nossel, H. L., and LaGamma, K. S.,** Activation of factor IX bound to cultured bovine aortic endothelial cells, *Proc. Natl. Acad. Sci. U.S.A.*, 81, 913, 1984.
33. **Fuchs, H. E. and Pizzo, S. V.,** Regulation of factor Xa in vitro in human and mouse plasma and in vivo in mouse; role of the endothelium and plasma proteinase inhibitors, *J. Clin. Invest.*, 72, 2041, 1983.
34. **Rodgers, G. M. and Schuman, M. A.,** Characterization of the interaction between factor Xa and bovine aortic endothelial cells, *Biochim. Biophys. Acta*, 844, 320, 1985.
35. **Becker, C. G. and Harpel, P. C.,** Alpha 2-macroglobulin on human vascular endothelium, *J. Exp. Med.*, 144, 1, 1976.
36. **Bartha, K., Kovács, T., Léránt, I., Papp, B., Kolev, K., Csonka, E., and Machovich, R.,** Interaction of antithrombin III and thrombin-antithrombin III complex with cultured aortic endothelial cells, *Thromb. Res.*, submitted.
37. **Bauer, P. I., Machovich, R., Arányi, P., Büki, K., Csonka, E., and Horváth, I.,** Mechanism of thrombin binding to endothelial cells, *Blood*, 61, 368, 1983.
38. **Karnovsky, M. J. and Leventhal, M. M.,** Some aspects of the structural basis for permeability of small blood vessels, in *Small Vessel Angiography*, Hilal, S. K., Ed., C. V. Mosby, St. Louis, 1973.
39. **Simionescu, M., Simionescu, N., and Palade, G. E.,** Chracteristic endothelial junctions in different segments of the vascular system, *Thromb. Res.*, 8(Suppl. II), 247, 1976.
40. **Biempica, L., Morecki, R., Wu, C. H., Gimbrone, M. A., and Rojkind, M.,** Immunocytochemical localization of type B collagen. A component of basement membrane in human liver, *Am. J. Pathol.*, 98, 591, 1980.
41. **Birdwell, C. R., Gospodarovicz, D., and Nicolson, G.,** Identification, localization and role of fibronectin in cultured bovine endothelial cells, *Proc. Natl. Acad. Sci. U.S.A.*, 75, 3273, 1978.
42. **Cohen, M. P. and Ciborowski, C. J.,** Presence of glycosaminoglycans in retinal capillary basement membrane, *Biochim. Biophys. Acta*, 674, 400, 1981.
43. **Howard, B. V., Macarak, E. J., Gunson, D., and Kefalides, N. A.,** Characterization of the collagen synthesized by endothelial cells in culture, *Proc. Natl. Acad. Sci. U.S.A.*, 73, 2361, 1976.
44. **Jaffe, E. A. and Mosher, D. F.,** Synthesis of fibronectin by cultured human endothelial cells, *J. Exp. Med.*, 147, 1779, 1978.
45. **Kanwar, Y. S. and Farquhar, M. G.,** Presence of heparan sulfate in the glomerular basement membrane, *Proc. Natl. Acad. Sci. U.S.A.*, 76, 1303, 1979.
46. **Ruoslahti, E. and Engvall, E.,** Complexing of fibronectin, glycosaminoglycans and collagen, *Biochim. Biophys. Acta*, 631, 350, 1980.
47. **Forbes, M. S., Rennels, M. L., and Nelson, E.,** Ultrastructure of pericytes in mouse heart, *Am. J. Anat.*, 149, 47, 1977.
48. **Tilton, R. G., Kilo, C., and Williamson, J. R.,** Pericyte-endothelial relationships in cardiac and skeletal muscle capillaries, *Microvasc. Res.*, 18, 325, 1979.

49. **Simionescu, N. and Simionescu, M.,** The cardiovascular system, in *Histology,* Weiss, L., Ed., Elsevier, New York, 1983, 371.
50. **Stensas, L. J.,** Pericytes and perivascular microglial cells in the basal forebrain of the neonatal rabbit, *Cell Tissue Res.,* 158, 517, 1975.
51. **Weibel, E. R.,** On pericytes, particularly their existence on lung capillaries, *Microvasc. Res.,* 8, 218, 1974.
52. **Van Deurs, B.,** Observations on the blood-brain barrier in hypertensive rats, with particular reference to phagocytic pericytes, *J. Ultrastruct. Res.,* 56, 65, 1976.
53. **Tilton, R. G., Kilo, G. C., Williamson, J. R., and Murch, D. W.,** Differences in pericyte contractile function in rat cardiac and skeletal muscle microvasculatures, *Microvasc. Res.,* 18, 336, 1979.
54. **Blose, S. H.,** Ten-nanometer filaments and mitosis: maintenance of structural continuity in dividing endothelial cells, *Proc. Natl. Acad. Sci. U.S.A.,* 76, 3372, 1979.
55. **Becker, C. G. and Nachman, R. L.,** Contractile proteins of endothelial cells, platelets and smooth muscle, *Am. J. Pathol.,* 71, 1, 1973.
56. **Majno, G., Shea, S. M., and Leventhal, M.,** Endothelial contraction induced by histamine-type mediators, an electron microscopic study, *J. Cell Biol.,* 42, 647, 1969.
57. **Simionescu, N., Heltianu, C., Antohe, F., and Simionescu, M.,** Endothelial cell receptors for histamine, *Ann. N.Y. Acad. Sci.,* 401, 132, 1982.
58. **Weibel, E. R. and Palade, G. E.,** New cytoplasmic components in arterial endothelia, *J. Cell Biol.,* 23, 101, 1964.
59. **Santolaya, R. C. and Bertini, F.,** Fine structure of endothelial cells of vertebrates. Distribution of dense granules, *Z. Anat. Entwicklungsgesch.,* 131, 148, 1970.
60. **Sholley, M. M., Cavallo, T., and Cotran, R. S.,** Endothelial proliferation in inflammation. I. Autoradiographic studies following thermal injury to the skin of normal rats, *Am. J. Pathol.,* 89, 277, 1977.
61. **Ausprunk, D. H. and Folkman, J.,** Migration and proliferation of endothelial cells in preformed and newly formed blood vessels during tumor angiogenesis, *Microvasc. Res.,* 14, 53, 1977.
62. **Ericson, L. E. and Wollman, S. H.,** Increase in the rough endoplasmatic reticulum in capillary endothelial cells and pericytes in hyperplastic rat thyroid glands, *Endocrinology,* 107, 732, 1980.
63. **Palade, G. E. and Bruns, R. R.,** Structural modulations of plasmalemmal vesicles, *J. Cell Biol.,* 37, 633, 1968.
64. **Simionescu, N., Simionescu, M., and Palade, G. E.,** Structural basis of permeability in sequential segments of the microvasculature. I. Bipolar microvascular fields in the diaphragm, *Microvasc. Res.,* 15, 1, 1978.
65. **Simionescu, N., Simionescu, M., and Palade, G. E.,** Structural basis of permeability in sequential segments of the microvasculature. II. Pathways followed by microperoxidase across the endothelium, *Microvasc. Res.,* 15, 17, 1978.
66. **Tomllin, S. G.,** Vesicular transport across endothelial cells, *Biochim. Biophys. Acta,* 13, 559, 1969.
67. **Palade, G. E., Simionescu, M., and Simionescu, N.,** Structural aspects of the permeability of the microvascular endothelium, *Acta Physiol. Scand. Suppl.,* 463, 11, 1979.
68. **Simionescu, N., Simionescu, M., and Palade, G. E.,** Permeability of muscle capillaries to small hemepeptides. Evidence for the existence of patent transendothelial channels, *J. Cell Biol.,* 64, 586, 1975.
69. **Casley-Smith, J. R. and Carter, D. B.,** The passage of macromolecules across inflamed capillary endothelium via large vacuoles, *Microvasc. Res.,* 18, 319, 1979.
70. **Michel, C. C.,** The flow of water through the capillary wall, in *Water Transport Across Epithelial Barriers, Gradients, and Mechanisms,* Ussing, H. H., Bindslev, N. B., Lassen, N. A., and Sten-Knudsen, O., Eds., Munksgaard, Copenhagen, 1981, 268.
71. **Wisse, E.,** An electron microscopic study of the fenestrated endothelial lining of rat liver sinusoids, *J. Ultrastruct. Res.,* 31, 125, 1970.
72. **De Bruyn, P. P. H., Michelson, S., and Becker, R. P.,** Endocytosis, transfer tubules, and lysosomal activity in myeloid sinusoidal endothelium, *J. Ultrastruct. Res.,* 53, 133, 1975.
73. **Vasile, E., Simionescu, M., and Simionescu, N.,** Visualization of the binding, endocytosis and transcytosis of low density lipoprotein in the arterial endothelium *in situ, J. Cell Biol.,* 96, 1677, 1983.
74. **Vlodavsky, I., Fielding, P. E., Fielding, C. J., and Gospodarowicz, D.,** Role of contact inhibition in the regulation of receptor-mediated uptake of low density lipoprotein in cultured vascular endothelial cells, *Proc. Natl. Acad. Sci: U.S.A.,* 75, 356, 1978.
75. **Friederici, H. H. R.,** On the diaphragm across fenestrae of capillary endothelium, *J. Ultrastruct. Res.,* 27, 373, 1969.
76. **Simionescu, N., Simionescu, M., and Palade, G. E.,** Sulfated glycosaminoglycans are major components of the anionic sites of fenestral diaphragms in capillary endothelium, *J. Cell Biol.,* 83(Abstr.), 78, 1979.
77. **Casley-Smith, J. R.,** Endothelial fenestrae in intestinal villi: differences between the arterial and venous ends of the capillaries, *Microvasc. Res.,* 3, 49, 1971.

78. **Folkman, J., Haudenschild, C. C., and Zetter, B. R.,** Long-term culture of capillary endothelial cells, *Proc. Natl. Acad. Sci. U.S.A.,* 76, 5217, 1979.
79. **Landis, E. M. and Pappenheimer, J. R.,** Exchange of substances through the capillary walls, in *Handbook of Physiology, Circulation,* Vol. 2, Sect. 2, Hamilton, W. F., Ed., American Physiology Society, Washington, D.C., 1963, 961.
80. **Crone, C. and Christensen, O.,** Transcapillary transport of small solutes and water, in *Cardiovascular Physiology III,* Vol. 18, Guyton, A. C. and Young, D. B., Eds., University Park Press, Baltimore, 1978, 149.
81. **Simionescu, N.,** Transcytosis and traffic of membranes in the endothelial cell, in *International Cell Biology,* Schweiger, H. G., Ed., Springer-Verlag, Berlin, 1981, 657.
82. **Hausmann, K., Wulfhekel, U., Düllmann, J., and Kuse, R.,** Iron storage in macrophages and endothelial cells. Histochemistry, ultrastructure and clinical significance, *Blut,* 32, 289, 1976.
83. **Van Deurs, B.,** Endocytosis in high-endothelial venules. Evidence for transport of exogenous material to lysosomes by uncoated "endothelial" vesicles, *Microvasc. Res.,* 16, 28, 1978.
84. **Van Deurs, B., Ropke, C., and Westergaard, E.,** Permeability properties of the postcapillary high-endothelial venules in lymph nodes of the mouse, *Lab. Invest.,* 32, 201, 1975.
85. **Goldstein, J. L., Anderson, R. G. W., and Brown, M. S.,** Coated pits, coated vesicles, and receptor-mediated endocytosis, *Nature (London),* 279, 679, 1979.
86. **Johansson, B. R.,** Capillary permeability to interstitial microinjections of macromolecules and influence of capillary hydrostatic pressure on endothelial ultrastructure, *Acta Physiol. Scand.,* 463, 45, 1979.
87. **Simionescu, N. and Palade, G. E.,** Dextrans and glycogens as particulate tracers for studying capillary permeability, *J. Cell Biol.,* 50, 616, 1971.
88. **Suzuki, Y., Ookawara, S., and Ooneda, G.,** Increased permeability of the arteries in hypertensive rats: an electron-microscopic study, *Exp. Mol. Pathol.,* 15, 198, 1971.
89. **Wolff, J. R.,** Ultrastructure of the terminal vascular bed as related to function, in *Microcirculation,* Vol. 1, Kaley, G. and Altura, B. M., Eds., University Park Press, Baltimore, 1977, 95.
90. **Curry, F. E. and Michel, C. C.,** A fiber matrix model of capillary permeability, *Microvasc. Res.,* 20, 96, 1980.
91. **Bundgaard, M. and Frøkjaer-Jensen, J.,** Functional aspects of the ultrastructure of terminal blood vessels: a quantitative study of consecutive segments of frog mesenteric vasculature, *Microvasc. Res.,* 23, 1, 1982.
92. **Curry, F. E.,** Effect of albumin on the structure of the molecular filter at the capillary wall, *Fed. Proc.,* 44, 2610, 1985.
93. **Frederickson, D. S., Levy, R. I., and Lees, R. S.,** Fat transport in lipoproteins — an integrated approach to mechanisms and disorders, *N. Engl. J. Med.,* 276, 34, 1967.
94. **Robinson, D. S.,** The function of the plasma triglycerides in fatty acid transport, in *Comprehensive Biochemistry,* Vol. 18, Florkin, M. and Stotz, E. H., Eds., Elsevier, Amsterdam, 1970, 51.
95. **Scow, R. O., Blanchette-Mackie, E. J., and Smith, L. C.,** Role of capillary endothelium in the clearance of chylomicrons. A model for lipid transport from blood by lateral diffusion in cell membranes, *Circ. Res.,* 39, 149, 1976.
96. **Spector, A. A. and Fletcher, J. E.,** Transport of fatty acids in the circulation, in *Disturbances in Lipid and Metabolism,* Dietschy, J. M., Gotto, A. M., and Ontko, J. A., Eds., American Physiology Society, Bethesda, Md., 1978, 229.
97. **Scow, R. O., Blanchette-Mackie, E. J., and Smith, L. C.,** Transport of lipid across capillary endothelium, *Fed. Proc.,* 39, 2610, 1980.
98. **Betz, A. L.,** Epithelial properties of brain capillary endothelium, *Fed. Proc.,* 44, 2614, 1985.
99. **Bradbury, M. W. B. and Stulcová, B.,** Efflux mechanism contributing to the stability of the potassium concentration in cerebrospinal fluid, *J. Physiol.,* 208, 415, 1970.
100. **Betz, A. L., Firth, J. A., and Goldstein, G. W.,** Polarity of the blood-brain barrier: distribution of enzymes between the luminal and antiluminal membranes of brain capillary endothelial cells, *Brain. Res.,* 192, 17, 1980.
101. **Betz, A. L.,** Sodium transport from blood to brain: inhibition by furosemide and amiloride, *J. Neurochem.,* 41, 1158, 1983.
102. **Sage, H.,** Collagen synthesis by endothelial cells in culture, in *Biology of Endothelial Cells,* Jaffe, E. A., Ed., Martinus-Nijhoff, Boston, 1984, 161.
103. **Sage, H., Priztl, P., and Bornstein, P.,** Secretory phenotypes of endothelial cells in culture: comparison of aortic, venous, capillary, and corneal endothelium, *Arteriosclerosis,* 1, 427, 1981.
104. **Sage, H., Pritzl, P., and Bornstein, P.,** A unique, pepsin-sensitive collagen synthesized by aortic endothelial cells in culture, *Biochemistry,* 19, 5747, 1980.
105. **Gross, J. L., Moscatelli, D., Jaffe, E. A., and Rifkin, D. B.,** Plasminogen activator and collagenase production by cultured capillary endothelial cells, *J. Cell Biol.,* 95, 974, 1982.
106. **Kalebic, T., Garbisa, S., Glaser, B., and Liotta, L. A.,** Basement membrane collagen: degradation by migrating endothelial cells, *Science,* 221, 281, 1983.

107. **Mecham, R. P., Madaras, J., McDonald, J. A., and Ryan, U.,** Elastin production by cultured calf pulmonary artery endothelial cells, *J. Cell. Physiol.*, 116, 282, 1983.
108. **Carnes, W. H., Abraham, P. A., and Buonassisi, V.,** Biosynthesis of elastin by an endothelial cell culture, *Biochem. Biophys. Res. Commun.*, 90, 1393, 1979.
109. **Cantor, J. O., Keller, S., Parshley, M. S., Darnule, T. V., Darnule, A. T., Cerreta, J. M., Turino, G. M., and Mandl, I.,** Synthesis of cross-linked elastin by an endothelial cell culture, *Biochem. Biophys. Res. Commun.*, 95, 1381, 1980.
110. **Sage, H. and Bornstein, P.,** Endothelial cells from umbilical vein and a hemangioendothelioma secrete basement membrane largely to the exclusion of interstitial collagens, *Arteriosclerosis*, 2, 27, 1982.
111. **Mosher, D. F., Doyle, M. J., and Jaffe, E. A.,** Synthesis and secretion of thrombospondin by cultured endothelial cells, *J. Cell Biol.*, 93, 343, 1982.
112. **McPherson, J., Sage, H., and Bornstein, P.,** Isolation and characterization of a glycoprotein secreted by aortic endothelial cells in culture. Apparent identity with platelet thrombospondin, *J. Biol. Chem.*, 256, 11330, 1981.
113. **Gospodarowicz, D., Greenburg, G., Foidart, J. M., and Savion, N.,** The production and localization of laminin in cultured vascular and corneal endothelial cells, *J. Cell. Physiol.*, 107, 171, 1981.
114. **Buonassisi, V.,** Sulfated mucopolysaccharide synthesis and secretion in endothelial cell cultures, *Exp. Cell Res.*, 76, 363, 1973.
115. **Sampson, P., Parshley, M. S., Mandl, I., and Turino, G. M.,** Glycosaminoglycans produced in tissue culture by rat lung cells. Isolation from a mixed cell line and a derived endothelial clone, *Connect. Tissue Res.*, 4, 41, 1975.
116. **Bihari-Varga, M., Csonka, E., and Jellinek, H.,** Endothelial glycosaminoglycans — in vitro studies, *Artery*, 8, 355, 1980.
117. **Oohira, A., Wight, T. N., and Bornstein, P.,** Sulfated proteoglycans synthesized by vascular endothelial cells in culture, *J. Biol. Chem.*, 258, 2014, 1983.
118. **Gamse, G., Fromme, H. G., and Cresse, H.,** Metabolism of sulfated glycosaminoglycans in cultured endothelial cells from bovine aorta, *Biochim. Biophys. Acta*, 544, 514, 1978.
119. **Chiang, T. M., Mainardi, C. L., Seyer, J. M., and Kang, A. H.,** Collagen platelet interaction. Type V (A-B) collagen induced platelet aggregation, *J. Lab. Clin. Med.*, 95, 99, 1980.
120. **Barnes, M. J., Bailey, A. J., Gordon, J. L., and Macintyre, D. E.,** Platelet aggregation by basement membrane-associated collagens, *Thromb. Res.*, 18, 375, 1980.
121. **Tryggrason, K., Oikarinen, J., Viinikka, L., and Ylikorkala, O.,** Effect of laminin, proteoglycan, type IV collagen, and components of basement membranes on platelet aggregation, *Biochem. Biophys. Res. Commun.*, 100, 233, 1981.
122. **Fauvel, F., Grant, M. E., Legrand, Y. J., Souchon, H., Tobelem, G., Jackson, D. S., and Caen, J. P.,** Interaction of blood platelets with a microfibrillar extract from adult bovine aorta: requirement for von Willebrand factor, *Proc. Natl. Acad. Sci. U.S.A.*, 80, 551, 1983.
123. **Wiggins, R. C., Loskutoff, D. J., Cochrane, C. G., Griffin, J. H., and Edgington, T. S.,** Activation of rabbit Hageman factor by homogenates of cultured rabbit endothelial cells, *J. Clin. Invest.*, 65, 197, 1980.
124. **Wagner, D. D. and Marder, V. J.,** Biosynthesis of von Willebrand protein by human endothelial cells. Identification of a large precursor polypeptide chain, *J. Biol. Chem.*, 258, 2065, 1983.
125. **Lynch, D. C., Williams, R., Zimmerman, T. S., Kirby, E. P., and Livingston, D. M.,** Biosynthesis of the subunits of factor VIIIR by bovine aortic endothelial cells, *Proc. Natl. Acad. Sci. U.S.A.*, 80, 2738, 1983.
126. **Meyer, D. and Baumgartner, H. R.,** Role of von Willebrand factor in platelet adhesion to the subendothelium, *Br. J. Haematol.*, 54, 1, 1983.
127. **Kao, K. J., Pizzo, S. V., and McKee, P. A.,** Demonstration and characterization of specific binding sites of factor VIII-von Willebrand factor on human platelets, *J. Clin. Invest.*, 63, 656, 1979.
128. **Morisato, D. K. and Gralnick, H.,** Selective binding of the factor VIII-von Willebrand factor protein to human platelets, *Blood*, 55, 9, 1980.
129. **Tchopp, T. B., Weiss, H. J., and Baumgartner, H. R.,** Decreased adhesion of platelets to subendothelium in von Willebrand's disease, *J. Lab. Clin. Med.*, 83, 296, 1974.
130. **Weiss, H. J., Baumgartner, H. R., Tschopp, T. B., Turitto, V. T., and Cohen, D.,** Correction by factor VIII of the impaired platelet adhesion to subendothelium in von Willebrand's disease, *Blood*, 51, 267, 1978.
131. **De Groot, P. G., Gonsalves, M. D., Loesberg, C., van Buul-Wortelboer, M. F., van Aken, W. G., and van Mourik, J. A.,** Thrombin-induced release of von Willebrand factor from endothelial cells is mediated by phospholipid methylation, *J. Biol. Chem.*, 259, 13329, 1984.
132. **Harrison, R. L. and McKee, P. A.,** Estrogen stimulates von Willebrand factor production by cultured endothelial cells, *Blood*, 63, 657, 1984.

133. **Maynard, J. R., Dreyer, B. E., Stemerman, M. B., and Pitlick, F. A.,** Tissue-factor coagulant activity of cultured human endothelial and smooth muscle cells and fibroblasts, *Blood,* 50, 387, 1977.
134. **Rodgers, G. M., Greenberg, C. S., and Shuman, M. A.,** Characterization of the effects of cultured vascular cells on the activation of blood coagulation, *Blood,* 61, 1155, 1983.
135. **Cerveny, T. J., Fass, D. N., and Mann, K. G.,** Synthesis of coagulation factor V by cultured aortic endothelial cells, *Blood,* 63, 1467, 1984.
136. **Johnsen, U. L. H., Lyberg, T., Galdal, K. S., and Prydz, H.,** Platelets stimulate thromboplastin synthesis in human endothelial cells, *Thromb. Haemost.,* 49, 69, 1983.
137. **Brox, J. H., Osterud, B., Bjorklid, E., and Fenton, J. W.,** Production and availability of thromboplastin in endothelial cells: the effects of thrombin, endotoxin, and platelets, *Br. J. Haematol.,* 57, 239, 1984.
138. **Stern, D. M., Drillings, M., Nossel, H. L., Hurlet-Jensen, A., Lagamma, K., and Owen, J.,** Binding of factors IX and IXa to cultured vascular endothelial cells, *Proc. Natl. Acad. Sci. U.S.A.,* 80, 4119, 1983.
139. **Heimark, R. L. and Schwartz, S. M.,** Binding of coagulation factors IX and X to the endothelial cell surface, *Biochem. Biophys. Res. Commun.,* 111, 723, 1983.
140. **Chan, V. and Chan, T. K.,** Antithrombin III in fresh and cultured human endothelial cells: a natural anticoagulant from vascular endothelium, *Thromb. Res.,* 15, 209, 1979.
141. **Isaacs, J., Savion, N., Gospodarowicz, D., and Schuman, M. A.,** Effect of cell density on thrombin binding to a specific site on bovine vascular endothelial cells, *J. Cell Biol.,* 90, 670, 1981.
142. **Knauer, D. J. and Cunningham, D. D.,** Protease nexins: cell-secreted proteins which regulate extracellular serine proteinases, *Trends Biochem. Sci.,* 9, 231, 1984.
143. **Loskutoff, D. J. and Edgington, T. S.,** Synthesis of a fibrinolytic activator and inhibitor by endothelial cells, *Proc. Natl. Acad. Sci. U.S.A.,* 74, 3903, 1977.
144. **Levin, E. G. and Loskutoff, D. J.,** Cultured bovine endothelial cells produce both urokinase and tissue-type plasminogen activators, *J. Cell Biol.,* 94, 631, 1982.
145. **Booyse, F. M., Osikowicz, G., Feder, S., and Scheinbuks, J.,** Isolation and characterization of a urokinase-type plasminogen activator (Mr = 54,000) from cultured human endothelial cells indistinguishable from urinary urokinase, *J. Biol. Chem.,* 259, 7138, 1984.
146. **van Mourik, J. A., Lawrence, D. A., and Loskutoff, D. J.,** Purification of an inhibitor of plasminogen activator (antiactivator) synthesized by endothelial cells, *J. Biol. Chem.,* 259, 14,914, 1984.
147. **Sprengers, E. D., Verheigen, J. H., van Hinsbergh, V. W., and Emeis, J. J.,** Evidence for the presence of two different fibrinolytic inhibitors in human endothelial cell conditioned medium, *Biochim. Biophys. Acta,* 801, 163, 1984.
148. **Loskutoff, D. J., van Mourik, J. A., Erickson, L. A., and Lawrence, D.,** Detection of an unusually stable fibrinolytic inhibitor produced by bovine endothelial cells, *Proc. Natl. Acad. Sci. U.S.A.,* 80, 2956, 1983.
149. **Levin, E. G. and Loskutoff, D. J.,** Comparative studies of the fibrinolytic activity of cultured vascular cells, *Thromb. Res.,* 15, 869, 1979.
150. **Levin, E. G., Marzec, U., Anderson, J., and Harker, L. A.,** Thrombin stimulates tissue plasminogen activator release from cultured human endothelial cells, *J. Clin. Invest.,* 74, 1988, 1984.
151. **Moncada, S., Gryglewski, R., Bunting, S., and Vane, J. R.,** An enzyme isolated from arteries transforms prostaglandin endoperoxides to an unstable substance that inhibits platelet aggregation, *Nature (London),* 263, 663, 1976.
152. **Gryglewski, R., Bunting, S., Moncada, S., and Vane, J. R.,** Arterial walls are protected against deposition of platelet thrombi by a substance (prostaglandin x) which they make from prostaglandin endoperoxides, *Prostaglandins,* 12, 685, 1976.
153. **Czervionke, R. L., Smith, J. B., Fry, G. L., Hoak, J. C., and Haycraft, D. L.,** Inhibition of prostacyclin by treatment with aspirin. Correlation with platelet adherence, *J. Clin. Invest.,* 63, 1089, 1979.
154. **Raz, A., Isakson, P. C., Minkes, M. S., and Needleman, P.,** Characterization of a novel metabolic pathway of arachidonate in coronary arteries which generates a potent coronary vasodilator, *J. Biol. Chem.,* 252, 1123, 1977.
155. **Weksler, B. B., Marcus, A. J., and Jaffe, E. A.,** Synthesis of prostaglandin I_2 (prostacyclin) by cultured human and bovine endothelial cells, *Proc. Natl. Acad. Sci. U.S.A.,* 74, 3922, 1977.
156. **Marcus, A. J., Weksler, B. B., and Jaffe, E. A.,** Enzymatic conversion of prostaglandin endoperoxide H_2 and arachidonic acid to prostacyclin by cultured human endothelial cells, *J. Biol. Chem.,* 253, 7138, 1978.
157. **Ingerman-Wojenski, C., Silver, M. J., Smith, J. B., and Macarak, E.,** Bovine endothelial cells in culture produce thromboxane as well as prostacyclin, *J. Clin. Invest.,* 67, 1292, 1981.
158. **Weksler, B. B., Ley, C. W., and Jaffe, E. A.,** Stimulation of endothelial prostacyclin production by thrombin, trypsin, and the ionophore A 23187, *J. Clin. Invest.,* 62, 923, 1978.
159. **Hong, S. L.,** Effect of bradykinin and thrombin on prostacyclin synthesis in endothelial cells from calf and pig-aorta and human umbilical vein, *Thromb. Res.,* 18, 787, 1980.

160. **Baenziger, N. L., Force, L. E., and Becherer, P. R.,** Histamine stimulates prostacyclin synthesis in cultured human endothelial cells, *Biochim. Biophys. Res. Commun.*, 92, 1435, 1980.
161. **Baenziger, N. L., Fogerty, F. J., Mertz, L. F., and Chernuta, L. F.,** Regulation of histamine-mediated prostacyclin synthesis in cultured human vascular endothelial cells, *Cell*, 24, 915, 1981.
162. **Fleisher, L. N., Tall, A. R., Witte, L. D., Miller, R. W., and Cannon, P. J.,** Stimulation of arterial endothelial cells prostacyclin synthesis by high-density lipoproteins, *J. Biol. Chem.*, 257, 6653, 1982.
163. **Coughlin, S. R., Moskowitz, A. M., Zetter, B. R., Antoniades, H. N., and Levine, L.,** Platelet-dependent stimulation of prostacyclin synthesis by platelet-derived growth factor, *Nature (London)*, 288, 600, 1980.
164. **Pearson, J. D., Slakey, L. L., and Gordon, J. L.,** Stimulation of prostaglandin production through purinergic receptors on endothelial cells and macrophages, *Biochem. J.*, 214, 273, 1983.
165. **Boogaerts, M. A., Vermylen, A. J., Deckmyn, H., Roelant, C., Verwilgen, R. L., Jacob, H. S., and Moldow, C. F.,** Enkephalins modify granulocyte-endothelial interactions by stimulating prostacyclin production, *Thromb. Haemost.*, 50, 572, 1983.
166. **Cramer, E. B., Pologe, L., Pawlowski, N. A., Cohn, Z. A., and Scott, W. A.,** Leukotriene C promotes prostacyclin synthesis by human endothelial cells, *Proc. Natl. Acad. Sci. U.S.A.*, 80, 4109, 1983.
167. **Busacca, M., Dejana, E., Balconi, G., Olivieri, S., Pietra, A., Vergara-Dauden, M., and De Gaetano, G.,** Reduced prostacyclin production by cultured endothelial cells from umbilical arteries of babies born to women who smoke, *Lancet*, 2, 609, 1982.
168. **Jaffe, E. A. and Weksler, B. B.,** Recovery of endothelial cell prostacyclin production after inhibition by low doses of aspirin, *J. Clin. Invest.*, 63, 532, 1979.
169. **Prescott, S. M., Zimmerman, G. A., and McIntyre, T. M.,** Human endothelial cells in culture produce platelet-activating factor (1-alkyl-2-acetyl-sn-glycero-3-phosphocholine) when stimulated with thrombin, *Proc. Natl. Acad. Sci. U.S.A.*, 81, 3514, 1984.
170. **Vanhoutte, P. M., Rimele, T. J., and Rooke, T. W.,** Calcium entry and the contraction of vascular smooth muscle, in *Advances in Cyclic Nucleotide and Protein Phosphorylation Research*, Vol. 17, Greengard, P., Ed., Raven Press, New York, 1984, 569.
171. **Burnstock, G.,** Neurohumoral control of blood vessels: some future directions, *J. Cardiovasc. Pharmacol.*, 7, 5137, 1985.
172. **Burnstock, G.,** Do some nerve cells release more than one transmitter?, *Neuroscience*, 1, 239, 1976.
173. **Furchgott, R. F. and Zawadzki, J. V.,** The obligatory role of endothelial cells in the relaxation of arterial smooth muscle by acetylcholine, *Nature (London)*, 288, 373, 1980.
174. **De Mey, J. G. and Vanhoutte, P. M.,** Role of the intima in cholinergic and purinergic relaxation of isolated canine femoral arteries, *J. Physiol.*, 316, 347, 1981.
175. **Furchgott, R. F.,** Role of endothelium in responses of vascular smooth muscle, *Circ. Res.*, 53, 557, 1983.
176. **Furchgott, R. F.,** The role of endothelium in the responses of vascular smooth muscle to drugs, *Annu. Rev. Pharmacol. Toxicol.*, 24, 175, 1984.
177. **Griffith, T. M., Edwards, D. H., Lewis, M. J., Newby, A. C., and Henderson, A. H.,** The nature of endothelium-derived vascular relaxant factor, *Nature (London)*, 308, 645, 1984.
178. **Förstermann, U., Trogisch, G., and Busse, R.,** Species-dependent differences in the nature of endothelium-derived vascular relaxing factor, *Eur. J. Pharmacol.*, 106, 639, 1985.
179. **Furchgott, R. F.,** The requirement for endothelial cells in the relaxation of arteries by: acetylcholine and some other vasodilators, *Trends Pharmacol. Sci.*, 2, 173, 1981.
180. **Van de Voorde, J. and Leusen, J.,** Role of endothelium in the vasodilator response of rat thoracic aorta to histamine, *Eur. J. Pharmacol.*, 87, 113, 1983.
181. **Furchgott, R. F., Cherry, P. D., and Zawadzki, J. V.,** Endothelium dependent relaxation of arteries by acetylcholine, bradykinin and other agents, in *Vascular Neuroeffector Mechanisms*, Bevan, J., Ed., Raven Press, New York, 1983, 37.
182. **Cherry, P. D., Furchgott, R. F., Zawadzki, J. V., and Jothianandan, D.,** The role of endothelial cells in the relaxation of isolated arteries by bradykinin, *Proc. Natl. Acad. Sci. U.S.A.*, 79, 2106, 1982.
183. **DeMey, J. G., Claeys, M., and Vanhoutte, P. M.,** Endothelial-dependent inhibitory effects of acetylcholine, adenosine triphosphate, thrombin and arachidonic acid in the canine femoral artery, *J. Pharmacol. Exp. Ther.*, 222, 166, 1982.
184. **DeMey, J. G. and Vanhoutte, P. M.,** Heterogenous behavior of the canine arterial and venous wall, *Circ. Res.*, 51, 439, 1982.
185. **Blumberg, A. L., Denny, S. E., Marshall, G. R., and Needleman, P. A.,** Blood vessel-hormone interactions: angiotensin, bradykinin and prostaglandin, *Am. J. Physiol.*, 232, H305, 1977.
186. **Cohen, R. A., Shepherd, J. T., and Vanhoutte, P. M.,** Inhibitory role of the endothelium in the response of isolated coronary arteries to platelets, *Science*, 221, 273, 1983.
187. **Burnstock, G.,** A basis for distinguishing two types of purinergic receptor, in *Cell Membrane Receptors for Drugs and Hormones: a Multidisciplinary Approach*, Balis, L. and Straub, R. W., Eds., Raven Press, New York, 1978, 107.

188. **Vizi, E. S.,** Presynaptic modulation of neurochemical transmission, *Prog. Neurobiol.,* 12, 181, 1979.
189. **DiCorleto, P. E. and Bowen-Pope, D. F.,** Cultured endothelial cells produce a platelet-derived growth factor-like protein, *Proc. Natl. Acad. Sci. U.S.A.,* 80, 1919, 1983.
190. **Kazlauskas, A. and DiCorleto, P. E.,** Cultured endothelial cells do not respond to a platelet-derived growth-factor-like protein in an autocrine manner, *Biochim. Biophys. Acta,* 846, 405, 1985.
191. **Gajdusek, C. M. and Schwartz, S. M.,** Ability of endothelial cells to condition culture medium, *J. Cell. Physiol.,* 110, 35, 1982.
192. **Castellot, J. J., Addonizo, M. L., Rosenberg, R., and Karnovsky, M. J.,** Cultured endothelial cells produce a heparin-like inhibitor of smooth muscle cell growth, *J. Cell Biol.,* 90, 372, 1981.
193. **Machovich, R.,** Choices among the possible reaction routes catalyzed by thrombin, *Ann. N.Y. Acad. Sci.,* 485, 170, 1986.
194. **Smith, G. F.,** Fibrinogen — the specific thrombin substrate, in *The Thrombin,* Vol. 1, Machovich, R., Ed., CRC Press, Boca Raton, Fla., 1984, 55.
195. **White, G. C., Knupp, C. L., and Lundblad, R. L.,** The interaction of thrombin with platelets, in *The Thrombin,* Vol. 2, Machovich, R., Ed., CRC Press, Boca Raton, Fla., 1984, 25.
196. **Muszbek, L. and Laki, K.,** Interaction of thrombin with proteins other than fibrinogen. Activation of Factor XIII, in *The Thrombin,* Vol. 1, Machovich, R., Ed., CRC Press, Boca Raton, Fla., 1984, 83.
197. **Machovich, R.,** Thrombin and hemostasis, in *The Thrombin,* Vol. 1, Machovich, R., Ed., CRC Press, Boca Raton, Fla., 1984, 1.
198. **Machovich, R.,** Inactivation of thrombin by plasma proteinase inhibitors, in *The Thrombin,* Vol. 2, Machovich, R., Ed., CRC Press, Boca Raton, Fla., 1984, 1.
199. **Awbrey, B. J., Hoak, J. C., and Owen, W. G.,** Binding of human thrombin to cultured human endothelial cells, *J. Biol. Chem.,* 254, 4092, 1979.
200. **Lollar, P., Hoak, J. C., and Owen, W. G.,** Binding of thrombin to cultured human endothelial cells: nonequilibrium aspects, *J. Biol. Chem.,* 255, 10279, 1980.
201. **Lollar, P. and Owen, W. G.,** Clearance of thrombin from circulation in rabbits by high affinity binding sites on endothelium, *J. Clin. Invest.,* 66, 1222, 1980.
202. **Marcum, J. A., McKennay, J. B., and Rosenberg, R. D.,** Acceleration of thrombin-antithrombin complex formation in rat hindquarters via heparin-like molecules bound to the endothelium, *J. Clin. Invest.,* 74, 341, 1984.
203. **Esmon, C. T. and Owen, W. G.,** Identification of an endothelial cell cofactor for thrombin-catalyzed activation of protein C, *Proc. Natl. Acad. Sci. U.S.A.,* 78, 2249, 1981.
204. **Jakubowski, H. V. and Owen, W. G.,** Effect of bovine thrombomodulin on thrombin specificity, *Thromb. Haemostas.,* 54, 119, 1985.
205. **Gebremedhin, D., Ballagi-Pordany, G., Hadhazi, P., Magyar, K., and Machovich, R.,** Species specificity of thrombin-induced changes in vascular tone, *Eur. J. Pharmacol.,* 132, 71, 1986.
206. **Kisiel, W., Canfield, W. M., Ericsson, L. A., and Davie, E. W.,** Anticoagulant properties of bovine plasma protein C following activation by thrombin, *Biochemistry,* 16, 5824, 1977.
207. **Walker, F. J., Sexton, P. W., and Esmon, C. T.,** The inhibition of blood coagulation by activated protein C through the selective inactivation of activated factor V, *Biochim. Biophys. Acta,* 571, 333, 1979.
208. **Esmon, C. T., Esmon, N. L., and Harris, K. W.,** Complex formation between thrombin and thrombomodulin inhibits both thrombin-catalyzed fibrin formation and factor V activation, *J. Biol. Chem.,* 257, 7944, 1982.
209. **Esmon, N. L., Carrel, R. C., and Esmon, C. T.,** Thrombomodulin blocks the ability of thrombin to activate platelets, *J. Biol. Chem.,* 258, 12238, 1983.
210. **Maruyama, I. and Majerus, P. W.,** The turnover of thrombin-thrombomodulin complex in cultured human umbilical vein endothelial cells and A 549 lung cancer cells, endocytosis and degradation of thrombin, *J. Biol. Chem.,* 260, 15432, 1985.
211. **Savion, N., Isaacs, J. D., Gospodarowicz, D., and Schuman, M. A.,** Internalization and degradation of thrombin and up regulation of thrombin-binding sites in corneal endothelial cells, *J. Biol. Chem.,* 256, 4514, 1981.
212. **Hatton, M. W. C. and Mour, S.,** Uptake and catabolism of ^{125}I-thrombin by the rabbit thoracic aorta in vitro: permeability of the endothelium, intima-media and adventitial layers, *Thromb. Haemost.,* 52, 105, 1984.
213. **Payling-Wright, H.,** Endothelial turnover, in *Vascular Factors and Thrombosis,* Koller, F., Ed., Schattauer, Stuttgart, 1970, 79.
214. **Schwartz, S. M. and Benditt, E. P.,** Cell replication in the aortic endothelium: a new method for study of the problem, *Lab. Invest.,* 28, 699, 1973.
215. **Engerman, R. L., Pfaffenbach, D., and Davis, M. D.,** Cell turnover of capillaries, *Lab. Invest.,* 17, 738, 1967.
216. **Björkerud, S.,** Injury and repair in arterial tissue, *Angiology,* 25, 636, 1974.

217. **Ross, R. and Harker, L.,** Hyperlipidemia and atherosclerosis, *Science,* 193, 1044, 1976.
218. **Stemermas, M. B., Spaet, T. H., Pitlick, F., Cintron, J., Lejnieks, I., and Tiell, M. L.,** Intimal healing: the patterns of reendothelialization and intimal thickening, *Am. J. Pathol.,* 87, 125, 1977.
219. **Poole, J. C. F., Cromwell, S. B., and Benditt, E. P.,** Behavior of smooth muscle cells and formation of extracellular structures in the reaction of arterial wall cells to injury, *Am. J. Pathol.,* 62, 391, 1970.
220. **Schwartz, S. M. and Benditt, E. P.,** Clustering of replicating cells in aortic endothelium, *Proc. Natl. Acad. Sci. U.S.A.,* 73, 651, 1976.
221. **Schwartz, S. M., Gajdusek, C. M., Reidy, M. A., Selden, S. C., and Haudenschild, C. C.,** Maintenance of integrity in aortic endothelium, *Fed. Proc.,* 39, 2618, 1980.
222. **James, R. and Bradshaw, R. A.,** Polypeptide growth factors, *Annu. Rev. Biochem.,* 53, 259, 1984.
223. **Widmann, J. J. and Fahimi, H. D.,** Proliferation of endothelial cells in oestrogen-stimulated rat liver. A light and electron microscopic cytochemical study, *Lab. Invest.,* 34, 141, 1976.
224. **Maca, R. D., Fry, G. L., and Hoak, J. C.,** The effect of glucocorticoids on cultured human endothelial cells, *Br. J. Haematol.,* 38, 501, 1978.
225. **Nichols, N. R., Lloyd, C. J., Mendelsohn, F. A. D., and Funder, J. W.,** Glucocorticoid-induced proteins in bovine endothelial cells, *Mol. Cell. Endocrinol.,* 32, 245, 1983.
226. **Hoshi, H. and McKeehan, W. L.,** Brain- and liver cell-derived factors are required for growth of human endothelial cells in serum-free culture, *Proc. Natl. Acad. Sci. U.S.A.,* 81, 6413, 1984.
227. **Maciag, T., Hoover, G. A., and Weinstein, R.,** High and low molecular weight forms of endothelial cell growth factor, *J. Biol. Chem.,* 257, 5333, 1982.
228. **Schreiber, A. B., Kenney, J., Kowalski, W. J., Friesel, R., Mehlman, T., and Maciag, T.,** Interaction of endothelial cell growth factor with heparin: characterization by receptor and antibody recognition, *Proc. Natl. Acad. Sci. U.S.A.,* 82, 6138, 1985.
229. **Thomas, K. A., Rios-Candelore, M., Gimenez-Gallego, G., DiSalvo, J., Bennett, C., Rodkey, J., and Fitzpatrick, S.,** Pure brain-derived acidic fibroblast growth factor is a potent angiogenic vascular endothelial cell mitogen with sequence homology to interleukin 1, *Proc. Natl. Acad. Sci. U.S.A.,* 82, 6409, 1985.
230. **Macarak, E. J., Howard, B. V., and Kefalides, A. N.,** Properties of calf endothelial cells in culture, *Lab. Invest.,* 36, 62, 1977.
231. **Schwartz, S. M.,** Selection and characterization of bovine aortic endothelial cells, *In Vitro,* 14, 966, 1978.
232. **Gospodarowicz, D. and Mecher, A. L.,** The control of cellular proliferation by the fibroblast and epidermal growth factors, *Natl. Cancer Inst. Mongr.,* 48, 109, 1978.
233. **Gospodarowicz, D., Moran, J., Braun, D., and Birdwell, C.,** Clonal growth of bovine vascular endothelial cells: fibroblast growth factor as a survival agent, *Proc. Natl. Acad. Sci. U.S.A.,* 73, 4120, 1976.
234. **McAuslan, B. R., Hannan, G. N., and Reilly, W.,** Signals causing change in morphological phenotype, growth mode, and gene expression of vascular endothelial cells, *J. Cell. Physiol.,* 112, 96, 1982.
235. **Malczak, H. T. and Buck, R. C.,** Regeneration of endothelium in rat aorta after local freezing, *Am. J. Pathol.,* 86, 133, 1977.
236. **Barnhart, M. I. and Baechler, C. A.,** Endothelial cell physiology, perturbations and responses, *Sem. Thromb. Hemost.,* 5, 50, 1978.
237. **Schwartz, S. M., Haudenschild, C. C., and Eddy, E. M.,** Endothelial regeneration I: quantitative analysis of initial stages of endothelial regeneration in rat aortic intima, *Lab. Invest.,* 38, 568, 1978.
238. **Haudenschild, C. and Schwartz, S. M.,** Endothelial regeneration. II. Restitution of endothelial continuity, *Lab. Invest.,* 41, 407, 1979.
239. **Minick, C. R., Stemerman, M. B., and Insull, W., Jr.,** Effect of regenerated endothelium on lipid accumulation in the arterial wall, *Proc. Natl. Acad. Sci. U.S.A.,* 74, 1724, 1977.
240. **Folkman, J. and Haudenschild, C.,** Angiogenesis in vitro: implications for tumor biology, in *Pathobiology of the Endothelial Cell,* Nossel, H. L. and Vogel, H. J., Eds., Academic Press, New York, 1982, 79.
241. **Folkman, J.,** The vascularization of tumors, *Sci. Am.,* 234, 58, 1976.
242. **Folkman, J.,** Tumor angiogenesis, *Adv. Cancer Res.,* 19, 331, 1974.
243. **Folkman, J. and Haudenschild, C.,** Angiogenesis in vitro, *Nature (London),* 288, 551, 1980.
244. **McAuslan, B. R., Reilly, W. G., Hannan, G. N., and Gole, G. A.,** Angiogenic factors and their assay: activity of formyl methionyl leucyl phenylalanine, adenosine diphosphate, heparin, copper, and bovine endothelium stimulating factor, *Microvasc. Res.,* 26, 323, 1983.
245. **McAuslan, B. R. and Hoffman, H.,** Endothelium stimulating factor from Walker carcinoma cells: relation to tumor angiogenic factor, *Exp. Cell Res.,* 119, 181, 1979.
246. **Weiss, J. B., Brown, R. A., Kumar, S., and Phillips, P.,** An angiogenic factor isolated from tumors: a potent low molecular weight compound, *Br. J. Cancer,* 40, 493, 1979.
247. **Fenselau, A., Watt, S., and Mello, R. J.,** Tumor angiogenic factor. Purification from the Walker 256 rat tumor, *J. Biol. Chem.,* 256, 9605, 1981.
248. **Zetter, B. R.,** Migration of capillary endothelial cells is stimulated by tumor-derived factors, *Nature (London),* 285, 41, 1980.

249. **McAuslan, B. R. and Reilly, N.,** Endothelial cell phagokinesis in response to specific metal ions, *Exp. Cell Res.,* 130, 147, 1980.
250. **Taylor, S. and Folkman, J.,** Protamine is an inhibitor of angiogenesis, *Nature (London),* 297, 307, 1982.
251. **Ziche, M., Jones, J., and Gullino, P. M.,** Role of prostaglandin E_1 and copper in angiogenesis, *J. Natl. Cancer Inst.,* 69, 475, 1982.
252. **Goodwin, J. S., Husby, G., and Williams, R. C.,** Prostaglandin E_2 and cancer growth, *Cancer Immunol. Immunother.,* 8, 3, 1980.
253. **Ungar-Waron, H., Gluckman, A., Spira, E., Waron, M., and Trainin, Z.,** Ceruloplasmin as a marker of neoplastic activity in rabbits bearing the VX-2 carcinoma, *Cancer Res.,* 38, 1296, 1978.
254. **Raju, K. S., Alessandri, G., Ziche, M., and Gullino, P. M.,** Ceruloplasmin, copper ions, and angiogenesis, *J. Natl. Cancer Inst.,* 69, 1183, 1982.
255. **Folkman, J.,** Angiogenesis: initiation and control, *Ann. N.Y. Acad. Sci.,* 401, 212, 1982.
256. **Azizkhan, R. G., Azizkhan, J. C., Zetter, B. R., and Folkman, J.,** Mast cell heparin stimulates migration of capillary endothelial cells in vitro, *J. Exp. Med.,* 152, 931, 1980.
257. **Fromer, C. H. and Klintworth, G. K.,** An evaluation of the role of leukocytes in the pathogenesis of experimentally induced corneal neovascularization. II. Studies on the effect of leukocyte elimination on corneal vascularization, *Am. J. Pathol.,* 81, 531, 1975.
258. **McAuslan, B. R. and Gole, G. A.,** Cellular and molecular mechanisms in angiogenesis, *Trans. Ophthalmol. Soc. U.K.,* 100, 354, 1980.
259. **Shing, Y., Folkman, J., Sullivan, R., Butterfield, C., Murray, J., and Klagsbrun, M.,** Heparin affinity: purification of a tumor-derived capillary endothelial cell growth factor, *Science,* 223, 1296, 1984.
260. **Fishman, A. P.,** Endothelium: a distributed organ of diverse capabilities, *Ann. N.Y. Acad. Sci. U.S.A.,* 401, 1, 1982.
261. **Jaffe, E. A., Nachman, R. L., Becker, C. G., and Minick, C. R.,** Culture of human endothelial cells derived from umbilical veins, Identification by morphological and immunological criteria, *J. Clin. Invest.,* 52, 2745, 1973.
262. **Gimbrone, M. A., Cotran, R. S., and Folkman, J.,** Human vascular endothelial cells in culture: growth and DNA synthesis, *J. Cell Biol.,* 60, 673, 1974.
263. **Galdal, K. S. and Evensen, S. A.,** Effects of divalent cations and various vasoactive and hemostatically active agents on the integrity of monolayers of cultured human endothelial cells, *Thromb. Res.,* 21, 273, 1981.
264. **Maciag, T., Hoover, G. A., Spek, J., Stemerman, M. B., and Weinstein, R.,** Growth and differentiation of human umbilical-vein endothelial cells in culture, in *Growth of Cells in Hormonally Defined Media,* Vol. 9A, Sato, G. H., Pardee, A. B., and Sirbasku, D. A., Eds., Cold Spring Harbor Laboratory, Cold Spring Harbor, N.Y., 1982, 525.
265. **Fitzgerald, L. A., Charo, I. F., and Phillips, D. R.,** Human and bovine endothelial cells synthesize membrane proteins similar to human platelet glycoproteins IIb and IIIa, *J. Biol. Chem.,* 260, 10893, 1985.
266. **van Buul-Wortelboer, M. F., Brinkman, J. J. M., Dingemans, K. P., De Groot, Ph. G., van Aken, W. G., and van Mourik, J. A.,** Reconstitution of the vascular wall in vitro. A novel model to study interactions between endothelial and smooth muscle cells, *Exp. Cell Res.,* 162, 151, 1986.
267. **Booyse, F. M., Sedlock, B. J., and Rafelson, M. E.,** Culture of arterial endothelial cells. Characterization and growth of bovine aortic cells, *Thromb. Diath. Haemorrh.,* 34, 825, 1975.
268. **Levin, E. G. and Loskutoff, D. J.,** Serum-mediated suppression of cell-associated plasminogen activator activity in cultured endothelial cells, *Cell,* 22, 701, 1980.
269. **Hagiwara, H., Ohtsu, Y., Shimonaka, M., and Inada, Y.,** Ca^{2+}- or Mg^{2+}-dependent ATPase in plasma membrane of cultured endothelial cells from bovine carotid arteries, *Biochim. Biophys. Acta,* 734, 133, 1983.
270. **Csonka, E., Szemenyei, K., Miskulin, M., and Robert, A. M.,** Morphological examination of aortic endothelial and smooth muscle cells grown in vitro on collagen membranes, *Artery,* 8, 253, 1980.
271. **Junod, A. F., Clément, A., Jornot, L., and Petersen, H.,** Differential effects of hyperoxia and hydrogen peroxide on thymidine kinase and adenosine kinase activities of cultured endothelial cells, *Biochim. Biophys. Acta,* 847, 20, 1985.
272. **Csonka, E., Kerényi, T., Koch, A. S., and Jellinek, A.,** In vitro cultivation and identification of aortic endothelium from miniature pig, *Arterial Wall,* 3, 31, 1975.
273. **Csonka, E., Kádár, A., Kerényi, T., and Jellinek, H.,** Morphology of cultured endothel and smooth muscle cells of different origin, *Acta Morphol.,* 14, 18, 1973.
274. **DeBault, L. E., Esmon, N. L., and Esmon, C. T.,** The relationship between thrombomodulin expression and cell cycle stages in cultured rabbit endothelial cells, *Cytometry,* 5, 386, 1984.
275. **Hirsch, E. Z., Martino, W., Orr, C. H., White, H., and Chisolm, G. M.,** A simple rapid method for the preparation of en face endothelial (Häutchen) monolayers from rat and rabbit aortas, *Atherosclerosis,* 37, 539, 1980.

276. **Parshley, M. S., Cerreta, J. M., Mandl, I., Fierer, J. A., and Turino, G. U.,** Characteristics of a clone of endothelial cells derived from a line of normal adult rat lung cells, *In Vitro,* 15, 709, 1979.
277. **Picciano, P. T., Johnson, B., Walenga, R. W., Donovan, M., Borman, B. J., Douglas, W. H. J., and Kreutzer, D. L.,** Effect of D-valine on pulmonary artery endothelial cell morphology and function in cell culture, *Exp. Cell Res.,* 151, 134, 1984.
278. **Blomhoff, R., Smedsrød, B., Eskild, W., Granum, P. E., and Berg, T.,** Preparation of isolated liver endothelial cells and Kupffer cells in high yield by means of an enterotoxin, *Exp. Cell Res.,* 150, 194, 1984.
279. **Ford, J. B., Burkel, W. E., and Kahn, R. H.,** Isolation of adult canine venous endothelium for tissue culture, *In Vitro,* 17, 44, 1981.
280. **Bowman, P. D., Betz, A. L., Ar, D., Wolinsky, J. S., Penney, J. B., Shivers, R. R., and Goldstein, G. W.,** Primary culture of capillary endothelium from rat brain, *In Vitro,* 17, 353, 1981.
281. **DeBault, L. E., Henriquez, E., Hart, M. N., and Cancilla, P. A.,** Cerebral microvessels and derived cells in tissue culture. II. Establishment, identification and preliminary characterization of an endothelial cell line, *In Vitro,* 17, 480, 1981.
282. **Folkman, J., Haudenschild, C., and Zetter, B.,** Capillary endothelial cells: growth control and differentiation, in *Growth of Cells in Hormonally Defined Media,* Vol. 1A, Sato, G. H., Pardee, A. B., and Sirbasku, D. A., Eds., Cold Spring Harbor Laboratory, Cold Spring Harbor, N.Y., 1982, 509.
283. **Banerjee, D. K., Ornberg, R. L., Youdim, M. B. H., Heldman, E., and Pollard, H. B.,** Endothelial cells from bovine adrenal medulla develop capillary-like growth pattern in culture, *Proc. Natl. Acad. Sci. U.S.A.,* 82, 4702, 1985.
284. **Gibofsky, A., Jaffe, E. A., Fotino, M., and Becker, C. G.,** The identification of HL-A antigens on fresh and cultured human endothelial cells, *J. Immunol.,* 115, 730, 1975.
285. **Buonassisi, V. and Root, M.,** Enzymatic degradation of heparin-related mucopolysaccharides from the surface of endothelial cell cultures, *Biochim. Biophys. Acta,* 385, 1, 1975.
286. **Polgar, J., Lerant, I., Muszbek, L., and Machovich, R.,** Thrombomodulin inhibits the activation of Factor XIII by thrombin, *Thromb. Res.,* 43, 585, 1986.
287. **Machovich, R.,** Role of the blood coagulation-fibrinolytic system and endothelial cells in malignancy, in *Hemostasis* and Cancer, Muszbek, L., Ed., CRC Press, Boca Raton, Fla., 1987, 1.
288. **Machovich, R. and Owen, G. W.,** unpublished data.

Chapter 5

THE STRUCTURE AND FUNCTION OF VASCULAR SMOOTH MUSCLE*

B. Lowell Langille and Avrum I. Gotlieb

TABLE OF CONTENTS

* This paper received the Toronto General Hospital's Gordon N. Fisher Prize for 1987.

I. INTRODUCTION

Vascular smooth muscle cells are the only cells found in the media of the normal adult blood vessel wall. As such, their functions are not limited to the regulation of contractile tone, but also involve the maintenance of arterial wall integrity. This is accomplished by the synthesis and secretion of connective tissue elements and associated extracellular substances. In addition, following vascular injury that involves endothelium, smooth muscle cells migrate to the luminal surface and carry out many functions of the endothelium, including thromboresistance, and thereby contribute to a complex and highly integrated repair process.

This chapter begins with a consideration of smooth muscle cell ultrastructure, including the relation of structure to contractile function. Some consideration will be given to the relation of smooth muscle cells to contiguous wall elements, but, for the most part, the reader is referred to Chapter 2 for a discussion of the integration of vessel wall constituents. Contractile behavior then will be examined with emphasis on excitation-contraction coupling. Particular attention will be paid to the initiation of contraction or vasospasm following vessel injury, including the direct effect of tissue injury and the influence of extravascular blood.

The synthesis of extracellular proteins and the factors that control this synthesis will be considered in conjunction with interactions between the cell and the matrix. Finally, we will examine control of smooth muscle cell proliferation and migration within the arterial wall and their relation to vascular injury and repair in both normal and disease states.

II. CONTRACTILE BEHAVIOR

A. Structure of Vascular Smooth Muscle

1. Cell Ultrastructure: Relation to Function

About 85% of the volume of the vascular smooth muscle cells consists of myofilaments, intermediate filaments, and dense bodies (Figure 1; for review, see Reference 1). The rest is made up of the nucleus, microtubules, mitochondria, Golgi apparatus, and the rough and smooth endoplasmic reticulum, which are often close to the nucleus. The cell membrane exhibits many caveolae (Figure 2) which increase the surface area of the cell by about 70%. Both adherens-type junctions and gap junctions are present between cells and a basal lamina is also present external to the cell coat.

The myofilaments consist of 7-nm actin filaments and larger 15-nm myosin filaments. There are also actin-associated proteins in smooth muscle, including α-actinin, filamin, and tropomyosin. Compared to those of skeletal muscle, the myosin filaments are more irregular in diameter and thickness. The molar ratio of actin to myosin is about 2.7, i.e., 12 times larger than that of the skeletal muscle,[2] and the ratio of the number of actin to myosin filaments in rabbit aorta is 15:1.[3] There is no organized pattern of sarcomeres between actin and myosin filaments as there is in skeletal muscle. Thin filaments insert into cytoplasmic densities (dense bodies),[5] both in the cytoplasm (Figure 1B) and along the cytoplasmic side of the cell membrane where they appear as very prominent bands or patches (Figure 2). The precise role of the dense bodies is not known; it is postulated that they may anchor thin filaments in a manner similar to that of the Z-disk of striated muscle. α-Actinin is localized in the dense bodies[4] and may be involved in such anchoring. The force transmission from the contractile apparatus to the cell membrane appears to be mediated by the actin filaments which insert into the dense bands along the cell membrane. Vinculin, the 130,000 dalton protein associated with adherens junctions, is present in these bands.[6]

2. The Contractile Apparatus

The normal function of smooth muscle cells is to maintain vascular tone and it is assumed that the actin-myosin myofilament system provides this function. Recently, studies using

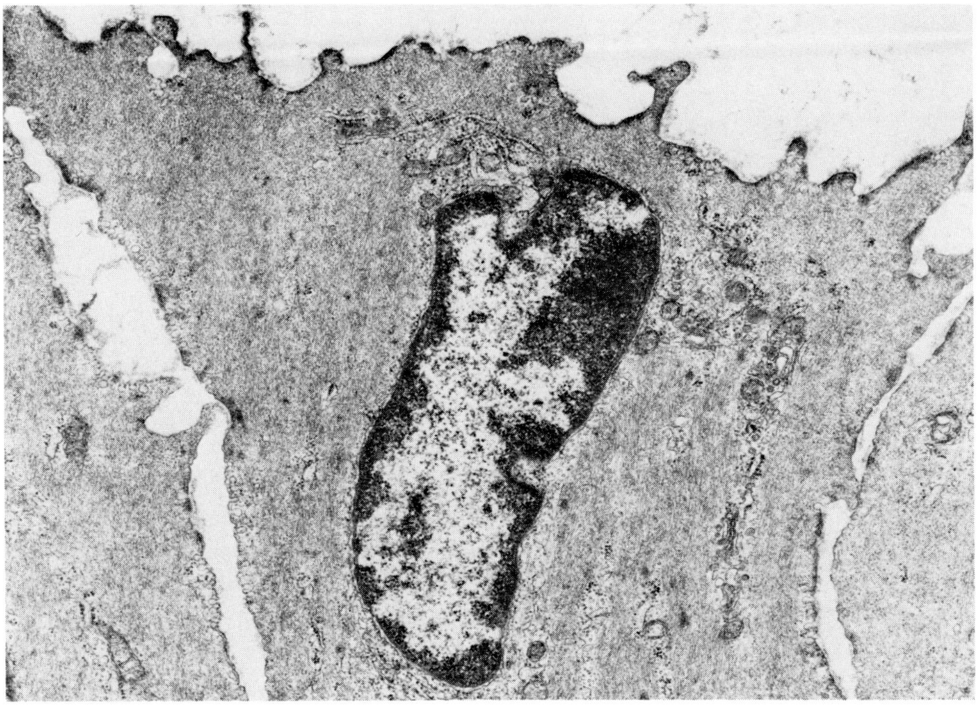

A

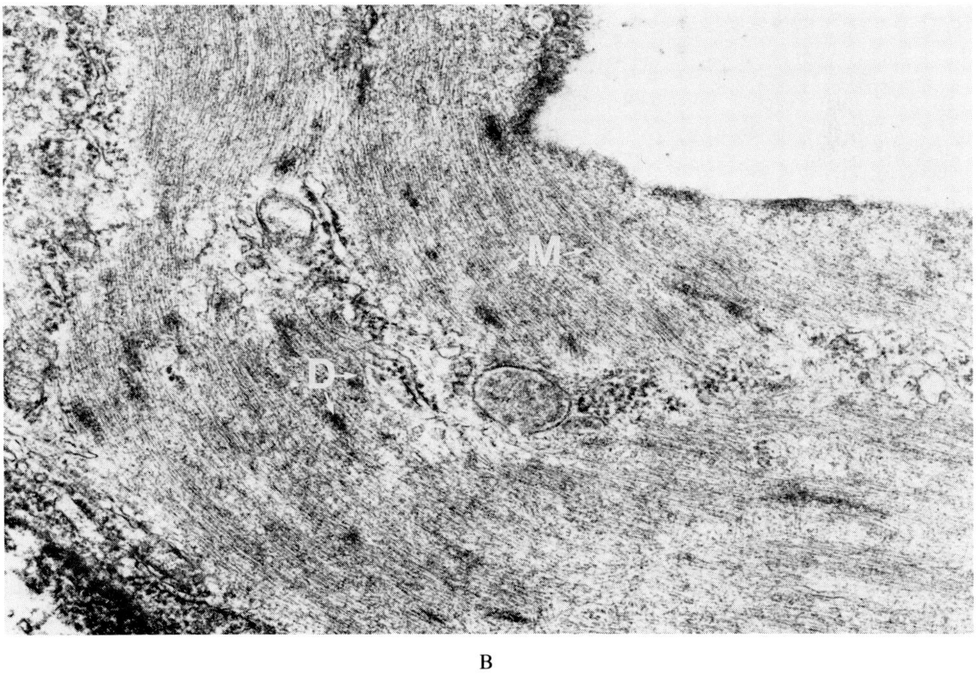

B

FIGURE 1. Electron micrographs of normal aortic medial smooth muscle cells. (A) Note sparse organelles. (Magnification ×17,940.) (B) Note cytoplasmic dense bodies (D) and myofilaments (M); N, nucleus. (Magnification × 33,856.)

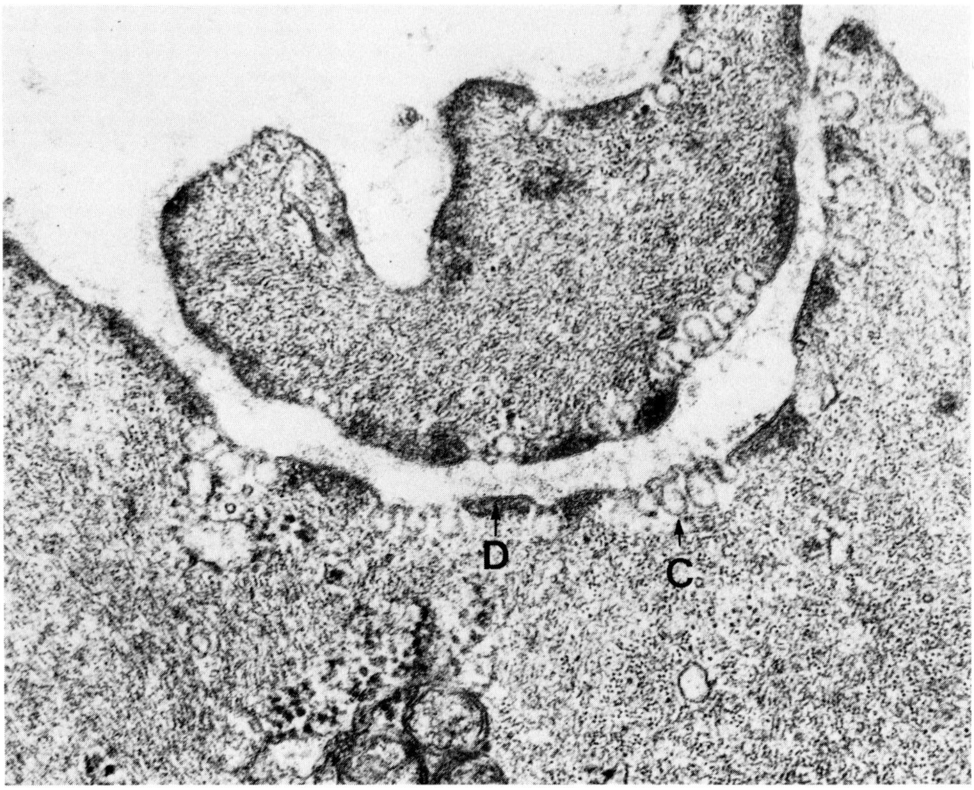

FIGURE 2. Electron micrograph of a normal aortic medial smooth muscle cell showing membrane associated dense bands (D) and caveolae (C). Caveolae are absent where the dense band is associated with the membrane. (Magnification × 63,000.)

electron microscope immunocytochemistry with colloidal gold probes[7] have shown that guinea pig taenia coli smooth muscle cells contain separate actomyosin domains and actin-intermediate filament domains. The former is made up of continuous longitudinal arrays of actin and myosin filaments and is thought to be responsible for contraction. The latter is made up of longitudinal, fibrillar, intermediate filament domains containing actin and α-actinin-rich dense bodies as well as filamin. This system may regulate slow relaxation and tone.

Vascular smooth muscle cells contain a predominance of α-actin, some β-actin, and very little γ-actin.[8] Smooth muscle cells of the neointima, which have undergone a change to a secretory (synthetic) phenotype following vascular injury, show both a decrease in the amount of actin and a change in the isotypes. β-Actin becomes the predominant type, while α-actin decreases and there is a significant increase in γ-actin.[8] These cells migrate and proliferate and it is possible that the change of actin isotype is related to the change in the functions of the cell.

Vascular smooth muscle myosin is antigenically distinct from cardiac, skeletal, and non-muscle myosin. Studies[9] have shown a heterogeneity of myosin antigenic expression in vascular smooth muscle. The functional significance of these observations is not known.

Medial smooth muscle cells also contain 10-nm intermediate filaments. Most medial smooth muscle cells contain vimentin while some contain both vimentin and desmin.[10] Following injury, the smooth muscle cells of the thickened intima contain increased amounts of vimentin and decreased amounts of desmin.[8] The functional significance is not known; however, it is possible that the vimentin-rich medial cells are the ones that migrate to the intima and proliferate.

B. Regulation of Vascular Smooth Muscle Tone

Contraction of vascular smooth muscle is regulated by a broad spectrum of factors including autonomic innervation, local metabolites, vessel wall distension, endocrine hormones, and paracrine and autocrine mediators. It is not surprising, therefore, that excitation processes are more complex than those involved in contraction of striated muscle. It appears that excitation of vascular smooth muscle, like skeletal muscle, is intimately linked to increases in intracellular Ca^{2+}, although Ca^{2+} release and the mechanisms by which this ion alters contractile state differ considerably. There also has been considerable controversy concerning the source(s) of activator Ca^{2+} in vascular smooth muscle, since the sarcoplasmic reticulum represents only 1.5 to 7.5% of cell volume. Other intracellular storage sites and transmembrane Ca^{2+} flux have been cited. Somlyo[11] recently reviewed studies in this area and argued that the SR acts as the primary source of Ca^{2+}, but this view is not universally accepted. Ratz and Murphy[12] argued that Ca^{2+} release from the sarcoplasmic reticulum and transmembrane fluxes serve different functions, the former initiating changes in tone and the latter supporting sustained "latch-bridge" formation.

1. Cell Membrane Electrical Activity

The relation between cell electrical activity, Ca^{2+} release, and contractile function in smooth muscle is not straightforward. First, resting transmembrane potential (E_m), which varies from -25 to -65 mV,[13] does not follow a simple Nernst relation for K^+, probably because of a significant permeability to Na^+. This assessment appears confirmed by measurements of a P_{Na}/P_k ratio of about 0.2,[14,15] which is an order of magnitude higher than in other excitable cells. Furthermore, the contribution of electrogenic active transport is variable. Casteels[16] observed a significant contribution to the resting membrane potential in guinea pig taenia coli, whereas no effect was reported for rat portal vein.[17] Interestingly, Hermsmeyer[18] reports that the electrogenic contribution to the membrane potential of rat arteries is enhanced in hypertensive animals.

The production of action potentials is tightly linked to contractile behavior in many vessels, although vasoactive substances can modulate excitation-contraction coupling.[19] Action potentials may follow prepotentials, may be linked to oscillations in E_m, and may exhibit extended plateaus.[13] In other vessels, such as the sheep carotid artery[20] or the rabbit ear and pulmonary arteries,[21,22] contractile activity appears independent of production of action potentials. Accordingly, Johansson and Somlyo's proposal may be the most meaningful way of classifying vascular smooth muscle. They make the distinction between vascular smooth muscle that exhibits action potentials which synchronize contraction in a population of cells and nonspike-generating cells that regulate tone via graded depolarization.[13]

It also appears that under some conditions, smooth muscle excitation by agonists may be decoupled from membrane electrical events. Invoking such "pharmacomechanical coupling" is required to explain why contractile responses to agonists frequently do not match contractile responses to K^+ that produce equal depolarizations or why agonists can induce responses in depolarized preparations.[23] Pharmacomechanical coupling is discussed further in Section II.B.3.

2. Activation of the Contractile Apparatus

In striated muscle, the liberation of Ca^{2+} from intracellular stores triggers contraction through "disinhibition" of the troponin-tropomyosin system, i.e., Ca^{2+} binding to troponin C causes a conformational change of the thin filaments that permits cross-bridge attachment and cycling. In smooth muscle, sensitivity of activation to Ca^{2+} is not abolished in purified actomyosin, i.e., in the absence of tropomyosin.[24,25] Instead Ca^{2+} regulation is associated with myosin and is mediated through the activation of a myosin light chain kinase. A Ca^{2+}-calmodulin complex binds to, and activates, the kinase and the subsequent phosphorylation of a myosin light chain reverses an inhibition of actin-induced actomyosin ATPase activity.[26]

A second mechanism proposed for Ca^{2+} regulation of contraction[27] involves the protein leitonin, which is associated with thin filaments. Leitonin has Ca^{2+} binding and regulatory moieties. Its mode of action is unclear since there appears to be too little leitonin associated with each actin filament to permit the type of conformational changes that the troponin-tropomyosin system initiates in skeletal muscle to allow cross-bridge attachment.[28]

3. Physiological Regulation of Vascular Tone

Vascular smooth muscle contraction is regulated by neural, hormonal, and local factors that subserve both central homeostatic controls (fluid balance, baroreceptor function, etc.) and local tissue requirements. The former involves regulation via the autonomic nervous system, the renin-angiotensin system, and adrenal hormones. The latter involves local by-products of metabolism that adjust blood flow to energy consumption. In addition, prostanoids and bradykinin mediate many specialized local responses, including those associated with inflammation and vessel injury. Biophysical factors also exert fundamental controls over vascular tone. Obvious examples include the effects of temperature on vascular perfusion and myogenic regulation, through which distension of the vessel wall induces smooth muscle contraction so that a net ''autoregulation'' occurs.[29]

Recently, there has been increasing interest in the influence of local shear forces transmitted to the vessel wall from intraluminal blood flow. Large arteries adjust, both acutely and chronically, to changes in blood flow by corresponding adjustments in vessel diameter (Figure 3). The response is purely local and independent of arterial pressure changes; therefore shear stress, the force directly attributable to blood flow, is implicated. The striking feature about such responses is that this force is extremely small, i.e., bulk shear deformation of the artery wall at physiological blood flow rates is well below 1%. It is unlikely that important physiological controls are mediated by such small tissue deformations and for this reason the possibility that endothelial cells, which are in direct contact with blood flow, mediate the response has been raised.[30,31,34] Holtz et al.[32] and Pohl et al.[33] presented evidence that acute responses were endothelium-mediated and Langille and O'Donnell[34] have reported that chronic adjustments to altered flow are abolished by endothelial denudation (Figure 4). The acute response appears to be regulated by a product of the lipoxygenase pathway for arachidonic acid metabolism, although the plethora of vasoactive substances released or controlled by endothelium, including prostaglandins,[35] angiotensin,[36] histamine,[37] and endothelium-derived relaxing factor,[38] plus the existence of gap junctions between endothelial and some smooth muscle cells,[39] indicates that sorting out all potential mediators may prove difficult. The fact that chronic responses involve structural modification as well as contraction[125] further complicates this phenomenon; however, its potential significance in determining adaptations to developmental, physiological, and pathological changes in blood flow provides considerable stimulus for further work.

The diversity of factors controlling vessel tone and the complex nature of the activation process are reflected in multiple mechanisms through which regulators can act. For example, some agents, including norepinephrine can act on cell membrane properties to adjust transmembrane potential.[40] β-Adrenergic receptor mechanisms appear to increase cyclic AMP (cAMP) levels which in turn activate a protein kinase. Subsequent phosphorylation of internal membrane (SR) proteins may then enhance Ca^{2+} sequestration and inhibit contraction. There is also increasing interest in the potential role of cyclic GMP (cGMP) in regulating contraction. Nitroprusside[41,42] is thought to induce dilation by increasing guanylate cyclase activity and cGMP production, and more recent studies implicate this secondary messenger in endothelium-dependent relaxation.[43]

Pharmacomechanical coupling, i.e., regulation of tone not dependent on membrane potential changes, may be mediated by intracellular release of inositol 1,4,5-trisphosphate ($InsP_3$)[44] which then controls Ca^{2+} release from sarcoplasmic reticulum. This messenger is

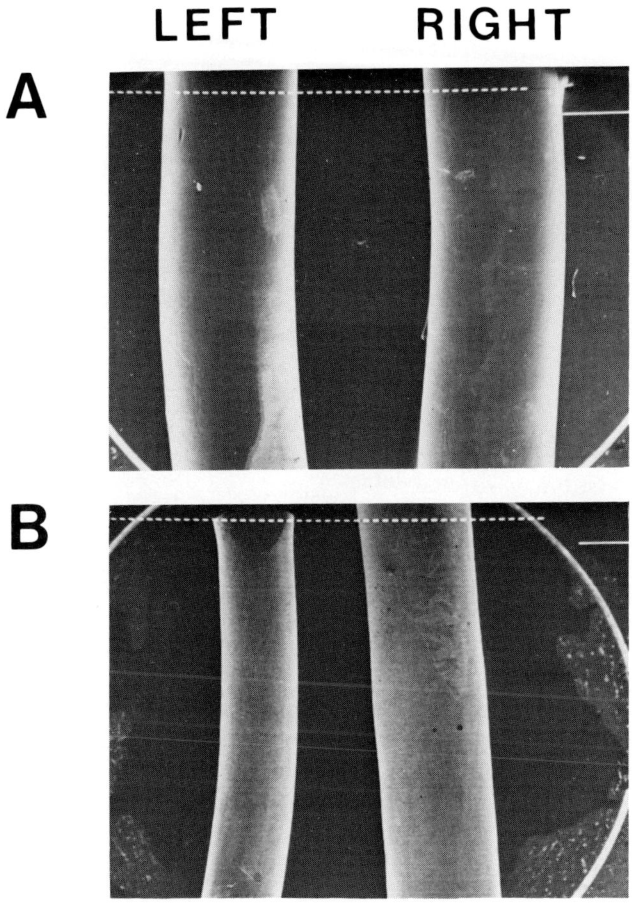

FIGURE 3. Low-power scanning electron micrographs of infusion casts of left and right common carotid arteries from a normal rabbit (A) and from a rabbit 2 weeks after 70% flow reduction in the left common carotid artery. Flow reduction induces relative narrowing of the left carotid. (From Langille, B. L. and O'Donnell, F., *Science*, 231, 405, 1986. With permission.)

produced in many cells by the hydrolysis of phosphotidylinositol 4,5-bisphosphate, an inositol lipid found in the inner leaflet of the plasma membrane, subsequent to agonist binding to cell surface receptors.[45] $InsP_3$ may then bind to a second receptor on the sarcoplasmic reticulum and thereby trigger Ca^{2+} release. In the experiments of Somlyo et al.,[44] $InsP_3$ induced both Ca^{2+} release and contraction in rabbit pulmonary artery, however, the mediation of agonist-induced activation through this agent remains to be demonstrated.

Myogenic regulation, i.e., the influence of vessel wall stretch on contractile tone may involve multiple mechanisms. Johansson and Mellander[46] demonstrated altered electrical activity and increased spike generation in the guinea pig portal vein. On the other hand, Pieper and Laven[47] recorded responses to stretch in totally depolarized preparations. Price[48] has shown that stretch induces increased sensitivity to agonists, as indicated by a reduced EC_{50} (effective concentration producing 50% of maximal contraction), and that this effect is observed above and below the optimal length for isometric contraction. The latter observation indicates that this effect of stretch is not a reflection of the degree of filament overlap, which primarily affects the maximal response to agonist. Striated muscle exhibits ''length-

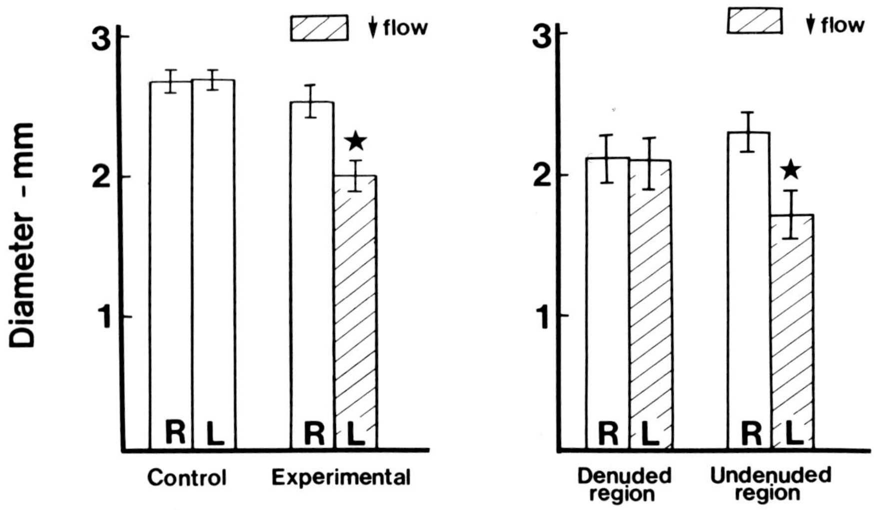

FIGURE 4. Graph on left shows diameter reduction of the left carotid artery 2 weeks after 70% flow reduction. Graph on right shows that this diameter reduction is abolished over segments of the vessel that have been denuded of endothelium, but the response persists in the undenuded region. (From Langille, B. L. and O'Donnell, F., *Science,* 231, 405, 1986. With permission.)

dependent activation'' that has been attributed to a direct effect of stretch on Ca^{2+} release from the sarcoplasmic reticulum and a similar mechanism in smooth muscle may mediate the effects of stretch.

C. Contractile Responses to Vessel Injury

1. Contraction Induced by Blood Constituents — Role in Hemostasis

Classical responses to vessel wall injury include platelet activation and release of potent vasoconstrictor substances, especially thromboxane A_2 and serotonin. Subsequent local contraction of the vessel wall may persist for hours and can play a major role in hemostasis. These agonists induce much more effective constriction of inner layers of the vessel wall than outer layers (see Reference 49, pages 93 and 94); therefore, maximal constriction during hemorrhage may be localized at the immediate site of injury where platelet release is at the luminal surface.

Platelet activation may contribute to acute responses; however, prolonged and severe constriction that results from extravasation of blood probably is of other origins. Such vasospasm can be of critical clinical importance following subarachnoid or other hemorrhagic events; nonetheless, the etiology of this vasospasm is controversial. Eicosanoids,[50-52] serotonin,[53,54] and epinephrine and norepinephrine[55,56] have been implicated, but there is also considerable interest in products of red cell degradation in extravascular space.[57] These agents can induce vessel contraction[58] or inhibit normal vasodilator mechanisms.[59] The recent observation that platelet-derived growth factor is vasoactive[60] raises the interesting possibility that this agent influences both contractile responses and the modulation of tissue proliferation following vascular injury.

2. Contractile Responses to Nonhemorrhagic Vascular Injury

Constriction can also be induced as a direct by-product of vessel injury in the absence of bleeding. Graham and Keatinge[61] used a blunt needle to injure the media of sheep carotid arteries and observed annular constriction of the vessel near the site of injury. Focal (1-mm-diameter) crushing injuries in vitro also induced contraction; furthermore, sucrose-gap records

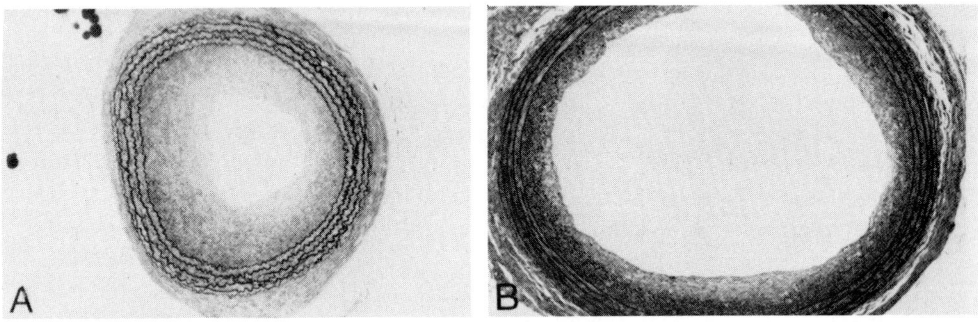

FIGURE 5. Intimal tissue proliferation and luminal narrowing in the rat carotid artery 2 weeks after the vessel was injured with a balloon catheter. Vessel on right (B) was dilated with papaverine, confirming that part of the luminal narrowing seen in A was due to active contraction. (From Clowes, A. W., Reidy, M. A., and Clowes, M. M., *Lab. Invest.*, 49, 208, 1983. With permission.)

demonstrated membrane depolarization without spikes, that decayed abruptly (within less than 1 mm) in the longitudinal direction and more gradually, i.e., with a space constant of 2.66 mm, in the circumferential direction. Thus, annular constriction appears to result from cell-to-cell conduction of depolarization that radiates from the site of injury. Preferential propagation in the circumferential direction may reflect the nature and location of cell-cell junctions. Alternatively, a nearly circumferential orientation of smooth muscle cells implies that more cells must be traversed during conduction along the length of the vessel; therefore, a lower space constant should not be surprising.

More recently, Clowes et al.[62] injured rat carotid arteries by inserting a balloon embolectomy catheter and repeatedly drawing the inflated balloon along the vessel. This technique, used to totally remove endothelium, also caused significant injury to medial smooth muscle cells, due presumably to hyperdistension of the vessel. Luminal narrowing occurred due to intimal proliferation of smooth muscle cells (Section IV) and also due to an active constrictor mechanism (Figure 5). This active constriction persisted for at least 8 weeks and was reversible using topical application of papaverine after 2 weeks.[62] Initial platelet adhesion and activation at the de-endothelialized surface may have contributed to the early phase of the response, but much of the platelet interaction with denuded vessel is a transient phenomenon.[63] Endothelial denudation may also abolish tonic effects of vasodilator release by these cells, including PGI_2 and endothelium-derived relaxing factor. It is also possible that medial smooth muscle injury initiated constriction through the release of unspecified vasoconstrictor agents.

III. SYNTHETIC BEHAVIOR

A. Normal Expression of Extracellular Material

The resting adult smooth muscle cells produce Type III collagen as well as Type I, IV, and V.[65] Elastin is produced from proelastin[66] in young aortic smooth muscle cells, but not in cells of the normal adult artery. The cell basal lamina consists of surface glycoproteins and the matrix of the media contains a variety of glycoproteins including fibronectin the 220,000-dalton molecular weight glycoprotein which mediates adhesion of cells to matrix. Glycoproteins produced by the smooth muscle cells also include heparan sulfate, chondroitin sulfate, and dermatin sulfate.[68]

B. Smooth Muscle Cell-Matrix Interactions

The arterial media is made up of relatively discrete lamellar units that can be resolved further into "musculo-elastic fascicles".[69] These consist of elongated smooth muscle cells demarcated by elastic fibers oriented in the same direction as the cells.[69] The cells are surrounded by a matrix consisting of the basal lamina and a fine meshwork of collagen fibrils, the 11-nm microfibrils extending from the basal lamina to extracellular collagen and elastin. Clark and Glagov[69] suggest that the microarchitecture of these subunits reflects the distribution and magnitude of local tensile stresses.

It is now becoming apparent that the extracellular matrix is important in modulating a variety of cell processes including those important to vascular wall cells. For example, both collagen and proteoglycan metabolism are altered during migration and proliferation of endothelial cells.[70,71] Furthermore, heparan sulfate proteoglycan is reduced markedly at the tips of growing capillaries.[72] Since heparan sulfate may modulate cell adhesion,[73] it is possible that changes in this proteoglycan facilitate cell migration.

IV. PROLIFERATIVE RESPONSE TO INJURY

Trauma to the vascular wall is followed by a complex repair process that involves interactions between blood cells and other blood constituents, endothelial cells and smooth muscle cells. Smooth muscle exhibits a proliferative response in which a subpopulation of these cells undergoes significant ultrastructural modulation, migrates to the intima, and replicates. This "response to injury" mechanism, which is characterized by both proliferation and a concomitant synthesis of extracellular matrix, is a fundamental component of the restoration of vessel integrity.

A. Initiation and Characterization of the Proliferative Response

A critical initiator of this process may be loss of endothelium. Endothelial denudation induces platelet attachment and the subsequent release of platelet-derived growth factor (PDGF) which is both mitogenic[74] and chemotactic[75] for smooth muscle cells. However, platelets alone may not be totally responsible, since proliferation continues for weeks,[62] whereas the initial massive platelet interaction with the denuded vessel is transient.[63] Furthermore, endothelial denudation, without medial injury, may not induce intimal proliferation.[64] It is of interest that smooth muscle cells[76] and endothelial cells[77] also release PDGF. It is possible, therefore, that both platelets and wall cells initiate a response that is sustained, in a positive feedback manner by the latter.[76]

Other factors including LDL from hypercholesterolemic animals[78] and macrophage derived growth factor[79] are mitogenic for smooth muscle cells. In addition, heparin-like products from endothelial cells,[80] exogenous heparin,[81] and heparan sulfate proteoglycans synthesized by postconfluent smooth muscle cells have potent antiproliferative activity.[82] The latter finding further suggests that smooth muscle cells may be able to regulate their own growth.

Clowes and co-workers have carefully examined the kinetics of smooth muscle proliferation after balloon catheter injury of the rat carotid artery. Ballooning removed all endothelium and significant loss of medial smooth muscle also was noted.[83] The initial injury was followed by a proliferative response in which cells throughout the vessel wall participated. By 4 days, smooth muscle cells migrated into the intima and were actively proliferating. Only the innermost intimal cells continued to replicate after 4 weeks, but turnover of these cells continued for at least 12 weeks and possibly only arrested if and when endothelium recovered the injury. Intimal cell number did not increase despite this persistent replication, i.e., cell replication was matched by cell loss; nonetheless, intimal thickening continued through synthesis of connective tissue.[62] In an interesting follow-up study, Clowes and Schwartz[84] demonstrated that only 50% of the cells that initially migrated into the intima participated in the intimal proliferative response. The nonproliferating cells were ultimately greatly outnumbered by their dividing neighbors, but their existence raises interesting questions concerning regulation of cell proliferation and the heterogeneity of the smooth muscle

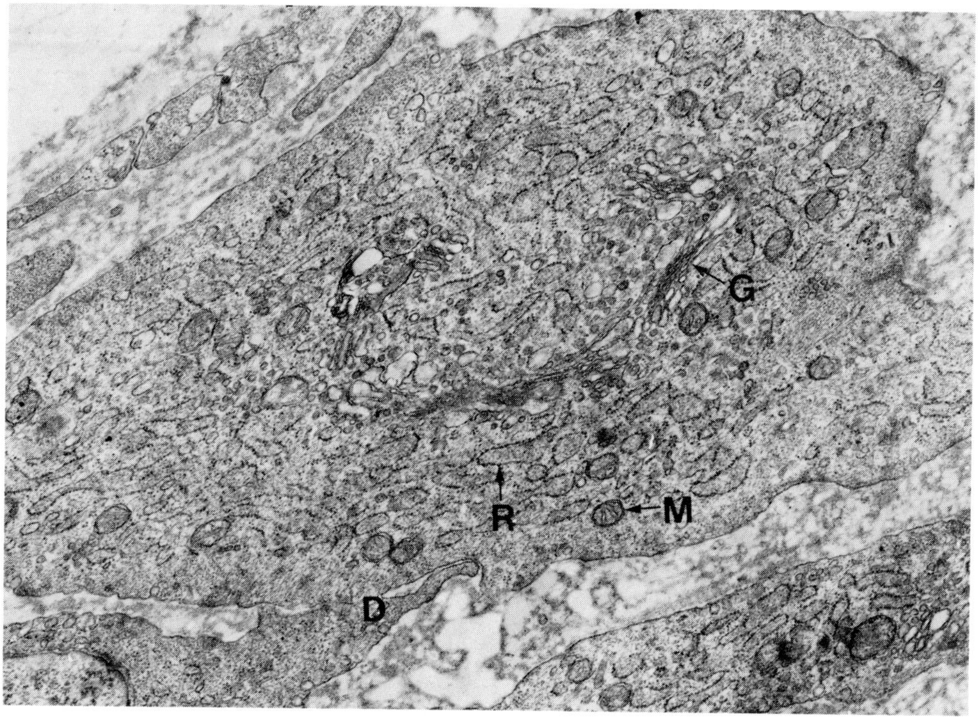

FIGURE 6. Electron micrograph of a smooth muscle cell from an aortic atherosclerotic plaque. The cell contains numerous organelles including rough endoplasmic reticulum (R), Golgi complex (G), and mitochondria (M) with few myofilaments and dense bodies (D). (Magnification × 44,528.)

cells that have migrated. Haudenschild and Grunwald[85] showed that smooth muscle cells from undisturbed vessels are more heterogeneous in proliferative behavior than those from the neointima of an injured vessel.

B. Modulation of Smooth Muscle Cell Characteristics

The proliferation and expression of extracellular protein by smooth muscle cells that characterize tissue repair differ greatly from the contractile behavior that normally characterizes smooth muscle. Consequently, there has been much interest in defining the modulation of functions of these cells. Given the divergent demands imposed on cell organelles, it is not surprising that this modulation has a structural counterpart. Although a spectrum of cell structural properties is observed, Campbell and Campbell[86] and their co-workers have defined two phenotypes, "contractile" (Figure 1) and "synthetic" (Figure 6), which represent the extremes of this spectrum. The table shown below categorizes the important functions of these extreme phenotypes.

Contractile	Synthetic
Contract	Noncontractile
Do not migrate or divide	Migrate and divide
Minimal collagen, GAG synthesis	Synthesize collagen, GAG
Degrade LDL	Degrade LDL
	Degrade VLDL
	Esterify and accumulate cholesterol
	Bind and accumulate β-VLDL

Consistent with these functions, contractile cells contain extensive myofilaments, but minimal Golgi apparatus, ribosomes, and rough endoplasmic reticulum. In contrast, synthetic cells have few contractile filaments, but larger amounts of the organelles associated with protein synthesis (Figure 6). Examination of smooth muscle cells at sites of injury indicates high cell proliferation and also cell ultrastructure characteristic of the synthetic phenotype, i.e., results are consistent with the suggestion that injury induces phenotypic modulation toward the synthetic state at the onset of repair.

Smooth muscle cell differentiation and modulation may, however, be more complex. Owens et al.[87] has shown that those myosin isoforms which have been associated with contractile activity are extensive in secretory- (synthetic) type cells and that significant amounts of α-smooth muscle actin were indeed present at the onset of cell replication. In addition, secretory-type cells display characteristics of contractile behavior.[87]

Smooth muscle proliferation in the media may be critical for reestablishing structural integrity of injured arteries. As described above, injury that denudes endothelium can induce intimal proliferation of smooth muscle cells. Although much interest has been focused on the potential pathologic implications of this proliferation if the source of injury is chronic (Section V.A), such a response to transient injury may have considerable adaptive significance. Specifically, intimal smooth muscle proliferation generates a new cellular intima on the lumen of the vessel through very modest translocation of medial smooth muscle. This relining of the injured vessel can be accomplished much more rapidly than reendothelialization from large wound margins. Indeed, studies by Reidy and co-workers[88] suggest that reendothelialization never recovers some large denudations. It follows that any capacity of smooth muscle cells to assume endothelial functions under these conditions may be critical to subsequent repair, and perhaps the ultimate viability, of the vessel. In this regard, it is noteworthy that vessel wall production of prostacylcin, normally synthesized primarily by endothelium, returns to control levels within about 1 week of denudation, about the time it takes smooth muscle to invade the intima. It is also of interest that luminal smooth muscle cells can even take on a morphology that resembles endothelial cells (Figure 7), at least in some species, a factor that may significantly obscure the identity of cells at the intimal surface.[89] There is no evidence, however, that neointima can assume many other functions of normal endothelium, e.g., the formation of a highly selective permeability barrier. Also, the neointima and endothelium respond differently to injury.[90] Denudation of the endothelium is followed by adherence of a layer of platelets while injury to neointima is followed by a prominent appearance of fibrin as well as adherence of platelets. Thus, the end product of the coagulation system is prominent on the surface of an injured neointima.

V. THE SMOOTH MUSCLE CELL IN VASCULAR DISEASE

A. Atherosclerosis

Atherosclerosis is a disease of the arterial intima characterized by the development of focal fibrofatty or atheromatous plaques in large elastic arteries and large- and medium-size muscular arteries. The smooth muscle cells are the most common cell type in the fibrofatty plaque. The smooth muscle cells, together with macrophages, can take up extensive amounts of lipids to become the ''foam cells'' characteristic of these lesions. The smooth muscle cells also produce the bulk of the matrix of the fibrofatty plaque,[91-93] but the connective tissue elements of the lesion are different from those secreted by medial SMC in normal media. Collagen makes up as much as 30% of the plaque by dry weight.[94] A total of 70% of the collagen in the normal aorta is type III, while in plaques type III makes up 35% and type I makes up 65%.[95] The plaque also contains larger amounts of collagen B chain.[96] Glycosaminoglycans[97] and elastins[98] found in the plaque bind lipoproteins and this may contribute to the prominent lipid component of plaques.

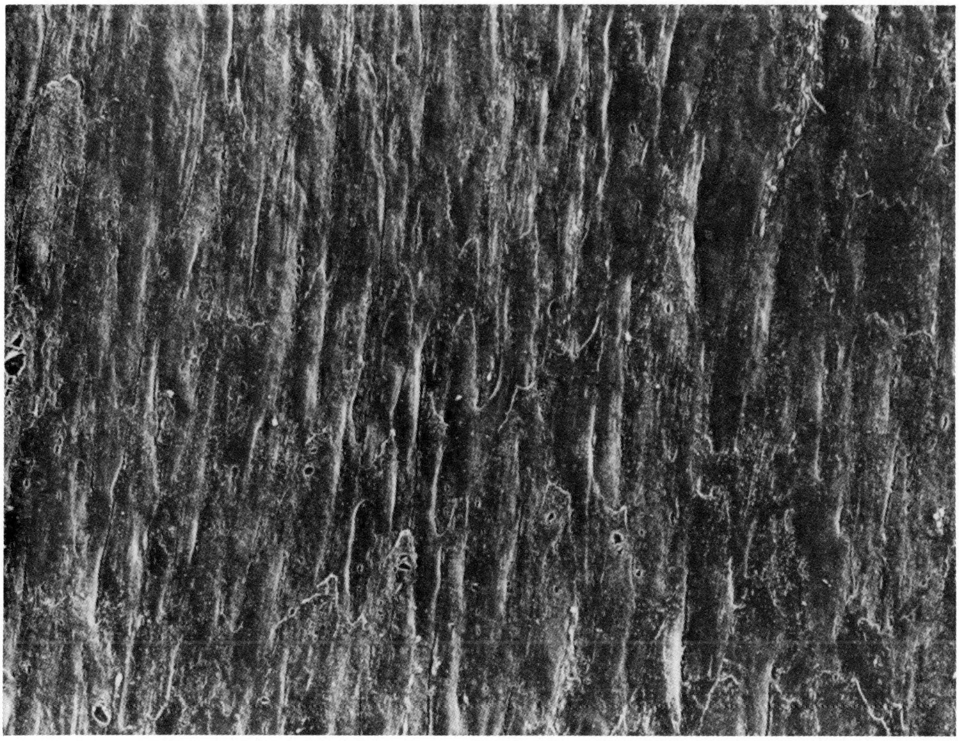

FIGURE 7. Intimal smooth muscle cells on the luminal surface of a rat carotid artery 12 months after endothelial denudation. Cell morphology resembles that of normal endothelium, i.e., cells are long and thin and oriented in the direction of blood flow (top to bottom). (From Clowes, A. W., Clowes, M. M., and Reidy, M. A., *Lab. Invest.*, 54, 295, 1986. With permission.)

Proteoglycans are probably important in atherogenesis. Proteoglycan-rich matrix accumulates in reendothelialized regions of aortas injured with balloon catheters, but not in noninjured or de-endothelialized areas.[99] In addition, these former areas are rich in lipids and lipoproteins which suggests that the proteoglycans trap the lipid thus enhancing atherogenesis.[100]

During atherogenesis the profile of proteoglycans produced is changed. Dermatan sulfate is most prominent in atheromas,[101] although others found mainly chondroitin sulfate and heparan sulfate.[102] Yla-Herttuala et al.[103] reported that in normal coronary arteries the contents of dermatan sulfate and chondroitin sulfates A and C increased significantly with age, but not as much as the very large increases seen in atherosclerotic vessels.

The most popular hypothesis to account for intimal smooth muscle cell proliferation in atherogenesis derives from a response of medial cells to chronic injury, specifically injury to the endothelium.[104] This hypothesis gained much support from studies described in Section IV in which endothelial injury induced massive intimal smooth muscle cell proliferation. More recently, failure to observe extensive and denuding injury to endothelium during atherogenesis[105,106] and the observation that denudation alone may not be an adequate stimulus for intimal smooth muscle proliferation[64] have much modified this hypothesis.[107] Thus, the production of growth modulators by other cells, including endothelium,[108] smooth muscle,[109] and the monocyte/macrophage,[110] has shifted focus somewhat away from the platelet, at least in early lesions. Nonetheless, the response to injury hypothesis remains one of the most fruitful areas of atherosclerosis research. Other hypotheses are that the intimal smooth muscle cells may represent neoplastic growth of a monoclonal colony of medial smooth muscle cells[111] or that the disease involves the extensive elaboration of a few smooth muscle cells present in the intima since birth.[112]

B. Hypertension

Increases in blood pressure are accompanied by thickening and increased smooth muscle content of the arterial wall. This response has obvious adaptive significance during development[113] and may also help to ensure integrity of large arteries of hypertensive individuals. On the other hand, Folkow[114] has argued that a similar hypertrophic response in resistance vessels may cause proliferating tissue to encroach upon the vessel lumen and experimental evidence tends to support this argument.[115] Furthermore, increases in arteriolar smooth muscle mass imply greater contractile responses to any tonic level of constrictor agonist. Both of these sequelae to increased smooth muscle mass would exacerbate the primary cause of hypertension, i.e., increased peripheral vascular resistance. Folkow goes further and proposes that chronic hypertension is a result of transient physiologic increases in blood pressure that became entrenched by the arteriolar hypertrophic response.

Although morphological features of the vessel wall response to elevated pressure have been extensively described,[116,117] major aspects of the cellular response have only recently been elucidated. Thus, increased thymidine incorporation has been interpreted as evidence of vessel wall hyperplasia,[118] whereas morphometric studies implicated cellular hypertrophy.[119] Recent analyses by Owens and co-workers[120,121] resolved this apparent inconsistency by demonstrating an extensive increase in the number of large, tetraploid cells in the walls of arteries from hypertensive rats, at least from those animals with spontaneous or two-kidney Goldblatt hypertension. Thus, these models of hypertension apparently induce smooth muscle cell DNA replication without cell division. The story has been complicated by recent observations that hypertension induced by coarctation of the aorta between the renal arteries in rats induces hyperplasia, not hypertrophy and hyperploidy.[122]

The stimulus for smooth muscle alterations in hypertension is unknown, but a local response to vessel wall tension, involving unknown intracellular processes, may be involved. Alternatively, Schwartz[123] reviewed evidence of endothelial injury, as indicated primarily by permeability changes, during the acute phase of experimental hypertension. He suggested that such injury may increase exposure of smooth muscle to growth factors, including PDGF, released at the intimal surface. This attractive hypothesis opens some new avenues of research relevant both to hypertension and to normal arterial adaptations to tensile forces.

REFERENCES

1. **Gabella, G.,** Structural apparatus for force transmission in smooth muscle, *Physiol. Rev.*, 64, 455, 1984.
2. **Cohen, D. M. and Murphy, R. A.,** Differences in cellular contractile protein contents among porcine smooth muscles, *J. Gen. Physiol.*, 72, 369, 1978.
3. **Devine, C. E. and Somlyo, A. P.,** Thick filaments in vascular smooth muscle, *J. Cell Biol.*, 49, 63, 1971.
4. **Geiger, B., Dutton, A. H., Tikuyasu, K. T., and Singer, S. J.,** Immunoelectron microscope studies of membrane-microfilament interactions: distribution of α-actin, tropomyosin and vinculin in intestinal epithelial brush border and chicken gizzard smooth muscle cells, *J. Cell Biol.*, 91, 614, 1981.
5. **Bond, M. and Somlyo, A. V.,** Dense bodies and actin polarity in vertebrate smooth muscle, *J. Cell Biol.*, 95, 403, 1984.
6. **Geiger, B., Tokuyasyu, K. T., Dutton, A. H., and Singer, S. J.,** Vinculin, an intracellular protein localized at specialized sites where microfilament bundles terminate at cell membrane, *Proc. Natl. Acad. Sci. U.S.A.*, 77, 4127, 1980.
7. **Small, J. V., Furst, D. O., and DeMey, J.,** Localization of filamin in smooth muscle, *J. Cell Biol.*, 102, 210, 1986.

8. **Kocher, O., Skalli, O., Bloom, W. S., and Gabbiani, G.,** Cytoskeleton of rat aortic smooth muscle cells, *Lab. Invest.*, 50, 645, 1984.
9. **Larson, D. M., Fujiwara, K., Alexander, R. W., and Gimbrone, M. A.,** Heterogeneity of myosin antigenic expression in vascular smooth muscle, in vivo, *Lab. Invest.*, 84, 401, 1984.
10. **Schmid, E., Osborn, M., Rungger-Brandle, E., Gabbiani, G., Weber, K., and Franke, W. W.,** Distribution of vimentin and desmin filaments in smooth muscle tissue of mammalian and avian aorta, *Exp. Cell Res.*, 137, 329, 1982.
11. **Somlyo, A. P.,** Excitation-contraction coupling and the ultrastructure of smooth muscle, *Circ. Res.*, 57, 497, 1985.
12. **Ratz, P. H. and Murphy, R. A.,** Effects of altering calcium pools on stress (S), myosin phosphorylation (Mp), and maximal shortening velocity (Vo) in swine carotid media, *Fed. Proc.*, 45, 763, 1986.
13. **Johansson, B. and Somlyo, A. P.,** Electrophysiology and excitation contraction coupling, in *The Handbook of Physiology, The Cardiovascular System,* Vol. 2, Bohr, D. F., Somlyo, A. P., and Sparks, H. V., Eds., American Physiological Society, Washington, D.C., 1980, 301.
14. **Casteels, R., Kitamara, K., Kurryama, H., and Suzki, H.,** The membrane potential of the smooth muscle cells of the rabbit main pulmonary artery, *J. Physiol. (London),* 271, 41, 1977.
15. **Harder, D. R. and Sperelakis, N.,** Membrane electrical properties of vascular smooth muscle from the guinea pig superior mesenteric artery, *Pfluegers Arch.*, 378, 377, 1978.
16. **Casteels, R.,** Calculation of the membrane potential in smooth muscle cells of the guinea pig's taenia coli by the Goldman equation, *J. Physiol. (London),* 205, 193, 1968.
17. **Wahlstrom, B. A.,** Ionic fluxes in the rat portal vein and the applicability of the Goldman equation in predicting the membrane potential from flux data, *Acta Physiol. Scand.*, 89, 436, 1973.
18. **Hermsmeyer, K.,** Electrogenesis of increased norepinephrine sensitivity of arterial vascular muscle in hypertension, *Circ. Res.*, 38, 362, 1976.
19. **Cuthbert, A. W. and Sutter, M. C.,** The effects of drugs on the relation between the action potential discharge and the tension in a mammalian vein, *Br. J. Pharmacol.*, 25, 592, 1965.
20. **Keatinge, W. R.,** Reversal of electrical response of arterial smooth muscle to noradrenaline in calcium-deficient solution, *J. Physiol. (London),* 198, 20P, 1968.
21. **Droogmans, G. L., Racymaekers, L., and Casteels, R.,** Electro- and pharmacomechanical coupling in the smooth muscle cells of the rabbit ear artery, *J. Gen. Physiol.*, 70, 129, 1977.
22. **Somylo, A. V., Vinall, P., and Somlyo, A. P.,** Excitation-contraction coupling and electrical events in two types of vascular smooth muscle, *Microvasc. Res.*, 1, 354, 1971.
23. **Bohr, D. F.,** Vascular smooth muscle, in *Peripheral Circulation,* Johnson, P. C., Ed., John Wiley & Sons, New York, 1978, 13.
24. **Lehman, W. J., Kendrick-Jones, J., and Szent-Gyorgyi, A. G.,** Myosin-linked regulatory systems: comparative studies, *Cold Spring Harbor Symp. Quant. Biol.*, 37, 319, 1972.
25. **Sparrow, M. P., Maxwell, L. C., Ruegg, J. C., and Bohr, D. F.,** Preparation and properties of a calcium ion-sensitive actomyosin from arteries, *Am. J. Physiol.*, 219, 1366, 1970.
26. **Webb, R. C. and Bohr, D. F.,** Regulation of vascular tone, molecular mechanisms, *Prog. Cardiovasc. Dis.*, 24, 213, 1981.
27. **Nonomura, Y. and Ebashi, S.,** Calcium regulation mechanisms in vertebrate smooth muscle, *Biochem. Res.*, 1, 1, 1980.
28. **Meisheri, K. D., Ruegg, J. C., and Paul, R. J.,** Studies on skinned fibre preparations, in *Calcium and Contractility,* Grover, A. K. and Daniel, E. E., Eds., Humana Press, Clifton, N.J., 1985, 191.
29. **Johnson, P. C.,** Principles of peripheral circulatory control, in *Peripheral Circulation,* Johnson, P. C., Eds., John Wiley & Sons, New York, 1978, 111.
30. **Rodbard, S.,** Vascular caliber, *Cardiology,* 60, 4, 1975.
31. **Kamiya, A. and Togawa, T.,** Adaptive regulation of wall shear stress to flow change in the canine carotid artery, *Am. J. Physiol.*, 239, H14, 1980.
32. **Holtz, J., Forstermann, U., Pohl, U., Gieshler, M., and Bassenge, E.,** Flow-dependent, endothelium-mediated dilation of epicardial coronary arteries in conscious dogs: effects of cyclooxygenase inhibition, *J. Cardiovasc. Pharmacol.*, 6, 1161, 1984.
33. **Pohl, U., Holtz, J., Busse, R., and Bassenge, E.,** Crucial role of endothelium in the vasodilator response to increased flow in vivo, *Hypertension,* 8, 37, 1986.
34. **Langille, B. L. and O'Donnell, F.,** Reductions in arterial diameter produced by chronic decreases in blood flow are endothelium dependent, *Science,* 231, 405, 1986.
35. **Moncada, S. and Vane, J. R.,** The role of prostaglandins in platelet-vessel wall interactions, in *Pathobiology of the Endothelial Cell,* Nossel, H. L. and Vogel, H. J., Eds., Academic Press, New York, 1982, 253.
36. **Ryan, J. W., Ryan, U. S., Schultz, D. R., Whitaker, C., Chung, A., and Dorer, F. R.,** Subcellular localization of pulmonary angiotensin-converting enzyme (Kininase II), *Biochem. J.*, 146, 497, 1975.

37. **Hollis, T. M., Gallik, S. G., Orlidge, A., and Yost, J. C.,** Aortic endothelial and smooth muscle histamine metabolism. Relationship to aortic ^{125}I-albumin accumulation in experimental diabetes, *Arteriosclerosis,* 3, 599, 1983.
38. **Furchgott, R. F.,** Role of endothelium in responses of vasular smooth muscle, *Circ. Res.,* 53, 557, 1983.
39. **Spagnoli, L. G., Villaschi, S., Neri, L., and Palmieri, G.,** Gap junctions in myo-endothelial bridges of rabbit carotid arteries, *Experientia,* 38, 124, 1982.
40. **Kreye, V. A. W., Kern, R., and Scheich, I.,** ^{36}Chloride efflux from noradrenaline-stimulated rabbit aorta inhibited by sodium nitropusside and nitroglycerine, in *Excitation-Contraction Coupling in Smooth Muscle,* Casteels, R., Godfraind, T., and Ruegg, J. C., Eds., Elsevier, Amsterdam, 1977, 145.
41. **Katsuki, S. and Murad, F.,** Regulation of adenosine cyclic 3′,5′-monophosphate and guanosine cyclic 3′,5′-monophosphate levels and contractility in bovine tracheal smooth muscle, *Mol. Pharmacol.,* 13, 330, 1977.
42. **Schultz, K. D., Schultz, K., and Schultz, G.,** Sodium nitroprusside and other smooth muscle relaxants increase cyclic GMP levels in rat ductus deferens, *Nature (London),* 256, 750, 1977.
43. **Rapoport, R. M. and Murad, F.,** Agonist-induced endothelium-dependent relaxation in rat thoracic aorta may be mediated througyh cGMP, *Circ. Res.,* 52, 352, 1983.
44. **Somlyo, A. V., Bond, M., Somlyo, A. P., and Scarpa, A.,** Inositol trisphosphate-induced calcium release and contraction in vascular smooth muscle, *Proc. Natl. Acad. Sci. U.S.A.,* 82, 5231, 1985.
45. **Berridge, M. J. and Irvine, R. F.,** Inositol trisphosphate, a novel second messenger in cellular signal transduction, *Nature (London),* 312, 315, 1984.
46. **Johansson, B. and Mellander, S.,** Static and dynamic changes in the vascular myogenic response to passive changes in length as revealed by electrical and mechanical recordings from the rat portal vein, *Circ. Res.,* 36, 76, 1975.
47. **Pieper, V. and Laven, R.,** The primary process of vascular smooth muscle contraction and the influence of stress, temperature, Ca+ +, H+, and norepinephrine, *Arzneim. Forsch.,* 26, 1235, 1976.
48. **Price, J. M.,** Length-dependent activation and sensitivity in arterial ring segments, *Ann. Biomed. Eng.,* 12, 481, 1984.
49. **Keatinge, W. R. and Harman, M. C.,** *Local Mechanisms Controlling Blood Vessels,* Academic Press, London, 1980.
50. **Sasaki, T., Murota, S., Wakai, S., Asano, T., and Sano, K.,** Evaluation of prostaglandin biosynthetic activity in canine basilar artery following subarachnoid injection of blood, *J. Neurosurg.,* 55, 771, 1981.
51. **Maeda, Y., Tani, E., and Mujamoto, T.,** Prostaglandin metabolism in experimental cerebral vasospasm, *J. Neurosurg.,* 55, 779, 1981.
52. **Walker, V., Pickard, J. D., Smythe, P., Eastwood, S., and Perry, S.,** Effects of subarachnoid haemorrhage on intracranial prostaglandins, *J. Neurol. Neurosurg. Psychiatry,* 46, 119, 1983.
53. **Allen, G. S. and Gross, C. J.,** Cerebral arterial spasm. I. In vitro contraction of vasoactive agents on canine basilar and middle cerebral arteries, *J. Neurosurg.,* 40, 433, 1974.
54. **Ragnor, R. B., McMurtry, J. G., and Pool, J. L.,** Cerebrovascular effects of topically applied serotonin in the cat, *Neurology,* 11, 190, 1961.
55. **Toda, N.,** Influence of dopamine and norepinephrine on isolated cerebral arteries of the dog, *Br. J. Pharmacol.,* 58, 121, 1976.
56. **Toda, N.,** Alpha adrenergic receptor subtype in human, monkey and dog cerebral arteries, *J. Pharmacol. Exp. Ther.,* 226, 861, 1983.
57. **Osaka, K.,** Prolonged vasospasm produced by the breakdown products of erythrocytes, *J. Neurosurg.,* 47, 403, 1977.
58. **Tanishima, T.,** Cerebral vasospasm: contractile activity of hemoglobin in isolated canine basilar arteries, *J. Neurosurg.,* 53, 787, 1980.
59. **Martin, V., Villani, G. M., Jothianandan, P., and Furchgott, R. F.,** Selective blockade of endothelium dependent and glycerol-trinitrate induced relaxation by hemoglobin and methylene blue in the rabbit aorta, *J. Pharmacol. Exp. Ther.,* 232, 708, 1985.
60. **Berk, B. C., Alexander, R. W., Brock, T. A., Gimbrone, M. A., Jr., and Webb, R. C.,** Vasoconstriction: a new activity for platelet-derived growth factor, *Science,* 232, 87, 1986.
61. **Graham, J. M. and Keatinge, W. R.,** Sensitivity of inner and outer muscle of the sheep carotid artery to injury, *J. Physiol.,* 247, 473, 1975.
62. **Clowes, A. W., Reidy, M. A., and Clowes, M. M.,** Mechanisms of stenosis after arterial injury, *Lab. Invest.,* 49, 208, 1983.
63. **Groves, H. M., Kinlough-Rathbone, R. L., Richardson, M., Moore, S., and Mustard, J. F.,** Platelet interaction with damaged rabbit aorta, *Lab. Invest.,* 40, 194, 1979.
64. **Reidy, M. A. and Silver, M.,** Endothelial regeneration. VII. Lack of intimal proliferation after defined injury to rat aorta, *Am. J. Pathol.,* 118, 173, 1985.
65. **Jander, R., Rauterberg, J., and Glanville, R. W.,** Further characterization of the three polypeptide chains of bovine and human short-chain collagen (intima collagen), *Eur. J. Biochem.,* 133, 39, 1983.

66. **Ross, R.,** The smooth muscle cell. II. Growth of smooth muscle in cell culture and formation of elastic fibres, *J. Cell Biol.*, 50, 172, 1971.
67. **Mills, A. J. T., Hoyle, M., Mann, D. M., and Brennan, M. J.,** Incorporation of cellular and plasma fibronectins into smooth muscle cell extracellular matrix in vitro, *Proc. Natl. Acad. Sci. U.S.A.*, 82, 2746, 1985.
68. **Wight, T. N. and Hascall, V. C.,** Proteoglycans in primate arteries. III. Characterization of the proteoglycans synthesized by arterial smooth muscle cells in culture, *J. Cell Biol.*, 96, 167, 1983.
69. **Clark, J. M. and Glagov, S.,** Transmural organization of the arterial media. The lamellar unit revisited, *Arteriosclerosis*, 5, 519, 1985.
70. **Madri, J. A. and Stenn, K. S.,** Aortic endothelial cell migration. I. Matrix requirements and composition, *Am. J. Pathol.*, 106, 80, 1982.
71. **Kinsilla, M. G. and Wight, T. N.,** Modulation of sulfated proteoglycan synthesis by bovine aortic endothelial cells during migration, *J. Cell Biol.*, 102, 679, 1986.
72. **Ausprunk, D. H., Boudreau, C. L., and Nelson, D. A.,** Proteoglycans in the microvasculature. I. Histochemical localization in microvessels of the rabbit eye, *Am. J. Pathol.*, 103, 353, 1981.
73. **Rapraeger, A. C. and Bernfield, M.,** Heparan sulfate proteoglycans of mouse mammary epithelial cells: a putative membrane proteoglycan associates quantitatively with lipid vesicles, *J. Biol. Chem.*, 258, 3632, 1983.
74. **Ross, R., Glomset, J., Kariya, B., and Harker, L.,** A platelet dependent serum factor that stimulates the proliferation of arterial smooth muscle cells in vitro, *Proc. Natl. Acad. Sci. U.S.A.*, 71, 1207, 1974.
75. **Grotendorst, G. R., Chang, T., Seppa, H. E. J., Kleinman, H. K., and Martin, G. R.,** Platelet-derived growth factor is a chemoattractant for vascular smooth muscle cells, *J. Cell. Physiol.*, 113, 161, 1982.
76. **Nilsson, J., Sjlund, M., Palmberg, L., Thyberg, J., and Heldin, C. H.,** Arterial smooth muscle cells in primary culture produce a platelet derived growth factor-like protein, *Proc. Natl. Acad. Sci. U.S.A.*, 82, 4418, 1985.
77. **DiCorleto, P. E. and Bowen-Pope, D. F.,** Cultured endothelial cells produce a platelet-derived growth factor-like protein, *Proc. Natl. Acad. Sci. U.S.A.*, 80, 1919, 1983.
78. **Fischer-Dzoga, K., Fraser, R., and Wissler, R. W.,** Stimulation of proliferation in stationary primary cultures of monkey and rabbit aortic smooth muscle cells. I. Effects of lipoprotein fractions of hyperlipemic serum and lymph, *Exp. Mol. Pathol.*, 24, 346, 1976.
79. **Martin, B. M., Gimbrone, M. A., Unanue, E. R., and Cotran, R. S.,** Stimulation of nonlymphoid mesenchymal cell proliferation by a macrophage-derived growth factor, *J. Immunol.*, 126, 1510, 1981.
80. **Guyton, J. R., Rosenberg, R. D., Clowes, A. W., and Karnovsky, M. J.,** Inhibition of rat arterial smooth muscle cell proliferation by heparin, *Circ. Res.*, 46, 625, 1980.
81. **Castellot, J. J., Beeler, D. L., Rosenberg, R. D., and Karnovsky, M. J.,** Structural determinants of the capacity of heparin to inhibit the proliferation of vascular smooth muscle cells, *J. Cell. Physiol.*, 120, 315, 1984.
82. **Fritze, L. M. S., Reilly, C. F., and Rosenberg, R. D.,** An antiproliferative heparan sulfate species produced by postconfluent smooth muscle cells, *J. Cell Biol.*, 100, 1041, 1985.
83. **Clowes, A. W., Reidy, M. A., and Clowes, M. M.,** Kinetics of cellular proliferation after arterial injury. I. Smooth muscle growth in the absence of endothelium, *Lab. Invest.*, 49, 327, 1983.
84. **Clowes, A. W. and Schwartz, S. M.,** Significance of quiescent smooth muscle migration in the injured rat carotid artery, *Circ. Res.*, 56, 139, 1985.
85. **Haudenschild, C. C. and Grunwald, J.,** Proliferative heterogeneity of vascular smooth muscle cells and its alteration by injury, *Exp. Cell Res.*, 157, 364, 1985.
86. **Campbell, G. R. and Campbell, J. H.,** Smooth muscle phenotypic changes in arterial wall homeostasis: implication for the pathogenesis of atherosclerosis, *Exp. Mol. Pathol.*, 42, 139, 1985.
87. **Owens, G. K., Loeb, A., Gordon, D., and Thompson, M. M.,** Expression of smooth muscle-specific isoactin in cultured vascular smooth muscle cells: relationship between growth and cytodifferentiation, *J. Cell Biol.*, 102, 343, 1986.
88. **Reidy, M. A., Clowes, A. W., and Schwartz, S. M.,** Endothelial regeneration. V. Inhibition of endothelial regrowth in arteries of rat and rabbit, *Lab. Invest.*, 49, 569, 1982.
89. **Reidy, M. A.,** A reassessement of endothelial injury and arterial lesion formation, *Lab. Invest.*, 53, 513, 1985.
90. **Mustard, J. F.,** The role of platelets and thrombosis in the development of atherosclerosis and its complications, *Am. R. Cell Ann. R. Coll. Phys. Surg. Can.*, 14, 22, 1981.
91. **Ross, R. and Klebanoff, S. J.,** The smooth muscle cell. I. In vivo synthesis of connective tissue proteins, *J. Cell Biol.*, 50, 159, 1971.
92. **Berenson, G. S., Radhakrishnamurthy, B., Dalferes, E. R., Jr., and Srinivasan, S. R.,** Carbohydrate macromolecules and atherosclerosis, *Hum. Pathol.*, 2, 57, 1971.

93. **Poole, J. C., Cromwell, B. S., and Benditt, E. P.,** Behavior of smooth muscle cells and formation of extracellular structures in the reaction of arterial walls to injury, *Am. J. Pathol.*, 62, 391, 1971.
94. **Bertelsen, S.,** Chemical studies of the arterial wall in relation to atherosclerosis, *Ann. N.Y. Acad. Sci. U.S.A.*, 149, 643, 1968.
95. **McCullagh, K. G., Duance, V. C., and Bishop, K. A.,** The distribution of collagen types I, III and V (AB) in normal and atherosclerotic human aorta, *J. Pathol.*, 130, 45, 1980.
96. **Ooshima, A.,** Collagen B chain: increased proportion in human atherosclerosis, *Science*, 213, 66, 1981.
97. **Vijayagopal, P., Radhakrishnamurthyu, B., Srinivasan, S. R., and Berenson, G. S.,** Studies of biological properties of proteoglycans from bovine aorta, *Lab. Invest.*, 42, 190, 1980.
98. **Kramsch, D. M., Franzblau, C., and Hollander, W.,** The protein and lipid composition of arterial elastin and its relationship to lipid accumulation in atherosclerotic plaque, *J. Clin. Invest.*, 50, 1666, 1971.
99. **Richardson, M., Ihnatowycz, I., and Moore, S.,** Glycosaminoglycan distribution in rabbit aortic wall following balloon catheter deendothelialization: an ultrastructural study, *Lab. Invest.*, 43, 509, 1980.
100. **Iverius, P. H.,** The interaction between plasma lipoproteins and connective tissue glycosaminoglycans, *J. Biol. Chem.*, 247, 2607, 1972.
101. **Stevens, R. L., Colombo, M., Gonzales, J. J., Hollander, W., and Schmid, K.,** The glycosaminoglycans of the human artery and their changes in atherosclerosis, *J. Clin. Invest.*, 58, 470, 1976.
102. **Srinivasan, S. R., Dolan, P., Radhakrishnamurthy, B., and Berenson, G. S.,** Isolation of lipoprotein-acid mucopolysaccharide complexes from fatty steaks of human aortas, *Atherosclerosis*, 16, 95, 1972.
103. **Yla-Herttuala, S., Sumuvuori, H., Karkola, K., Mottonen, M., and Nikkari, T.,** Glycosaminoglycans in normal and atherosclerotic human coronary arteries, *Lab. Invest.*, 54, 402, 1986.
104. **Ross, R. and Glomset, J.,** The pathogenesis of atherosclerosis, *N. Engl. J. Med.*, 295, 369, 1976.
105. **Faggiotto, A., Ross, R., and Harker, L.,** Studies of hypercholesterolemia in the nonhuman primate. I. Changes that lead to fatty streak formation, *Arteriosclerosis*, 4, 323, 1984.
106. **Faggiotto, A. and Ross, R.,** Studies of hypercholesterolemic in the nonhuman primate. II. Fatty streak conversion to fibrous plaque, *Arteriosclerosis*, 4, 341, 1984.
107. **Ross, R.,** The pathogenesis of atherosclerosis — an update, *N. Engl. J. Med.*, 314, 488, 1986.
108. **Gadjusek, C. M. and Schwartz, S. M.,** Ability of endothelial cells to condition culture medium, *J. Cell. Physiol.*, 110, 35, 1982.
109. **Seifert, R. A., Schwartz, S. M., and Bowen-Pope, D. F.,** Developmentally regulated production of platelet-derived growth factor-like molecules, *Nature (London)*, 311, 669, 1984.
110. **Martinet, Y., Bitterman, P. B., Mornex, J.-F., Grotendorst, G. R., Martin, F. R., and Criptal, R. G.,** Activated human monocytes express the c-sis proto-oncogene and release a mediator showing PDGF-like activity, *Nature (London)*, 319, 158, 1986.
111. **Benditt, E. P. and Benditt, J. M.,** Evidence for a monoclonal origin of human atherosclerotic plaques, *Proc. Natl. Acad. Sci. U.S.A.*, 70, 1753, 1973.
112. **Thomas, W. A. and Kem, D. N.,** Atherosclerosis as a hyperplastic and/or neoplastic process, *Lab. Invest.*, 48, 245, 1983.
113. **Leung, D. Y. M., Glagov, S., and Mathews, M. B.,** Elastin and collagen accummulation in rabbit ascending aorta and pulmonary trunk during postnatal growth, *Circ. Res.*, 41, 316, 1977.
114. **Folkow, B.,** Physiological aspects of primary hypertension, *Physiol. Rev.*, 62, 347, 1982.
115. **Mulvaney, M. J. and Halpern, W.,** Contractile properties of small artery resistance vessels in spontaneously hypertensive and normotensive rats, *Circ. Res.*, 41, 19, 1977.
116. **Wolinsky, H.,** Response of the rat aortic media to hypertension, *Circ. Res.*, 26, 507, 1970.
117. **Berry, C. L. and Greenwald, S. E.,** Effects of hypertension on the mechanical properties and chemical composition of the rat aorta, *Cardiovasc. Res.*, 10, 437, 1976.
118. **Bevan, R. D.,** An autoradiographic and pathologic study of cellular proliferation in rabbit arteries correlated with an increase in arterial pressure, *Blood Vessel*, 13, 100, 1976.
119. **Olivetti, G., Melissari, M., Marchette, G., and Anversa, P.,** Quantitative structural changes of the rat thoracic aorta in early spontaneous hypertension. Tissue composition, and hypertrophy and hyperplasia of smooth muscle cells, *Circ. Res.*, 51, 19, 1982.
120. **Owens, G. K., Rabinovitch, P. S., and Schwartz, S. M.,** Smooth muscle cell hypertrophy versus hyperplasia in hypertension, *Proc. Natl. Acad. Sci. U.S.A.*, 78, 7759, 1981.
121. **Owens, G. K. and Schwartz, S. M.,** Alterations in vascular smooth muscle mass in the spontaneously hypertensive rat. Role of cellular hypertrophy, hyperploidy and hyerplasia, *Circ. Res.*, 51, 280, 1982.
122. **Owens, G. K. and Reidy, M. A.,** Hyperplastic growth responses of vascular smooth muscle cells following induction of acute hypertension in rats by aortic coarctation, *Circ. Res.*, 57, 695, 1985.
123. **Schwartz, S. M.,** Hypertension as a vascular response to injury, *Hypertension*, 6, 33, 1984.
124. **Clowes, A. W., Clowes, M. M., and Reidy, M. A.,** Kinetics of cellular proliferation after arterial injury. III. Endothelial and smooth muscle growth in chronically denuded vessel, *Lab. Invest.*, 54, 295, 1986.
125. **Langille, B. L.,** unpublished results.

Chapter 6

STRUCTURE AND FUNCTION OF PLATELETS

László Muszbek and Róza Ádány

TABLE OF CONTENTS

I. INTRODUCTION

Primary hemostasis in a great extent is based on specific cellular elements of the blood that possess the ability of responding to certain physiological agents with a series of biochemical-structural changes. In highly developed organisms, thrombocytes, or in mammalians, their anucleated counterparts, platelets, represent the cellular component of the hemostatic system. Platelets or thrombocytes are functioning in close collaboration with vascular and humoral hemostatic mechanisms. They can undergo drastic changes within a short period of time and the final outcome of these events is the formation of primary hemostatic plug at the site of blood vessel injury that arrests bleeding. The electron microscopic structure of platelets as well as biochemical mechanisms leading to or involved in platelet activation and responsible for various platelet functions have been a subject of intensive research in the last two decades. A detailed discussion of the great many data accumulated in this field is beyond the scope of this book and in the following only the most essential information will be presented. For the same reason, an abundant list of references will be avoided; instead, concerning certain subjects we will refer to recent up-to-date reviews.

II. STRUCTURE OF THE PLATELET

Platelets are the tiniest cells of the human body, normally of 2- to 4-μm diameter. Circulating, unactivated ("resting") platelets possess a characteristic lentiform shape resembling a discus. Our knowledge concerning the morphology and structural organization of platelets is primarily based on electron microscopic investigations carried out in White's laboratory.[1-4] In order to simplify the complicated structural features of these cells, their anatomy was divided into the following four major structural-functional regions:

1. Peripheral zone
2. Sol-gel zone
3. Organelle zone
4. Membrane systems

The **peripheral zone** consists of three structural domains: (1) exterior coat (glycocalyx), (2) unit membrane, and (3) submembrane region. As estimated by electron-dense markers, the glycocalyx of platelets is thicker and denser than that of other cellular blood elements. Its dominant components are carbohydrate residues of peripheral and integral membrane glycoproteins (GP), some of which have an extremely important role in the process of platelet activation. The net negative charge of platelets at physiological pH is due to the negatively charged carbohydrate groups of the exterior coat.

The unit membrane, an asymmetric phospholipid bilayer, provides a physicochemical barrier between the extra- and intracellular space. The composition of the outer and the cytoplasmatic layer is different and phospholipids with significant procoagulant activity (especially phosphatidyl serine) are located in the internal layer.[5] Platelet phospholipids are unusually rich in arachidonic acid (AA), a fact in all probability related to the role of arachidonic derivatives in platelet activation. In addition to phospholipids, the unit membrane contains glycolipids and cholesterol, as well. A total of 35 to 40% of the platelet membrane is protein and 50 to 100 peripheral or integral membrane proteins can be differentiated by modern electrophoretic techniques. Among these proteins GP bear an outstanding importance.[6,7] The peripheral protein GPIb, the dominant membrane component, plays an important role in platelet adhesion, while the integral proteins GPIIb and GPIIIa are essential to the aggregation process. Important constituents of the platelet membrane are the receptors of activating and inhibitory agents (some of them also GP), as well as Na/K ATPase and anion pump which ensure appropriate transmembrane ionic gradients.

In the submembrane region the existence of a regular array of filaments has been verified[8-10] which together with the microtubular ring may participate in the maintenance of discoid shape and in the mechanism of extrusion and stabilization of pseudopodia.

In the **sol-gel zone**, two dynamic fiber systems, the microtubular and microfilamentous apparatus, are the dominant structures. In resting platelets, a circumferential ring of microtubules is located in the equatorial plane beneath the membrane and in close connection with filaments of the submembrane region.[11,12] An intact microtubular ring consisting of 8 to 24 circular profiles is essential in retaining the discoid shape and its disassembly results in the loss of a lentiform appearance. Microtubules are built up of polymerized tubulin and various associated proteins, while the basic component of the other fiber system, i.e., of microfilaments, is actin. The latter, like in the muscle, belongs to a contractile apparatus and the two together form the so-called cytoskeleton. Though according to various estimates actin and microfilament-associated proteins amount to 15 to 50% of the total platelet proteins, in resting platelets only a smaller portion of them exists in filamentous form.[1,10,16,17] The drastic changes in microtubular and microfilament systems during platelet activation and their involvement in the mechanism of the activation process will be discussed later in detail.

The cytoplasm of platelets is crowded with various subcellular organelles, different granules being the most numerous among them (a few mitochondria and remnants of Golgi apparatus can also be detected by electron microscopy). By modern electron microscopic techniques at least four types of granules can be differentiated:[3,18]

1. Dense bodies (δ-granules)
2. α-Granules
3. Lysosomes
4. Peroxisomes

Both dense bodies and α-granules have storage function. Calcium, pyrophosphate, serotonin, as well as the nonmetabolic pool of ADP and ATP are concentrated in dense bodies and their release during secretion is of high importance in the mechanism of second-wave aggregation. In contrast, α-granules are specialized for the storage of various platelet proteins.[18,19] A list of the most important α-granular proteins is provided below:

Proteins resembling or equivalent of plasma proteins:
- Fibrinogen
- Factor V (F-V)
- von Willebrand's factor (F-VIII_{vw} related antigen)
- Fibronectin
- Albumin

Platelet specific proteins:
- Platelet factor 4 (PF4)
- Low affinity PF4 (LA-PF4) and its proteolytic split product β-thromboglobulin (β-TG)
- Platelet basic protein (PBP)
- Platelet derived growth factors (PDGF)
- Vascular permeability factor
- Chemotactic factor
- Thrombospondin

As both clotting factors (fibrinogen and F-V) and proteins influencing the coagulation process (PF4, LA-PF4) are present in the α-granules, this list in itself emphasizes the close relationship of the cellular and humoral hemostatic mechanisms. The presence of classic lysosomes containing acid hydrolases and of catalase-containing peroxisomes has also been revealed and they can be clearly differentiated from storage granules by enzyme-cytochemical techniques.

In platelets two separate but not completely isolated membrane systems could be detected:[3,4] (1) surface connected open canalicular system (OCS) and (2) dense tubular system (DTS). Channels of OCS are invaginations of cell membrane transweaving the platelet cytoplasm and lending to it a sponge-like appearance. Their existence creates an intimate relationship between the platelet and its immediate plasma environment possible. In this way platelets have a contact with their surroundings through a large surface, various agents can easily reach the "interior" of the platelet body, and the contents of granules are secreted into an open surface-connected channel system. In addition, OCS might have an important role as a membrane store that provides a "new" surface membrane to pseudopode formation and other steps of the activation process requiring a rapid enlargement of surface area.

Due to its higher electron density DTS can be well distinguished from OCS by electron microscopy. Certain channels of DTS are connected to the circumferential microtubular ring. In other regions of the cytoplasm, elements of DTS and OCS are in close physical intimacy forming a morphological and perhaps also a functional entity.

DTS possesses a selective divalent cation binding capacity and by a Ca^{2+}/Mg^{2+} ATPase it can accumulate calcium ions.[20] Most of the Ca^{2+} released into the cytoplasm as a response to activating agents comes out of the DTS and in both morphological and functional points of view the OCS-DTS membrane complex resembles the transverse sarcotubular system in the muscle. Prostaglandin synthesis having a high importance in platelet activation also occurs in DTS.[21]

III. MECHANISM OF PLATELET ACTIVATION

A. Various Phases of the Activation Process

As mentioned earlier, subendothelial structures (collagen and other components of basal membrane) becoming available at vessel wall injury, ADP released by cell damage, and thrombin formed during the blood clotting process induce a series of changes resulting in the formation of hemostatic platelet plug. Consecutive events of this process, commonly termed as platelet activation, occur in the closest coordination and in reality they are manifestations of a progressing integrated biochemical mechanism. Nevertheless, due to didactic reasons, generally the following individual steps are separated.

1. Adhesion
2. Shape change
3. Aggregation, condensation of aggregate
4. Secretion (release reaction)
5. Availability of procoagulant activity
6. Clot retraction

In certain conditions or in response to a given activating agent, not necessarily all the above steps take place (e.g., epinephrine does not induce shape change; aggregation and secretion may occur independently; secretion is not a prerequisite for procoagulant activity; for retraction concordant activation of blood coagulation is also needed; in the case of soluble activating agents adhesion obviously does not occur; etc.). In the activation process when elicited by different agents, the order of consecutive events can be different. With collagen release reaction precedes aggregation, while in citrated platelet-rich plasma, thrombin, ADP, and epinephrine initiate aggregation before the release reaction.

Adhesion[22] means, in a broader sense, the ability of platelets to bind to an attractive surface. In physiological conditions such a surface is provided by collagen, the basal membrane, or other subendothelial structures. Adhesion could be divided into the following phases: (1) primary adhesion (adhesion of unstimulated platelets), contact, and spreading and (2) secondary adhesion of stimulated platelets.

In the first phase, the initial attachment of platelets occurs without any major shape change that is followed by a more intensive contact of spread platelets with the substrate. During spreading, an extensive shape change involving disc-sphere transformation and extrusion of pseudopodia occurs and the granular content is released. The free ''upper'' surface of fully spread, firmly attached platelets becomes thrombogenic and provides an adhesive surface for further platelets. The presence of both membrane components and plasma cofactors are essential to normal platelet adhesion. A membrane glycoprotein GPIb and a plasma protein von Willebrand's factor are both known to play an important role in the adhesion process and their inherited deficiency results in impaired adhesion and consequently, in bleeding diathesis. Fibronectin and perhaps fibronogen as well are also involved in platelet adhesion. Von Willebrand's factor, fibronectin, and fibrinogen are also found in the α-granules of platelets and become secreted into the surroundings during release reaction. In physiological conditions, contact to the damaged vessel wall is a Ca^{2+} requiring process.

Either following contact with adhesive surfaces or as a result of a direct effect of soluble activating agents, the originally discoid platelet becomes spheroid (this is the step missing at epinephrine-induced activation) and develops long spiny pseudopodia (disk to spiny sphere transition). This shape change does not only result in the enlargement of platelet surface, but also in definite alterations of membrane structure leading, among others, to the appearance of new membrane receptors (e.g., see the ADP-induced assembly of fibrinogen receptor).[23-26]

In case cell-to-cell contact is ensured (in vivo by the bloodstream or in vitro in the cuvette of an aggregometer by constant stirring) and appropriate conditions (e.g., Ca^{2+}, fibrinogen) are provided, platelets which have undergone shape change clump together and aggregates are formed. In the first phase, platelets adhere to each other in a rather loose configuration. At this phase, the aggregation is still reversible, which, using low concentrations of aggregating agents, can be well demonstrated in an aggregometer. In the later phase, more and more platelets become incorporated into the aggregates, large clumps consisting of tightly packed platelets are formed, they contract, and the aggregation process reaches an irreversible stage.

Aggregation is either preceded (collagen) or is accompanied by the so-called release reaction, a terminology commonly used for the secretion of granular content by exocytosis. It is to be noted that in some papers the term platelet activation is used as a synonym of release reaction which we find rather confusing and prefer to apply this terminology to the whole process elicited by an activating agent. During activation but prior to the release reaction, the granules become concentrated into the center of the cell; they are surrounded by a microtubular ring and get into close contact with the membrane of OCS. Following the fusion of granular and OCS membrane, the granular content is released into the OCS and into the immediate vicinity of the cells.[3,18] Not all activating agents induce the release of all types of granules; furthermore, in case of a given inducer, a dose dependence concerning the granules involved in the secretion process could be observed. For example, only α-granular and dense body release can be induced by ADP, epinephrine, or thromboxane A_2 (TXA_2), while thrombin, collagen, and the Ca^{2+} ionophore A23187 elicit also the secretion of lysosomal content.[18] A relatively low dose of thrombin releases α-granules selectively, but in a somewhat higher concentration, it also induces the secretion of dense bodies. An even further increase in thrombin concentration results in the release of all three types of granules including lysosomes. A similar dose dependence could be demonstrated with collagen as well. In contrast to thrombin and collagen, ADP in itself should not be considered as a direct release inducing agent since, unless intensive cell to cell contact is ensured (in

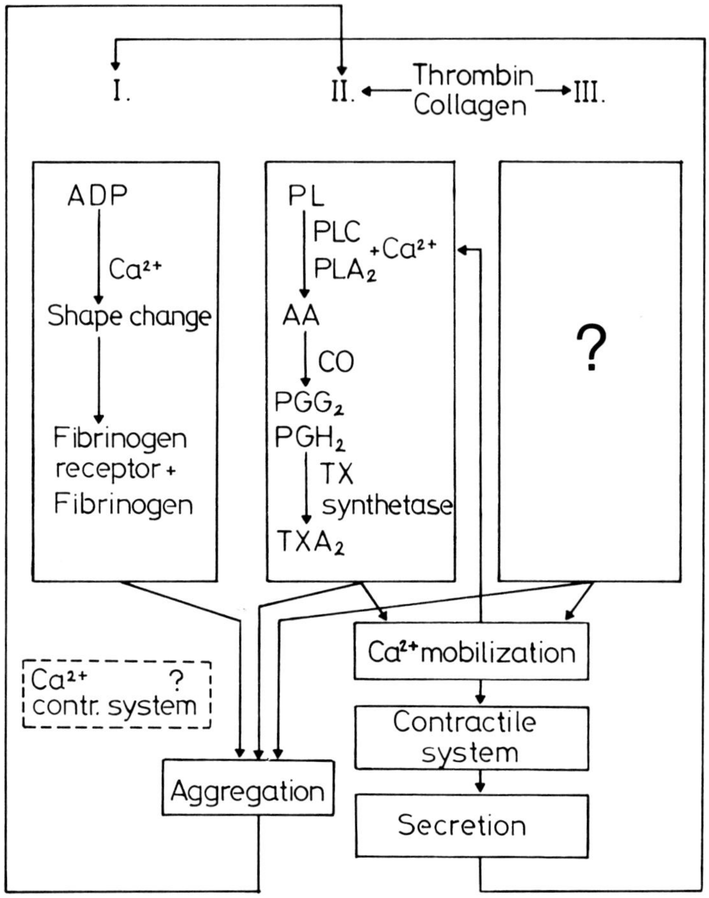

FIGURE 1. Biochemical pathways of platelet aggregation. Abbreviations: ADP, adenosine-5′-diphosphate; PL, phospholipid; PLA_2, phospholipase A_2; PLC, phospholipase C; AA, arachidonic acid; CO, cyclooxygenase; PGG_2, prostaglandin G_2; PGH_2, prostaglandin H_2; TX, thromboxane; TXA_2, thromboxane A_2.

vitro by thorough mixing or centrifugation), it cannot elicit per se a secretory response.[18,27-29] Release reaction has an essential role in the propagation and amplification of the aggregation process. In this respect, ADP (and in a smaller extent serotonin) secreted from dense bodies and fibrinogen released from α-granules are of primary importance.

B. Biochemical Pathways Leading to Activation

A schematic representation of the biochemical mechanisms responsible for platelet activation is shown in Figure 1. Three interrelated and in certain cases parallel ongoing biochemical mechanisms could be differentiated.[29] One of the mechanisms is induced by fibrinogen following the preparatory action of ADP. Binding of ADP to its receptor on the platelet membrane results in a structural reorganization, one of the consequences of which is the appearance of fibrinogen receptor (or an increase in their number by several magnitudes) on the membrane surface.

The receptor-signal relationship and the mechanism of membrane reorganization is not fully understood. It has been shown that within seconds following the addition of ADP the phosphatidyl-inositol 4′,5′-diphosphate (PIP_2) content of the membrane is decreased.[30] PIP_2 can chelate Ca^{2+} [31] and may constitute part of the Ca^{2+} pool of the internal membrane surface. The breakdown of PIP_2 could induce a local release of Ca ions and consequently depolymerization of microtubular ring as well as the activation of submembranous, presumably membrane GP-associated contractile-filamentous systems. (The role a phosphatidyl inositol metabolism plays in platelet activation will be discussed later in detail.) This would then result in shape change and reorganization of membrane GP, leading, among others, to the appearance of newly assembled fibrinogen receptors. The fibrinogen receptor of platelets is a complex of GPIIb, GPIIIa, and extracellular Ca^{2+}.[32,33] In case intensive cell-to-cell contact occurs, fibrinogen bound to its membrane receptor can bridge stimulated platelets and bring about reversible clumping. The contractile systems activated by Ca^{2+} released from intracellular sources other than the plasma membrane may participate in further regrouping of membrane receptors during aggregation and in the consolidation of the aggregate. This pathway is not restricted to the ADP-initiated response, but is involved in every type of activation that induces the secretion of dense bodies. Thus, ADP released from dense bodies (nonmetabolic nucleotide pool) is of great importance in the propagation of aggregatory response elicited by other agents through different pathway(s). As mentioned earlier, ADP is not a direct release inducer. The release of α-granules and dense bodies observed during ADP aggregation is brought about by cell-to-cell contact, i.e., by the aggregation process itself. It involves mechanism(s) other than the ADP-fibrinogen pathway and is, in all probability, mediated by TXA_2 formation. However, ADP-induced secretion occurs only at a physiologically low Ca^{2+} concentration and seems to be only an in vitro phenomenon.[29]

The main mediator of the second pathway is TXA_2. The activating agents here also release Ca^{2+} from submembranous sources which in turn activates membrane phospholipases resulting in the liberation of arachidonic acid.[34] The platelet membrane contains an unusually large amount of AA primarly in the sn-2 position of phosphatidyl-choline (PC) and phosphatidyl-ethanolamine (PE).[35] There are two main routes of AA release and it is accomplished by the concerted action of several phospholipases.[36] In resting platelets these phospholipases exist in a relatively inactive state and become activated by the local increase of Ca^{2+} availability. Phospholipase C (PLC) uses PI as a substrate and produces arachidonyl diglyceride which is further cleaved by diglyceride lipase and AA is released.[37-39] Another minor route of arachidonic acid liberation from PI derivatives is through the catabolism of PIP_2.[40] AA being on the second position may be stripped off from diacylglycerol (DG) or phosphatidic acid (PA), intermediates of PIP_2 catabolism, by a diacylglycerol lipase, or by a PA specific PLA_2. Though these mechanisms in all probability play a role in the early phase of activation,[41] a number of data suggest that PI or PI derivatives are not the major sources of AA supplied for the TXA_2 pathway.[36] The other route is initiated by PLA_2 which is associated to DTS membranes.[42] The primary substrates of PLA_2 are PC and PE. PLA_2 acts on the sn-2 position, thus liberating mainly AA[43-45] (Figure 2). Cyclization and oxidation of AA by cyclooxygenase (CO) then result in a cyclic endoperoxide, prostaglandin (PG) G_2, which is quickly transformed into PGH_2 by peroxidase activity. During activation, this process is accompanied by a highly increased oxygen consumption (''oxygen burst''). Cyclic endoperoxides themselves can exert an activating effect on platelets, however, in normal conditions they are rapidly converted into a labile but highly effective activating agent TXA_2 (for details, see References 36 and 46). As mentioned earlier, TXA_2 synthesis is located in the DTS.[21]

Certain activating agents like a high dose of thrombin or collagen can initiate a mechanism of platelet activation independent from ADP release or TXA_2 formation.[45,47] The biochemistry of this third pathway is not known. An earlier hypothesis suggesting platelet activating factor (PAF), chemically 1-0-alkyl-2-acetyl-*sn*-glycero-3-phosphocholine, as the mediator of the third pathway was not supported by experimental findings.[27,48,49]

C. Second Messengers: Phosphoinositide Metabolism, Ca^{2+}, and Cyclic Nucleotides

The fact that platelets respond to a certain stimulus with a series of changes and various

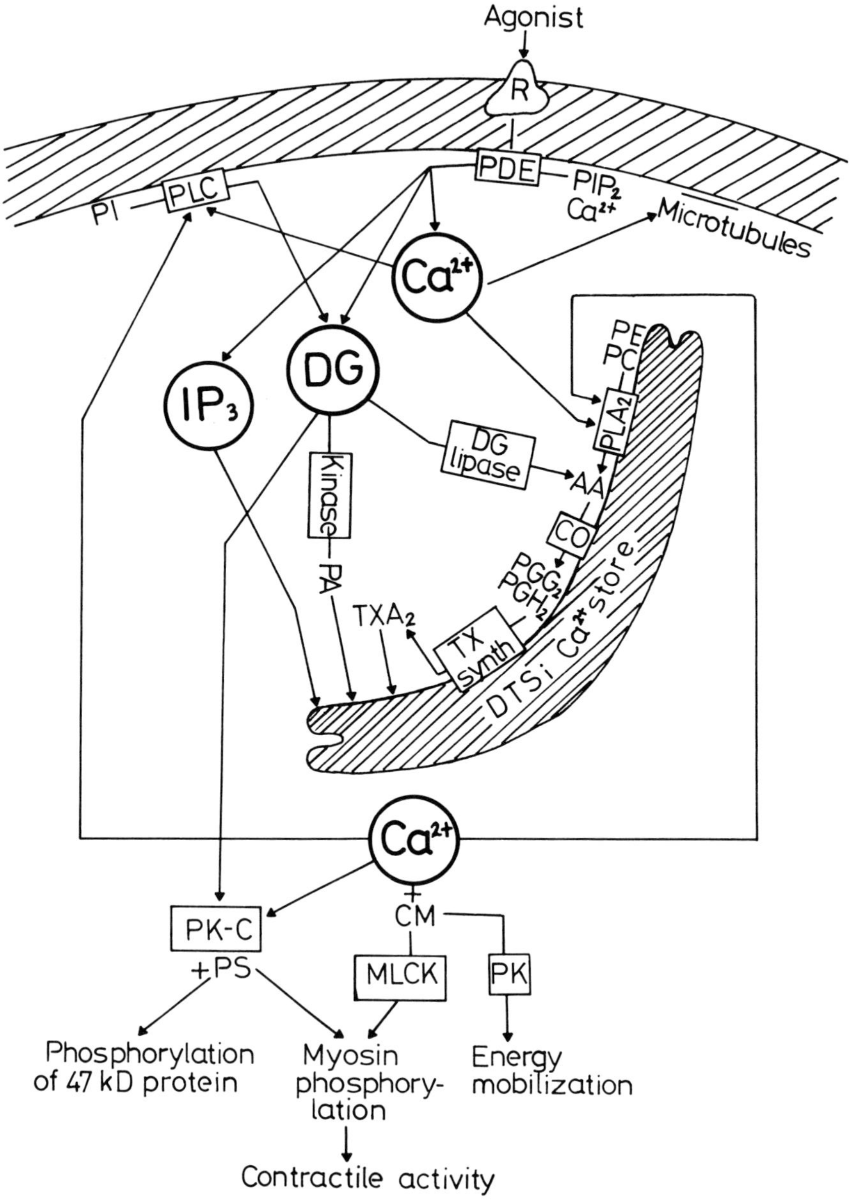

FIGURE 2. Biochemical mechanisms leading to platelet activation. Abbreviations: AA, arachidonic acid; CM, calmodulin, CO, cyclooxygenase; DG, diacyl glycerol; DTS, dense tubular system; IP_3, inositol-1,4,5-triphosphate; MLCK, myosin light chain kinase; PA, phosphatidic acid; PC, phosphatidyl choline; PDE, phosphodiesteratic activity that cleaves PIP_2/PLC/; PE, phosphatidyl ethanolamine; PGG_2, prostaglandin G_2; PGH_2, prostaglandin H_2; PI, phosphatidyl inositol; PIP_2, phosphatidyl inositol-4′,5′-diphosphate; PK, phosphorylase kinase; PK-C, proteinkinase C; PLA_2, phospholipase A_2; PLC, phospholipase C; PS, phosphatidyl serine; TX, thromboxane; TXA_2, thromboxane A_2.

stimuli may elicit the same response by different pathway(s) makes addressing the problem of second messengers in platelet activation extremely difficult. A further and frequently overlooked complication is that biochemical changes may be restricted to a certain platelet compartment and the same messenger released into different compartments and at different times in the course of activation will mediate different responses. Figure 2 summarizes the mechanism of formation, release, and action of second messengers involved in the activation process.

In the last few years, phosphoinositide metabolism has attracted much attention and two of the metabolic products of PIP_2, namely, inositol-1,4,5-triphosphate (IP_3) and diacylglycerol (DG), have been proposed as second messengers in platelet activation.[40] As perturbation of membrane phospholipids and alterations in its polyphosphoinositide composition seem to be the first changes elicited by an agonist,[50-54] we start discussing the question of second messengers of platelet activation by dealing with polyphosphoinositide metabolism. Polyphosphoinositides are formed by sequential phosphorylation of hydroxyl groups on the 4 and 5 positions of PI. Though they represent only a minor portion of membrane phosphoinositides, they have a highly active metabolic turnover and the kinases and phosphomonoesterases maintaining this dynamic equilibrium are among the most active cellular enzymes.[40]

IP_3 is removed from PIP_2 by a phosphodiesteratic (PLC) activity, leaving DG behind (Figure 2). The most crucial question concerning the second messenger nature of IP_3 and DG is if their release is independent from Ca^{2+} mobilization. Though purified human platelet PLC that hydrolyzes polyphosphoinositides shows Ca^{2+} sensitivity,[55] it has been shown in a number of cell types,[40] including platelets,[51,56] that the agonist dependent breakdown of polyphosphoinositides can occur independently of changes in cytosol calcium. In spite of a few contradictory examples,[57,58] the majority of data favor Michell's hypothesis[59] that hydrolysis of PIP_2 can occur at the calcium level of unactivated resting cell and is the direct consequence of receptor-agonist interaction.

The phospodiesteratic cleavage of PIP_2 results in the release of three active compounds: IP_3, DG, and Ca^{2+}. As mentioned, PIP_2 of the internal membrane surface might represent a membrane bound Ca^{2+} store which could be liberated when PIP_2 is hydrolyzed in the initial phase of platelet activation. Calculated from the total amount of PIP_2 in the platelet membrane the Ca^{2+} released from this storage site was found severalfold less than Ca^{2+} mobilized during the activation process induced by a strong stimulus. It is also questionable if in the presence of a much higher cytoplasmic Mg^{2+} concentration PIP_2 could really bind the above amount of Ca^{2+}.[60,61] From these data, it seems evident that Ca^{2+} released by PIP_2 breakdown does not significantly contribute to the increased Ca^{2+} concentration in the cytoplasm of activated platelets, however, it might well be involved in the induction of Ca^{2+} dependent local submembranous changes (dissassembly of microtubules, activation of submembranous filament system, etc.) during the initial phase of activation process.

An attractive new hypothesis concerning the role of PIP_2 metabolic products is that IP_3 might function as a second messenger for Ca^{2+} mobilization.[40,62] Findings showing that in permeabilized cells of various types IP_3 can release Ca^{2+} from nonmitochondrial intracellular sources provide strong experimental support of this idea.[40,63] Investigations carried out on platelets resulted in a similar conclusion and it was also shown that IP_3 can release Ca^{2+} from isolated DTS membrane vesicles.[64] The rapid rise in IP_3 concentration occurs at the early stage of thrombin activation[53] which suggests that it mediates Ca^{2+} release necessary to trigger mechanisms leading to activation.

The other metabolic product of phosphodiesteratic cleavage of phosphoinositides including PIP_2 is DG. DG is one of the sources of AA metabolized in the TXA_2 pathway. AA can be released directly from the 2-sn position by diglycerol lipase[38] or PA or following transformation into PA by a PLA_2.[65] The latter mechanism, however, seems to be too slow to account for much of the AA produced.[63,66] PA has also been proposed to act as an ionophore and by this way participate in Ca^{2+} mobilization.[67,68] Its ionophore nature has, however, been questioned[69] and its formation during thrombin activation is probably too slow to participate in the early rise of Ca^{2+} concentration.[63] In addition to being a substrate for PA and AA production, DG has been proposed to exert a second messenger function, as well.[40,63]

33. **Nachman, R. L. and Leung, L. L. R.,** Complex formation of platelet membrane glycoproteins IIb and IIIa with fibrinogen, *J. Clin. Invest.,* 69, 263, 1982.
34. **Feinstein, M. B. and Walenga, R.,** The role of calcium in platelet activation, in *Biochemistry of the Acute Allergic Reactions,* Becker, E. L., Simon, A. S., and Ansten, K. F., Eds., Alan R. Liss, New York, 1981, 279.
35. **Perret, B., Chap, H. J., and Douste-Blazy, L.,** Asymmetric distribution of arachidonic acid in the plasma membrane of human platelets. A determination using purified phospholipases and rapid method for membrane isolation, *Biochim. Biophys. Acta,* 56, 434, 1979.
36. **Longenecker, G. L.,** Platelet arachidonic acid metabolism, in *The Platelets. Physiology and Pharmacology,* Longenecker, G. L., Ed., Academic Press, New York, 1985, 159.
37. **Rittenhouse-Simmons, S.,** Production of diglyceride from phosphatidylinositol in activated human platelets, *J. Clin. Invest.,* 63, 580, 1979.
38. **Bell, R. L., Kennerly, D. A., Stanford, N., and Majerus, P. W.,** Diglyceride lipase: a pathway for arachidonate release from human platelets, *Proc. Natl. Acad. Sci. U.S.A.,* 76, 3238, 1979.
39. **Bell, R. L., Stanford, N., Kennerly, D. A., and Majerus, P. W.,** Diglyceride lipase: a pathway for arachidonate release from human platelets, *Adv. Prostaglandin Thromboxane Res.,* 6, 219, 1980.
40. **Berridge, J. M.,** Inositol triphosphate and diacylglycerol as second messengers, *Biochem. J.,* 220, 345, 1984.
41. **Bell, R. L. and Majerus, P. W.,** Thrombin-induced hydrolysis of phosphatidylinositol in human platelets, *J. Biol. Chem.,* 255, 1790, 1980.
42. **Lagarde, M., Menashi, S., and Crawford, N.,** Localisation of phospholipase A_2 and diglyceride lipase activities in human platelet intracellular membranes, *FEBS Lett.,* 124, 23, 1981.
43. **Bills, T. K., Smith, J. B., and Silber, M. J.,** Metabolism of ^{14}C-arachidonic acid by human platelets, *Biochim. Biophys. Acta,* 424, 303, 1976.
44. **Derksen, A. and Cohen, P.,** Patterns of fatty acid release from endogenous substrates by human platelet homogenates and membranes, *J. Biol. Chem.,* 250, 9342, 1975.
45. **Broekman, M. J., Ward, J. W., and Marcus, A. J.,** Phospolipid metabolism in stimulated human platelets. Changes in phosphatidylinositol, phosphatidic acid and lysophospholipids, *J. Clin. Invest.,* 66, 275, 1980.
46. **Marcus, J.,** Platelet lipids, in *Haemostasis and Thrombosis,* Colman, R. W., Hirsh, J., Marder, V. J., and Salzman, E. W., Eds., Lippincott, Philadelphia, 1982, 472.
47. **Packham, M. A., Kinlough-Rathbone, R. L., Reimers, H. J., Scott, S., and Mustard, J. F.,** Mechanisms of platelet aggregation independent of adenosine diphosphate, in *Prostaglandins in Haematology,* Spectrum, New York, 1977, 247.
48. **Sturk, A., Schaap, M. C. L., ten Cate, J. W., Roozendaal, K. J., Don, J. A., Haddeman, E., and Kloeze, J.,** Platelet function and arachidonic acid metabolism in the myeloproliferative syndrome: the role of lipoxygenase in platelet functioning, in *Hemostasis and Cancer,* Muszbek, L., Ed., CRC Press, Boca Raton, Fla., 1987, 215.
49. **Adams, G. A.,** Platelet aggregation, in *The Platelets. Physiology and Pharmacology,* Longenecker, G. L., Ed., Academic Press, New York, 1985, 1.
50. **Lloyd, J. V. and Mustard, J. F.,** Changes in ^{32}P-content of phosphatidic acid and the phosphoinositides of rabbit platelets during aggregation induced by collagen or thrombin, *Br. J. Haematol.,* 26, 243, 1974.
51. **Billah, M. M. and Lapetina, E. G.,** Rapid decrease of phosphatidylinositol 4,5-biphosphate in thrombin-stimulated platelets, *J. Biol. Chem.,* 257, 12,705, 1982.
52. **Shukla, S. D. and Hanahan, D. J.,** AGEPS (platelet activating factor) induced stimulations of rabbit platelets: effects on phosphatidic acid metabolism, *Biochem. Biophys. Res. Commun.,* 106, 697, 1982.
53. **Aggranoff, B. W., Murthy, P., and Segnin, E. B.,** Thrombin-induced phosphodiesteratic cleavage of phosphatidylinositol biphosphate in human platelets, *J. Biol. Chem.,* 258, 2076, 1983.
54. **Mauco, G., Chap, H., and Douste-Blazy, L.,** Platelet activating factor (PAF-acether) promotes an early degradation of phosphatidylinositol-4,5-biphosphate in rabbit platelets, *FEBS Lett.,* 153, 361, 1983.
55. **Rittenhouse, S. E.,** Human platelets contain phospholipase C that hydrolyzes polyphosphoinositides, *Proc. Natl. Acad. Sci. U.S.A.,* 80, 5417, 1983.
56. **Billah, M. M. and Lapetina, E. G.,** Degradation of phosphatidylinositol-4,5-biphosphate is insensitive to Ca^{2+} mobilization in stimulated platelets, *Biochem. Biophys. Res. Commun.,* 109, 217, 1982.
57. **Cockroft, S., Bennet, J. P., and Gonsperts, B. D.,** f-MetLeuPhe-induced phosphatidylinositol turnover in rabbit neutrophils is dependent on extracellular calcium, *FEBS Lett.,* 110, 115, 1980.
58. **Axen, K. V., Schubert, U. K., Blake, A. D., and Fleisher, N.,** Role of Ca^{2+} in secretagogue-stimulated breakdown of phosphatidylinositol in rat pancreatic islets, *J. Clin. Invest.,* 72, 13, 1983.
59. **Michell, R. H., Kirk, C. J., Jones, L. M., Downes, C., and Creba, J. A.,** The stimulation of inositol lipid metabolism that accompanies calcium mobilization in stimulated cells: defined characteristics and unanswered question, *Philos. Trans. R. Soc. London Ser. B,* 296, 123, 1981.

60. **Hendrickson, H. S. and Reinersten, J. L.,** Phosphoinositide interconversion: a model for control of Na^+ and K^+ permeability in the nerve axon membrane, *Biochem. Biophys. Res. Commun.*, 44, 1258, 1971.
61. **Downes, P. and Michell, R. H.,** Phosphatidylinositol 4-phosphate and phosphatidylinositol 4,5-biphosphate: lipids in search of a function, *Cell Calcium*, 3, 467, 1982.
62. **Berridge, M. J.,** Rapid accumulation of inositol triphosphate reveals that agonists hydrolyse polyphosphoinositides instead of phosphatidylinositol, *Biochem. J.*, 212, 849, 1983.
63. **Feinstein, M. B., Zavoico, G. B., and Halenda, S. P.,** Calcium and cyclic AMP: antagonistic modulators of platelet function, in *The Platelets: Physiology and Pharmacology*, Longenecker, G. L., Ed., Academic Press, New York, 1985, 237.
64. **O'Rourke, F., Halenda, S. P., Zavoico, G. B., and Feinstein, M. B.,** Inositol 1,4,5-triphosphate releases Ca^{2+} from a Ca^{2+}-transporting membranes vesicle fraction derived from human platelets, *J. Biol. Chem.*, 260, 956, 1985.
65. **Lapetina, E. G.,** Metabolism of inositides and the activation of platelets, *Life Sci.*, 32, 2069, 1983.
66. **Neufeld, E. J. and Majerus, P. W.,** Arachidonate release and phosphatidic acid turnover in stimulated human platelets, *J. Biol. Chem.*, 258, 2461, 1983.
67. **Serhan, C. N., Fridovich, J., Goetzl, E. J., Dunham, P. B., and Weissman, G.,** Leukotriene B4 and phosphatidic acid are calcium ionophores. Studies employing arsenazo III in liposomes, *J. Biol. Chem.*, 257, 4746, 1982.
68. **Gerrard, J. M., Butler, A. M., Peterson, D. A., and White, J. G.,** Phosphatidic acid releases calcium from a platelet membrane fraction in vitro, *Prostaglandins Med.*, 1, 387, 1978.
69. **Kaibuchi, K., Sano, K., Hoshijama, M., Takai, Y., and Nishizuka, Y.,** Phosphatidylinositol turnover in platelet activation, calcium mobilization and protein phosphorylation, *Cell Calcium*, 3, 323, 1982.
70. **Imaoka, T., Lynham, J. A., and Haslam, R. J.,** Purification and characterization of the 47,000-dalton protein phosphorylated during degranulation of human platelets, *J. Biol. Chem.*, 258, 11404, 1983.
71. **Rink, T. J., Sanchez, A., and Hallam, T. J.,** Diacylglycerol and phorbol ester stimulate secretion without raising cytoplasmic free calcium in human platelets, *Nature (London)*, 305, 317, 1983.
72. **White, J. G., Rao, G. H. R., and Estensen, R. D.,** Investigation of the release reaction in platelets exposed to phorbol myristate acetate, *Am. J. Pathol.*, 75, 301, 1974.
73. **Ware, J. A., Johnson, P. C., Smith, M., and Salzman, E. W.,** Aequorin detects increased cytoplasmic calcium in platelets stimulated with phorbol ester or diacylglycerol, *Biochem. Biophys. Res. Commun.*, 133, 98, 1985.
74. **Takai, Y., Kishimoti, A., Kawahara, Y., Minakuchi, R., Sano, K., Kikkawa, U., Mori, T., Yu, B., Kaibuchi, K., and Nishizuka, Y.,** Calcium and phosphatidylinositol turnover as signalling for transmembrane control of protein phosphorylation, *Adv. Cyclic Nucleotide Res.*, 14, 301, 1981.
75. **Kaibuchi, H., Takai, Y., Sawamura, M., Hoshijama, M., Fujikura, T., and Nishizuka, Y.,** Synergistic functions of protein phosphorylation and calcium mobilization in platelet activation, *J. Biol. Chem.*, 258, 6701, 1983.
76. **Knight, D. E. and Scrutton, M. C.,** Direct evidence that cyclic nucleotides and 1,2-diacylglycerol modulate the Ca^{2+} sensitivity of secretion in platelets, *J. Physiol.*, 349, 42, 1983.
77. **Steer, M. L. and Salzman, E. W.,** Intracellular regulatory processes in platelets, in *Hemostasis and Thrombosis*, Colman, R. W., Hirsh, J., Marder, V. J., and Salzman, E. W., Eds., Lippincott, Philadelphia, 1982, 486.
78. **Gerrard, J. M. and Carroll, R. C.,** Stimulation of platelet protein phosphorylation by arachidonic acid and endoperoxide analogs, *Prostaglandins*, 22, 81, 1981.
79. **Imai, A., Ishizuka, Y., Kawai, K., and Nozawa, Y.,** Evidence for coupling of phosphatidic acid formation and calcium influx in thrombin-activated human platelets, *Biochem. Biophys. Res. Commun.*, 108, 752, 1982.
80. **LeBreton, G. C., Venton, D. L., Euke, S. E., and Haluska, P. V.,** 13-Azaprostanoic acid: a specific antagonist of the human blood platelet thrombaxane/endoperoxide receptor, *Proc. Natl. Acad. Sci. U.S.A.*, 76, 4097, 1979.
81. **Massini, P. R., Kaser-Glanzmann, R., and Lüscher, E. F.,** Movement of calcium ions and their role in the activation of platelets, *Thromb. Haemostas.*, 40, 212, 1978.
82. **Jones, H. P.,** Calmodulin and platelet function, in *The Platelets, Physiology and Pharmacology*, Longenecker, G. L., Ed., Academic Press, New York, 1985, 221.
83. **Rao, G. H. R., Peller, J. D., Semba, C. P., and White, J. G.,** Influence of the calcium-sensitive fluorophore, quin 2, on platelet function, *Blood*, 67, 354, 1986.
84. **Gerrard, J. M., White, J. G., and Rao, G. H. R.,** Effects of the ionophore A23187 on blood platelets. II. Influence on ultrastructure, *Am. J. Pathol.*, 77, 151, 1974.
85. **Feinman, R. D. and Detwiler, T. C.,** Platelet secretion induced by divalent cation ionophores, *Nature (London)*, 249, 172, 1974.
86. **Massini, P. and Lüscher, E. F.,** Some effects of ionophores for divalent cations on blood platelets. Comparison with the effects of thrombin, *Biochim. Biophys. Acta*, 372, 109, 1974.

87. **White, J. G., Rao, G. H. R., and Gerrard, J. M.,** Effects of the ionophore A23187 on blood platelets. I. Influence on aggregation and secretion, *Am. J. Pathol.*, 77, 135, 1974.
88. **Charo, I. F., Feinman, R. D., and Detwiler, T. C.,** Inhibition of platelet secretion by an antagonist of intracellular calcium, *Biochem. Biophys. Res. Commun.*, 72, 1462, 1976.
89. **LeBreton, G. C., Dinerstein, R. J., Roth, L. J., and Feinberg, H.,** Direct evidence for intracellular divalent cation redistribution associated with platelet shape change, *Biochem. Biophys. Res. Commun.*, 71, 362, 1976.
90. **Tsien, R. Y.,** A non-disruptive technique for loading calcium buffers and indicators into cells, *Nature (London)*, 290, 527, 1981.
91. **Rink, T. J., Smith, S. W., and Tsien, R. Y.,** Intracellular free calcium in platelet shape change and aggregation, *J. Physiol.*, 324, 53P, 1982.
92. **Rink, T. J., Smith, S. W., and Tsien, R. Y.,** Cytoplasmic free Ca^{2+} in human platelets: Ca^{2+}-thresholds and Ca^{2+}-independent activation of shape change and secretion, *FEBS Lett.*, 148, 21, 1982.
93. **Hallam, T. J., Sauches, A., and Rink, T. J.,** Stimulus-response coupling in human platelets, *Biochem. J.*, 218, 819, 1984.
94. **Johnson, P. C., Ware, J. A., Cliveden, P., Smith, M., Dvorak, A. M., and Salzman, E. W.,** Measurement of ionized calcium in blood platelets with photoprotein aequorin: comparison with Quin 2, *J. Biol. Chem.*, 260, 2069, 1985.
95. **Knight, D. E., Hallam, T. J., and Scrutton, M. C.,** Agonist selectivity and second messenger concentration in Ca^{2+}-mediated secretion, *Nature (London)*, 296, 256, 1982.
96. **Mürer, E. H. and Holme, R.,** A study of the release of calcium from human platelets and its inhibition by metabolic inhibitors, N-ethylmaleimide and aspirin, *Biochim. Biophys. Acta*, 222, 197, 1970.
97. **Mills, D. C. B. and Macfarlane, D. E.,** Platelet receptors, in *Platelets in Biology and Pathology*, Gordon, J. L., Ed., North-Holland, Amsterdam, 1976, 159.
98. **LeBreton, G. C. and Feinberg, H.,** ADP-induced changes in intraplatelet Ca^{2+} ion concentration, *Pharmacologist*, 16, 313, 1974.
99. **Massini, P. and Lüscher, E. F.,** On the significance of the influx of calcium ions into stimulated human blood platelets, *Biochim. Biophys. Acta*, 436, 652, 1976.
100. **Grette, K.,** Studies on the mechanism of thrombin-catalyzed haemostatic reactions in blood platelets, *Acta Physiol. Scand.*, 56(Suppl. 195), 5, 1962.
101. **Mueller-Eckardt, C. H. and Lüscher, E. F.,** Immune reactions of human blood platelets. I. A comparative study on the effects on platelets of heterologous antiplatelet antiserum, antigen-antibody complexes, and thrombin, *Thromb. Diath. Haemorrh.*, 20, 155, 1968.
102. **Cohen, J. and de Vries, A.,** Platelet contractile regulation in an isometric system, *Nature (London)*, 246, 36, 1973.
103. **Menashi, S., Davis, C., and Crawford, N.,** Calcium uptake associated with an intracellular membrane fraction prepared from human blood platelets by high-voltage, free-flow electrophoresis, *FEBS Lett.*, 140, 298, 1982.
104. **Fauvel, J., Chap, H., Roques, V., Levy-Toledano, S., and Douste-Blazy, L.,** Biochemical characterization of plazma membranes and intracellular membranes isolated from human platelets using Percoll gradients, *Biochim. Biophys. Acta*, 856, 155, 1986.
105. **Borisy, G. G., Olmstead, J. B., Marcum, J. M., and Allen, C.,** Microtubule assembly in vitro, *Fed. Proc.*, 33, 167, 1974, 105.
106. **Crawford, N., Amos, L. A., and Castle, A. G.,** Platelet microtubule subunit proteins: assembly and disassembly factors, in *Platelets Cellular Response Mechanisms and their Biological Significance*, Rotman, A., Meyer, F. A., Gitler, C., and Silberberg, A., Eds., John Wiley & Sons, Chichester, England, 1980, 171.
107. **Pickett, W. C., Jesse, R. L., and Cohen, P.,** Initiation of phospholipase A_2 activity in human platelets by the calcium ionophore A_{23187}, *Biochim. Biophys. Acta*, 486, 209, 1977.
108. **Rittenhouse-Simmons, S. and Deykin, D.,** The mobilization of arachidonic acid in platelets exposed to thrombin or ionophore A_{23187}, *J. Clin. Invest.*, 60, 495, 1977.
109. **Chaiken, R., Pagano, D., and Detwiler, T. C.,** Regulation of platelet phosphorylase, *Biochim. Biophys. Acta*, 403, 315, 1975.
110. **Gear, A. R. L. and Schneider, W.,** Control of platelet glycogenolysis. Activation of phosphorylase kinase by calcium, *Biochim. Biophys. Acta*, 392, 111, 1975.
111. **Gergely, P., Castle, A. G., and Crawford, N.,** Platelet phosphorylase kinase activity and its regulation by the calcium dependent regulatory protein, calmodulin, *Biochim. Biophys. Acta*, 612, 50, 1980.
112. **Detwiler, T. C.,** Control of energy metabolism in platelets. The effects of thrombin and cyanide on glycolysis, *Biochim. Biophys. Acta*, 256, 163, 1972.
113. **Rodan, G. and Feinstein, M. B.,** Interrelationships between Ca^{2+} and adenylate and guanylate cyclases in the control of platelet secretion and aggregation, *Proc. Natl. Acad. Sci. U.S.A.*, 73, 1829, 1976.

114. **Feinstein, M. B., Rodan, G. A., and Cutler, L. S.,** Cyclic AMP and calcium in platelet function, in *Platelets in Biology and Pathology 2,* Gordon, J. L., Ed., Elsevier, Amsterdam, 1981, 437.
115. **Philips, D. R. and Jakabova, N.,** Ca^{2+}-dependent protease in human platelets. Specific cleavage of platelet polypeptides in the presence of added Ca^{2+}, *J. Biol. Chem.,* 252, 5602, 1977.
116. **Fox, J. E. B., Goll, D. E., Reynolds, C. C., and Philips, D. R.,** Identification of two proteins (actin-binding protein and P235) that are hydrolyzed by endogenous Ca^{2+} dependent protease during platelet aggregation, *J. Biol. Chem.,* 260, 1060, 1985.
117. **Smoake, J. A., Song, S. Y., and Cheung, W. Y.,** Cyclic 3′,5′-nucleotide phosphodiesterase distribution and developmental changes of the enzyme and its protein activator in mammalian tissue and cells, *Biochim. Biophys. Acta,* 341, 402, 1974.
118. **Muszbek, L., Kuznicki, J., Szabó, T., and Drabikowski, W.,** Troponin C like protein of blood platelets, *FEBS Lett.,* 80, 308, 1977.
119. **Kakincki, S., Sobue, K., Yamazaki, R., Kambayashi, J., Sakon, M., and Kosaki, G.,** Lack tissue specificity of calmodulin: a rapid and high-yield purification method, *FEBS Lett.,* 126, 203, 1981.
120. **Young, N., Gergely, P., and Crawford, N.,** Platelet and leucocyte calmodulins isolation and characterisation, *Eur. J. Biochem.,* 120, 303, 1981.
121. **White, G. C., Levine, S. N., and Steiner, A. N.,** Platelet calcium-dependent proteins: identification and localization of the calcium-dependent regulatory calmodulin, in platelets, *Am. J. Haematol.,* 10, 359, 1981.
122. **Dabrowska, R. and Hartshorne, D. J.,** Ca^{2+}- and modulator-dependent myosin light chain kinase from non-muscle cells, *Biochem. Biophys. Res. Commun.,* 85, 1352, 1978.
123. **McGowan, E. B.,** Comparison of cyclic nucleotide phosphodiesterase (PDE) activities from Triton-x100-and high- salt- disrupted platelets, *Fed. Proc.,* 38, 46, 1979.
124. **Wong, P. Y. K. and Cheung, W. K.,** Calmodulin stimulates human platelet phospholipase A_2, *Biochem. Biophys. Res. Commun.,* 90, 473, 1979.
125. **Welsh, M. J., Dedman, J. R., Brinkley, B. R., Means, A. R.,** Calcium-dependent regulator protein-localization in mitotic apparatus of eukaryotic cells, *Proc. Natl. Acad. Sci. U.S.A.,* 75, 1867, 1978.
126. **Kindness, G., Williamson, F. B., and Long, W. F.,** Inhibitory effect of trifluoperazine on aggregation of human platelets, *Thromb. Res.,* 17, 549, 1980.
127. **Kambayashi, J., Morimoto, K., Hakata, N., Kobayashi, T., and Kosaki, G.,** Involvement of calmodulin in platelet reaction, *Thromb. Res.,* 22, 553, 1983.
128. **Nishikawa, M., Tanaka, T., and Hidaka, K.,** Ca^{2+}-calmodulin-dependent phosphorylation and platelet secretion, *Nature (London),* 287, 863, 1980.
129. **Feinstein, M. B. and Hadjian, R. A.,** Effects of the calmodulin antagonist trifluoperazine on stimulus-induced calcium mobilization, aggregation, secretion, and protein phosphorylation in platelets, *Mol. Pharmacol.,* 21, 422, 1982.
130. **Schatzman, R. C., Wise, B. C., and Kuo, J. F.,** Phospholipid-sensitive calcium-dependent protein kinase: inhibition by anti-psychotic drugs, *Biochem. Biophys. Res. Commun.,* 98, 669, 1981.
131. **Walengo, R. W., Opas, E. E., and Feinstein, M. B.,** Differential effects of calmodulin antagonists on phospholipases A_2 and C in thrombin-stimulated platelets, *J. Biol. Chem.,* 256, 12523, 1981.
132. **Aktories, K. and Jakobs, K. H.,** Regulation of platelet cyclic AMP formation, in *The Platelets: Physiology and Pharmacology,* Longenecker, G. L., Ed., Academic Press, New York, 1985, 271.
133. **Steer, M. L. and Salzman, E. W.,** Cyclic nucleotides in hemostasis and thrombosis, *Adv. Cyclic Nucleotide Res.,* 12, 71, 1980.
134. **Wolfe, S. M. and Shulman, N. R.,** Adenylcyclase activity in human platelets, *Biochem. Biophys. Res. Commun.,* 35, 265, 1969.
135. **Robinson, G. A., Arnold, A., and Hartmann, R. C.,** Divergent effects of epinephrine and prostaglandin E_1 on the level of cyclic AMP in human blood platelets, *Pharmacol. Res. Commun.,* 1, 325, 1969.
136. **Ball, G., Brereton, G. G., Fulwood, M., Ireland, D. M., and Yates, P.,** Effect of prostaglandin E_1 alone and in combination with theophylline or aspirin or collagen-induced platelet aggregation and on platelet nucleotides including adenosine 3′,5′-monophosphate, *Biochem. J.,* 120, 709, 1970.
137. **Mills, D. and Smith, J. B.,** The influence on platelet aggregation of drugs that affect the accumulation of adenosine 3′,5′-cyclic monophosphate in rats, *Biochem. J.,* 121, 185, 1971.
138. **Mills, D. and Macfarlane, D.,** Stimulation of human platelet adenylate cyclase by prostaglandin D_2, *Thromb. Res.,* 5, 401, 1974.
139. **Michel, H., Caen, J. P., Born, G. V. R., Miller, R., d'Auriac, G. A., and Meyer, P.,** Relation between the inhibition of aggregation and the concentration of cAMP in human and rat platelets, *Br. J. Haematol.,* 33, 27, 1976.
140. **Gorman, R. R., Bunting, S., and Miller, O. V.,** Modulation of human platelet adenylate cyclase by prostacyclin (PGX), *Prostaglandins,* 13, 377, 1977.
141. **Haslam, R. J. and Lynham, J.,** Activation and inhibition of blood platelet adenylate cyclase by adenosine or by 2-chloroadenosine, *Life Sci.,* 11, 1143, 1972.

142. **Haslam, R. J. and Rosson, G. M.,** Effects of adenosine on levels of adenosine cyclic 3′,5′-monophosphate in human blood platelets in relation to adenosine incorporation and platelet aggregation, *Mol. Pharmacol.*, 11, 528, 1975.
143. **Insel, P. A., Stengel, D., Ferry, N., and Hanoune, J.,** Regulation of adenylate cyclase of human platelet membranes by forskolin, *J. Biol. Chem.*, 257, 7485, 1982.
144. **Salzman, E. W. and Levine, L.,** Cyclic 3′,5′-adenosine monophosphate in human blood platelets. II. Effect of NO-2′-O-dibutyryl cyclic 3′,5′-adenosine monophosphate on platelet function, *J. Clin. Invest.*, 50, 131, 1971.
145. **Gorman, R. R., Hamberg, M., and Samuelsson, B.,** Inhibition of basal and hormone-stimulated adenylate cyclase in adepocyte ghosts by the prostaglandin endoperoxide prostaglandin H_2, *J. Biol. Chem.*, 250, 6460, 1975.
146. **Miller, O. V. and Gorman, R. R.,** Modulation of platelet cyclic nucleotide content by PGE_1 and the prostaglandin endoperoxide PGG_2, *J. Cyclic Nucleotide Res.*, 2, 79, 1976.
147. **Miller, O. V., Johnson, R. A., and Gorman, R. R.,** Inhibition of PGE_1-stimulated cAMP accumulation in human platelets by thromboxane A_2, *Prostaglandins,* 13, 599, 1977.
148. **Salzman, E. W.,** Interrelation of prostaglandin endoperoxide (prostaglandin G_2) and cyclic 3′,5′-adenosine monophosphate in human blood platelets, *Biochim. Biophys. Acta,* 499, 48, 1977.
149. **Gorman, R. R., Fitzpatrick, F. A., and Miller, O. V.,** Reciprocal regulation of human platelet cAMP levels by thromboxane A_2 and prostacyclin, *Adv. Cyclic Nucleotide Res.*, 9, 597, 1978.
150. **Jakobs, K. H., Saur, W., and Schultz, G.,** Reduction of adenylate cyclase activity in lysates of human platelets by the alpha-adrenergic component of epinephrine, *J. Cyclic Nucleotide Res.*, 2, 381, 1976.
151. **Jakobs, K. H., Aktories, K., and Schultz, G.,** Inhibition of adenylate cyclase by hormones and neurotransmitters, *Adv. Cyclic Nucleotide Res.*, 17, 135, 1984.
152. **Cooper, D. M. F. and Rodbell, M.,** ADP is a potent inhibitor of human platelet plasma membrane adenylate cyclase, *Nature (London),* 282, 517, 1979.
153. **Mellwig, K. P. and Jakobs, K. H.,** Inhibition of platelet adenylate cyclase by ADP, *Thromb. Res.*, 18, 7, 1980.
154. **Lagarde, M. and Dechawanne, M.,** Thrombin decreases platelet cyclic AMP in the absence of prostaglandin synthesis, *Biomedicine,* 27, 110, 1977.
155. **Aktories, K. and Jakobs, K. H.,** N_i-mediated inhibition of human platelet adenylate cyclase by thrombin, *Eur. J. Biochem.*, 145, 333, 1984.
156. **Miller, O. V. and Gorman, R. R.,** Evidence for distinct prostaglandin-I_2 and prostaglandin-D_2 receptors in human platelets, *J. Pharmacol. Exp. Ther.*, 210, 134, 1979.
157. **Schafer, A. J., Cooper, B., O'Hara, D., and Handin, R. J.,** Identification of platelet receptors for prostaglandin I_2 and D_2, *J. Biol. Chem.*, 254, 2914, 1979.
158. **Leamon, K. B. and Daly, J. W.,** Forskolin: a unique diterpene activator of cyclic AMP generating systems, *J. Cyclic Nucleotide Res.*, 7, 201, 1981.
159. **Feinstein, M. B., Egan, J. J., Sha'afi, R. I., and White, J.,** The cytoplasmic concentration of free calcium in platelets is controlled by stimulators of cyclic AMP production (PGD_2, PGE_1, Forskolin), *Biochem. Biophys. Res. Commun.*, 113, 598, 1983.
160. **Yamanishi, J., Kawahara, Y., and Fukuzaki, H.,** Effect of cyclic AMP on cytoplasmic free calcium in human platelets stimulated by thrombin: direct measurement with QUIN2, *Thromb. Res.*, 32, 183, 1983.
161. **Statland, B. D., Heagan, B. M., and White, J. G.,** Uptake of calcium by platelet relaxing factor, *Nature (London),* 223, 521, 1969.
162. **Rolblee, L., Shepro, D., and Belamarich, F. A.,** Calcium uptake and associated adenosine triphosphatase activity of isolated platelet membranes, *J. Gen. Physiol.*, 61, 462, 1973.
163. **Cutler, L. S., Rhodan, G., and Feinstein, M. B.,** Cytochemical localization of adenylate cyclase and of calcium ion, magnesium ion-activated ATPase in the dense tubular system of human blood platelets, *Biochim. Biophys. Acta,* 542, 357, 1978.
164. **Cutler, L. S., Feinstein, M. B., Rhodan, G. A., and Christian, C. P.,** K^+-dependent para-nitrophenyl phosphatase in separate membrane compartments in human platelets, *Histochem. J.*, 13, 547, 1981.
165. **Kaser-Glanzmann, R., Jakabove, M., George, J. N., and Lüscher, E. F.,** Stimulation of calcium uptake in platelet membrane vesicles by adenosine 3′,5′-cyclic monophosphate and protein kinase, *Biochim. Biophys. Acta,* 466, 429, 1977.
166. **Haslam, R. J., Lynnam, J. A., and Fox, J. E. B.,** Effects of collagen ionophore A_{21387} and prostaglandin E_1 on the phosphorylation of specific proteins in blood platelets, *Biochem. J.*, 178, 397, 1979.
167. **Kaser-Glanzmann, R., Gerber, E., and Lüscher, E. F.,** Regulation of the intracellular calcium level in human blood platelet: cyclic adenosine 3′,5′ monophosphate dependent phosphorylation of a 22,000 dalton component in isolated Ca^{2+}-accumulating vesicles, *Biochim. Biophys. Acta,* 558, 344, 1979.
168. **LePench, C. J., LePench, D. A. M., Katz, S., DeMaille, J. G., Hincke, M. D., Bredoux, R., Enout, J., Levy-Toledano, S., and Caen, J.,** Regulation of calcium accumulation and efflux from platelet vesicles possible role for cyclic-AMP-dependent phosphorylation and calmodulin, *Biochim. Biophys. Acta,* 731, 456, 1983.

169. **Watson, S. P., McConnell, R. T., and Lapetina, E. G.,** The rapid formation of inositol phosphates in human platelets by thrombin is inhibited by prostacyclin, *J. Biol. Chem.*, 259, 13199, 1984.
170. **Gerrard, J. M., Peller, J. D., Kirck, T. P., and White, J. G.,** Cyclic AMP and platelet prostaglandin synthesis, *Prostaglandins*, 14, 39, 1977.
171. **Minkes, M., Stanford, N., Chi, M. M. Y., Roth, G. J., Raz, A., Needleman, P., and Majerus, P. W.,** Cyclic adenosine 3′,5′-monophosphate inhibits the availability of arachidonate to prostaglandin synthetase in human platelet suspensions, *J. Clin. Invest.*, 59, 449, 1977.
172. **Rittenhouse-Simmons, S. and Deykin, D.,** The activation by Ca^{2+} of platelet phospholipase A_2: effect of dibutyryl cyclic adenosine monophosphate and 8-(*N,N*-dimethylamino)-octyl-3,4,5-trimethoxybenzoate, *Biochim. Biophys. Acta*, 543, 409, 1978.
173. **Steiner, M.,** 3′,5′-Cyclic AMP binds to and promotes polymerization of platelet tubulin, *Nature (London)*, 272, 834, 1978.
174. **Bettex-Galland, M. and Lüscher, E. F.,** Extraction of an actomyosinlike protein from human thrombocytes, *Nature (London)*, 184, 276, 1959.
175. **Booyse, F. M. and Rafelson, M. E.,** Mechanism and control of platelet-platelet interaction. III. A relaxation contraction model for platelet aggregation, *Microvasc. Res.*, 4, 207, 1972.
176. **Gerrard, J. M. and White, J. G.,** The structure and function of platelets, with emphasis on their contractile nature, in *Pathobiology Annual*, Iochim, H. L., Ed., Appleton-Century-Crofts, New York, 1976, 31.
177. **Muszbek, L.,** Biochemical mechanism of platelet activation. Involvement of contractile proteins, *Folia Haematol.*, 106, 765, 1979.
178. **Harris, H.,** Regulation of motile activity in platelets, in *Platelets in Biology and Pathology 2*, Gordon, J. L., Ed., Elsevier, Amsterdam, 1981, 473.
179. **Cohen, J.,** Contractile platelet proteins, in *Haemostasis and Thrombosis*, Colman, R. W., Hirsh, J., Marder, V. J., and Salzman, E. W., Eds., Lippincott, Philadelphia, 1982, 459.
180. **Fox, J. E. B. and Philips, D. R.,** Polymerization and organization of actin filaments within platelets, *Sem. Haematol.*, 20, 243, 1983.
181. **Bettex-Galland, M., Portzehl, H., and Lüscher, E. F.,** Dissociation of thrombosthenin into two components comparable with actin and myosin, *Nature (London)*, 193, 777, 1962.
182. **Harris, H. E. and Weeds, A. G.,** Platelet actin: sub-cellular distribution and association with profilin, *FEBS Lett.*, 90, 84, 1978.
183. **Pollard, T. D.,** Functional implications of the biochemical and structural properties of cytoplasmic contractile proteins, in *Molecules and Cell Movement*, Inone, S. and Stephens, R. E., Eds., Raven Press, New York, 1975, 259.
184. **Castle, A. G. and Crawford, N.,** Isolation of tubulin from pig platelets, *FEBS Lett.*, 51, 195, 1975.
185. **Nachmias, V., Sallender, J., and Asch, A.,** Shape and cytoplasmic filaments in control and lidocaine treated human platelets, *Blood*, 50, 39, 1977.
186. **White, J. G. and Gerrard, J. M.,** Interaction of microtubules and microfilaments in platelet contractile physiology, in *The Cytoskeleton in Normal and Pathology Processes: Cell Physiopathology*, Vol. 9, Gabbiani, G., Ed., S. Karger, Basel, 1979, 1.
187. **Steiner, M. and Ikeda, Y.,** Quantitative assessment of polymerized and depolymerized platelet microtubules: changes caused by aggregating agents, *J. Clin. Invest.*, 63, 443, 1979.
188. **Nachmias, V. T.,** Platelet and megakaryocyte shape change: triggered alterations in the cytoskeleton, *Sem. Haematol.*, 20, 261, 1983.
189. **Maltson, J. C. and Zuicher, C. A.,** Elucidation of the platelet cytoskeleton, *Ann. N.Y. Acad. Sci.*, 11, 370, 1981.
190. **Behnke, O., Kristensen, B. I., and Nielsen, L. E.,** Electron microscopical observations on actinoid and myosinoid filaments in blood platelets, *J. Ultrastruct. Res.*, 37, 351, 1971.
191. **Niederman, R. and Pollard, T.,** Human platelet myosin. II. In vitro assembly and structure of myosin filaments, *J. Cell Biol.*, 67, 72, 1975.
192. **Tanaka, K., Onji, T., Okamoto, K., Matsusaka, T., Taniguchi, H., and Shibato, N.,** Reorganization of contractile elements in the platelet during clot retraction, 89, 98, 1984.
193. **Leven, R. M.,** Megakaryocyte Spreading: The Role of Sodium and of the Cytoskeleton, Thesis, University of Pennsylvania, Philadelphia, 1982.
194. **Muszbek, L., Ádány, R., Cjlukhova, M. A., Frid, M. G., Kabakov, A. E., and Koteliansky, V.,** The identification of vimentin in human platelets, *Eur. J. Cell Biol.*, 43, 501, 1987.
195. **Lazarides, E. and Lindberg, U.,** Actin is the naturally occurring inhibitor of deoxyribonuclease I, *Proc. Natl. Acad. Sci. U.S.A.*, 72, 4742, 1974.
196. **Blikstad, I., Markey, F., Carlsson, L., Persson, T., and Lindberg, U.,** Selective assay of monomeric and filamentous actin in cell extracts, using inhibition of deoxyribonuclease I, *Cell*, 15, 935, 1978.
197. **Fox, J. E. B., Dockter, M. E., and Philips, D. R.,** An improved method for determining the actin filament content of nonmuscle cells by the DNase I inhibition assay, *Anal. Biochem.*, 117, 170, 1981.

198. **Carlsson, L., Markey, F., Blikstad, I., Persson, T., and Lindberg, U.,** Reorganization of actin in platelets stimulated by thrombin as measured by DNase I inhibition assay, *Proc. Natl. Acad. Sci. U.S.A.*, 76, 6376, 1979.
199. **Pribluda, V., Laub, F., and Rotman, A.,** The state of actin in activated human platelets, *Eur. J. Biochem.*, 116, 293, 1981.
200. **Jennings, L. K., Fox, J. E. B., Edwards, H. H., and Philips, D. R.,** Changes in the cytoskeletal structure of human platelets following thrombin activation, *J. Biol. Chem.*, 256, 6927, 1981.
201. **Davies, G. E. and Palek, J.,** The state of actin polymerization in tetracaine-treated platelets, *Thromb. Haemostas.*, 48, 153, 1982.
202. **Gordon, D. J., Boyer, J. L., and Korn, E. D.,** Comparative biochemistry of non-muscle actins, *J. Biol. Chem.*, 252, 8300, 1977.
203. **Carlsson, L., Nyström, L. E., Sundkvist, J., Markey, F., and Lindberg, U.,** Actin polymerizability is influenced by profilin, a low molecular weight protein in non-muscle cells, *J. Mol. Biol.*, 115, 465, 1977.
204. **Harris, H. E. and Weeds, A. G.,** Platelet actin: subcellular distribution and association with profilin, *FEBS Lett.*, 90, 84, 1978.
205. **Markey, F., Lindberg, U., and Eriksson, L.,** Human platelets contain profilin, a potential regulator of actin polymerizability, *FEBS Lett.*, 88, 75, 1978.
206. **Markey, F., Persson, T., and Lindberg, U.,** Characterization of platelet extract before and after stimulation with respect to the possible role of profilactin as microfilament precursor, *Cell*, 23, 145, 1981.
207. **Wang, L. L. and Bryan, J.,** Isolation of calcium-dependent platelet proteins that interact with actin, *Cell*, 25, 637, 1981.
208. **Snabes, M. C., Boyd, A. E., and Bryan, J.,** Detection of actin binding proteins in human platelets by ^{115}I-actin overlay of polyacrylamide gels, *J. Cell Biol.*, 90, 809, 1981.
209. **Lind, S. E., Yin, H. L., and Stossel, T. P.,** Human platelets contain gelsolin, *J. Clin. Invest.*, 69, 1382, 1982.
210. **Tellam, R. and Frieden, C.,** Cytochalasin D and platelet gelsolin accelerate actin polymer formation. A model for regulation of the extent of actin polymer formation in vivo, *Biochemistry*, 21, 3207, 1982.
211. **Im, T., Kamitani, T., Tatsumi, N., Okuda, K., and Kusunose, M.,** Purification of calcium-sensitive regulatory protein of platelets which inhibits the gelation of actin, *Biochem. Biophys. Res. Commun.*, 107, 173, 1982.
212. **Kurth, M. C., Wang, L. L., Dingus, J., and Bryan, J.,** Purification and characterization of gelsolin-actin complex from human platelets, *J. Biol. Chem.*, 258, 10895, 1983.
213. **Olomucki, A., Huc, C., Lefebure, F., and Coue, M.,** Isolation and characterization of human blood platelet gelsolin, *FEBS Lett.*, 174, 80, 1984.
214. **Bryan, J. and Culuccio, L. M.,** Kinetic analysis of F-actin depolymerization in the presence of platelet gelsolin and gelsolin-actin complex, *J. Cell Biol.*, 101, 1236, 1985.
215. **Carrol, R. C., Butler, R. G., Morris, P. H., and Gerrard, J. M.,** Separable assembly of platelet pseudopodal and contractile cytoskeletons, *Cell*, 30, 385, 1982.
216. **Pribluda, V. and Rotman, A.,** Dynamics of membrane-cytoskeleton interactions in activated blood platelets, *Biochemistry*, 21, 2825, 1982.
217. **Imada, T., Kikuchi, T., Shimada, H., Inada, Y., and Saito, Y.,** Specific desensitization of actin polymerization of bovine platelets, *Biochem. Biophys. Res. Commun.*, 120, 846, 1984.
218. **Lin, D. C. and Lin, S.,** Actin polymerization induced by a motility related higher affinity cytochalasin binding complex from human erythrocyte membranes, *Proc. Natl. Acad. Sci. U.S.A.*, 76, 2345, 1979.
219. **Reichstein, E. and Korn, E. D.,** Acanthamoeba profilin. A protein of low molecular weight from *Acanthamoebe castellanii* that inhibits actin nucleation, *J. Biol. Chem.*, 254, 6174, 1979.
220. **Grumet, M. and Lin, S.,** Reversal of profilin inhibition of actin polymerization in vitro by erythrocyte cytochalasin binding complexes and crosslinked actin nuclei, *Biochem. Biophys. Res. Commun.*, 92, 1324, 1980.
221. **Cohen, J., Gerrard, J. M., Bergman, R. N., and White, J. G.,** The role of contractile filaments in platelet activation, in *Protides of the Biological Fluids*, Peeter, H., Ed., Pergamon Press, Oxford, 1979, 555.
222. **Lazarides, E. and Burridge, K.,** α-Actinin: immunofluorescent localization of a muscle structural protein in nonmuscle cells, *Cell*, 6, 289, 1975.
223. **Jokusch, B. M., Burger, M. M., Da Prada, M., Richards, J. G., Chaponnier, C., and Gabbiani, G.,** α-Actinin attached to membranes of secretory vesicles, *Nature (London)*, 270, 628, 1977.
224. **Gerrard, J. M., Schollmeyer, J. V., Philips, D. R., and White, J. G.,** α-Actinin deficiency in thrombosthenia, *Am. J. Pathol.*, 94, 509, 1979.
225. **Rosenberg, S., Stracher, A., and Burridge, K.,** Isolation and characterization of a calcium sensitive α-actinin-like protein from human platelet cytoskeleton, *J. Biol. Chem.*, 256, 12986, 1981.

226. **Landon, F. and Olomucki, A.,** Isolation and physico-chemical properties of blood platelet α-actinin, *Biochim. Biophys. Acta,* 742, 129, 1983.
227. **Lucas, R. C., Gallagher, M., and Stracher, A.,** Actin and actin binding protein in platelets, in *Contractile Systems in Non-Muscle Tissues,* Perry, S. V., Margreth, A., and Adelstein, R. S., Eds., Elsevier/North-Holland, Amsterdam, 1976, 133.
228. **Schollmeyer, J. V., Rao, G. H. R., and White, J. G.,** An actin binding protein in human platelets, *Am. J. Pathol.,* 93, 433, 1978.
229. **Muhlrad, A., Eldar, A., and Kahane, I.,** Distribution of myosin, actin and actin-binding protein in membrane and soluble fractions of human blood platelets, *FEBS Lett.,* 92, 85, 1978.
230. **Rosenberg, S., Stracher, A., and Lucas, R.,** Isolation and characterization of actin and actin-binding proteins from human platelets, *J. Cell Biol.,* 91, 201, 1981.
231. **Cohen, I. and Cohen, C.,** A tropomyosin-like protein from human platelets, *J. Mol. Biol.,* 68, 383, 1972.
232. **Cote, G., Lewis, W. G., and Smillie, L. B.,** Non-polymerizability of platelet tropomyosin and its NH_2- and COOH-terminal sequences, *FEBS Lett.,* 91, 237, 1978.
233. **Der Terrossian, E., Fullner, S. D., Stewart, M., and Weeds, A. G.,** Porcine platelet tropomyosin, *J. Mol. Biol.,* 153, 147, 1981.
234. **Cote, G. P. and Smillie, L. B.,** Preparation and some properties of equine platelet tropomyosin, *J. Biol. Chem.,* 256, 11004, 1981.
235. **Kakiuchi, R., Inui, M., Morimoto, K., Kanda, K., Sobue, K., and Kakiuchi, S.,** Caldesmon, a calmodulin binding, F-actin-interacting protein, is present in aorta, uterus and platelets, *FEBS Lett.,* 154, 351, 1983.
236. **Landon, F., Gache, Y., Toniton, H., and Olomucki, H.,** Properties of two isoforms: human blood platelet α-actinin *Eur. J. Biochem.,* 153, 231, 1985.
237. **Stromer, M. H. and Goll, D. E.,** Studies on purified α-actinin. Electron microscopic studies on the competitive binding of α-actinin and tropomyosin to Z-line extracted myofibrils, *J. Mol. Biol.,* 67, 489, 1972.
238. **Rosenberg, S. and Stracher, A.,** Effect of actin-binding protein on the sedimentation properties of actin, *J. Cell Biol.,* 94, 51, 1982.
239. **Zhuang, Q. Q., Rosenberg, S., Lawrence, J., and Stracher, A.,** Role of actin binding protein phosphorylation in platelet cytoskeleton assembly, *Biochem. Biophys. Res. Commun.,* 118, 508, 1984.
240. **Carrol, R. C. and Gerrard, J. M.,** Phosphorylation of platelet actin-binding protein during platelet activation, *Blood,* 59, 466, 1982.
241. **Nachmias, V. T., Sullender, J. S., and Fallon, J. R.,** Effects of local anesthetics on human platelets: filopodial suppression and endogenous proteolysis, *Blood,* 53, 63, 1979.
242. **Truglia, J. A. and Stracher, A.,** Purification and characterization of a calcium dependent sulfhydril protease in platelets, *Biochem. Biophys. Res. Commun.,* 100, 814, 1981.
243. **Sakon, M., Kambayaski, J., Ohno, N., and Kosaki, G.,** Two forms of Ca^{++}-activated neutral protease in platelets, *Thromb. Res.,* 24, 207, 1981.
244. **Tsujinaka, T., Sakon, M., Kambayashi, J., and Kosaki, G.,** Cleavage of cytoskeletal proteins by two forms of Ca^{2+} activated neutral proteases in human platelets, *Thromb. Res.,* 28, 149, 1982.
245. **Payne, M. R. and Rudnick, S. E.,** Tropomyosin as a modulator of microfilaments, *TIBS,* 9, 361, 1984.
246. **Cote, G. P. and Smillie, L. B.,** The interaction of equine platelet tropomyosin with skeletal muscle actin, *J. Biol. Chem.,* 256, 7257, 1981.
247. **Debus, E., Weber, K., and Osborn, M.,** The cytoskeleton of blood platelets viewed by immunofluorescence microscopy, *Eur. J. Cell Biol.,* 24, 45, 1981.
248. **Puszkin, E. G., Jenkins, C. S. P., Ores-Carton, C., and Zucker, M. B.,** Platelet cytoskeleton α-actinin in normal and thrombosthenic platelets: distribution and immunologic characterization, *J. Lab. Clin. Med.,* 105, 52, 1985.
249. **Pollard, T. D., Fujiwara, K., Handin, R., and Weiss, G.,** Contractile proteins in platelet activation and contraction, *Ann. N.Y. Acad. Sci.,* 283, 218, 1977.
250. **Jennings, L. K., Fox, J. E. B., Edwards, H. H., and Philips, D. R.,** Changes in the cytoskeletal structure of human platelets following thrombin activation, *J. Biol. Chem.,* 256, 6927, 1981.
251. **Gonella, P. A. and Nachmias, V. T.,** Platelet activation and microfilament bundling, *J. Cell Biol.,* 89, 146, 1981.
252. **Markey, F., Persson, T., and Lindberg, U.,** Characterization of platelet extract before and after stimulation with respect to the possible role of profilactin as microfilament precursor, *Cell,* 23, 145, 1981.
253. **Philips, D. R., Jennings, L. K., and Edwards, H. H.,** Identification of membrane proteins mediating the interaction of human platelets, *J. Cell Biol.,* 86, 77, 1980.
254. **Fox, J. E. B. and Phillips, D. R.,** Role of phosphorylation in mediating the association of myosin with the cytoskeleton structures of human platelets, *J. Biol. Chem.,* 257, 4120, 1982.
255. **Nachmias, V. T., Kavaler, J., and Jacubowitz, S.,** Reversible association of myosin with the platelet cytoskeleton, *Nature (London),* 313, 70, 1985.

256. **Muszbek, L., Fésüs, L., Szabó, T., and Hársfalvi, J.,** Procoagulant activity of thrombosthenin preparations, *Thromb. Res.*, 10, 635, 1977.
257. **Bennett, J. S., Vilaire, G., Colman, R. F., and Colman, R. W.,** Localization of human platelet membrane-associated actomyosin using the affinity label 5′-*p*-fluorosulfonylbenzoyl adenosine, *J. Biol. Chem.*, 256, 1185, 1981.
258. **Schick, P. K., Tuszynski, G. P., and Van der Voort, P. W.,** Human platelet cytoskeletons: specific content of glycolipids and phospholipids, *Blood,* 61, 163, 1983.
259. **Taylor, D. G., Mapp, R. L., and Crawford, N.,** Identification of actin in pig platelet membranes, *Biochem. Soc. Trans.*, 3, 161, 1975.
260. **Taylor, D. G. and Crawford, N.,** Enzymatic and chemical analysis of pig platelet membrane subfractions isolated by zonal centrifugation, *Biochim. Biophys. Acta,* 436, 349, 1976.
261. **Kinoshita, T., Nachman, R. L., and Minick, R.,** Isolation of human platelet plasma membranes with polylysine beads, *J. Cell Biol.*, 82, 688, 1979.
262. **Davies, G. E.,** Association of actin with the platelet membrane, *Biochim. Biophys. Acta,* 772, 149, 1984.
263. **Wu, M. P. and Stracher, A.,** Platelet cytoskeleton-membrane interaction, *Biochem. Biophys. Res. Commun.*, 126, 566, 1985.
264. **Rotman, A., Heldman, J., and Linder, S.,** Association of membrane and cytoplasmic proteins with the cytoskeleton in blood platelets, *Biochemistry,* 21, 1713, 1982.
265. **Fox, J. E. B.,** Identification of actin binding protein as the protein linking the membrane skeleton to glycoproteins on the platelet plasma membrane, *J. Biol. Chem.*, 260, 11970, 1985.
266. **Gogstad, G. O., Solum, N. O., and Hagen, I.,** Platelet glycoprotein III and α-actinin are different proteins, *Thromb. Res.*, 24, 157, 1981.
267. **Sixma, J. J., Schiphorst, M. E., Verhoecky, C., and Jockusch, B. M.,** Peripheral and integral proteins of human blood platelet membranes. α-Actinin is not identical to glycoprotein III, *Biochim. Biophys. Acta,* 704, 333, 1982.
268. **David-Pfeuty, T. and Singer, S. J.,** Altered distribution of the cytoskeletal proteins vinculin and actinin in cultured fibroblasts transformed by Rous sarcoma virus, *Proc. Natl. Acad. Sci. U.S.A.*, 77, 6687, 1980.
269. **Langer, B. G., Leung, L. L. K., Gonella, P. A., Nachmias, V. T., Nachman, R. L., and Pepe, F. A.,** α-Actinin and membrane glycoprotein IIIa are different proteins in human blood platelets, *Proc. Natl. Acad. Sci. U.S.A.*, 79, 432, 1982.
270. **Tokuyasu, K. T., Dutton, A. H., Geiger, B., and Singer, S. J.,** Ultrastructure of chicken cardiac muscle as studied by double immunolabelling in electron microscopy, *Proc. Natl. Acad. Sci. U.S.A.*, 78, 7619, 1981.
271. **Geiger, B., Dutton, A. H., Tokuyasu, K. T., and Singer, S. J.,** Immunoelectron microscope studies of membrane-microfilament interactions; distributions of α-actinin, tropomyosin and vinculin in intestinal epithelial brush border and chicken gizzard smooth muscle cells, *J. Cell Biol.*, 91, 614, 1981.
272. **Geiger, B.,** Microfilament-membrane interaction, *TIBS,* 10, 456, 1985.
273. **Geiger, B.,** A 130K protein from chicken gizzard: its localization at the termini of microfilament bundles in cultured chicken cells, *Cell,* 18, 193, 1979.
274. **Feramisco, J. R. and Burridge, K.,** A rapid purification of α-actinin, filamin and a 130,000-dalton protein from smooth muscle, *J. Biol. Chem.*, 255, 1194, 1980.
275. **Koteliansky, V. E., Gneushev, G. N., and Muszbek, L.,** Identification and isolation of vinculin from platelets, *Thromb. Haemost.*, 50, 188a, 1983.
276. **Koteliansky, V. E., Gneushev, G. N., Glukhova, M. A., Venyaminov, S. Y., and Muszbek, L.,** Identification and isolation of vinculin from platelets, *FEBS Lett.*, 165, 26, 1984.
277. **Asyee, G., Sturk, A., and Muszbek, L.,** Association of vinculin to the platelet cytoskeleton during thrombin induced aggregation, *Exp. Cell. Res.*, 168, 358, 1987.
278. **Horváth, A. R., Asyee, G. M., Sturk, A., and Muszbek, L.,** Association of vinculin to the platelet cytoskeleton during release reaction, *Thromb. Haemost.*, 58, 301a, 1987.
279. **Evans, R. R., Robson, R. M., and Stromer, M. A.,** Properties of smooth muscle vinculin, *J. Cell Biol.*, 259, 3916, 1984.
280. **Rosenfeld, G. C., Hou, D. C., Dingus, J., Meza, J., and Bryan, J.,** Isolation and partial characterization of human platelet vinculin, *J. Cell Biol.*, 100, 669, 1985.
281. **O'Hollaran, T., Beckerle, M. C., and Burridge, K.,** Identification of talin as a major cytoplasmic protein implicated in platelet activation, *Nature (London),* 317, 449, 1985.
282. **Collier, N. C. and Wang, K.,** Purification and properties of human platelet P235, *J. Biol. Chem.*, 257, 6937, 1982.
283. **Collier, N. C. and Wang, K.,** Human platelet P235: a high M_r protein which restricts the length of actin filaments, *FEBS Lett.*, 143, 205, 1982.
284. **D'Angelo Siliciani, J. and Craig, S. W.,** Meta-vinculin — a vinculin related protein with solubility properties of a membrane protein, *Nature (London),* 300, 533, 1982.

285. **Feramisco, J. R., Smart, J. E., Burridge, K., Helfman, D. M., and Thomas, G. P.,** Co-existence of vinculin and a vinculin-like protein of higher molecular weight in smooth muscle, *J. Biol. Chem.*, 25, 11,024, 1982.
286. **Bennet, V.,** Immunoreactive forms of human erythrocyte ankyrin are present in diverse cells and tissues, *Nature (London)*, 281, 597, 1979.
287. **McEver, R. P., Baezinger, N. L., and Majerus, P. W.,** Isolation and quantitation of the platelet membrane glycoproteins deficient in thrombasthenia using a monoclonal hybridoma antibody, *J. Clin. Invest.*, 66, 1311, 1980.
288. **Loftus, J. C. and Albrecht, R. M.,** Redistribution of the fibrinogen receptor of human platelets after surface activation, *J. Cell Biol.*, 99, 822, 1984.
289. **Rotman, A.,** Receptor and nonreceptor-mediated activation of blood platelets, effect on membrane-cytoskeleton interaction, *Biochem. Biophys. Res. Commun.*, 120, 898, 1984.
290. **Zucker, M. M. and Masiello, N. C.,** The Triton X-100-insoluble residue (''cytoskeleton'') of aggregated platelets contains increased lipid phosphorus as well as ^{125}I-labeled glycoproteins, *Blood*, 61, 676, 1983.
291. **Painter, R. G., Ginsberg, M., and Jaques, B.,** Concanavalin A induces interactions between surface glycoproteins and the platelet cytoskeleton, *J. Cell Biol.*, 92, 565, 1982.
292. **Tuszynski, G. P., Kornecki, E., Cierniewski, C., Knight, L. C., Koshy, A., Srivastava, S., Niewiarowski, S., and Walsh, P. N.,** Association of fibrin with the platelet cytoskeleton, *J. Biol. Chem.*, 259, 5247, 1984.
293. **George, J. N., Lyons, R. M., and Morgan, R. K.,** Membrane changes associated with platelet activation. Exposure of actin on the platelet surface after thrombin induced secretion, *J. Clin. Invest.*, 66, 1, 1980.
294. **Bouvier, C. A., Gabbiani, G., Ryan, G. B., Badonnel, M. C., Majno, G., and Lüscher, E. F.,** Binding of anti-actin autoantibodies to platelets, *Thromb. Haemostas.*, 37, 321, 1977.
295. **Diggle, T. A., Toh, B. H., Firkin, B. G., and Pfueller, S. L.,** Human platelet actin: surface expression after platelet activation, *Thromb. Haemost.*, 42, 799, 1979.
296. **Laki, K. and Muszbek, L.,** On the interaction of F-actin with fibrin, *Biochim. Biophys. Acta*, 371, 519, 1974.
297. **Tuszynski, G. P., Walsh, P. N., Piperno, J. R., and Koshy, A.,** Association of coagulation Factor V with the platelet cytoskeleton, *J. Biol. Chem.*, 257, 4557, 1982.
298. **Capitanio, A. M., Niewiarowski, S., Tuszynski, G. P., Korneczki, E., and Rao, A. K.,** *Blood*, 60(Suppl. 1), 709, 1982.
299. **Niewiarowska, J., Cierniewski, C. S., and Tuszynski, G. P.,** Association of fibronectin with the platelet cytoskeleton, *J. Biol. Chem.*, 259, 6181, 1984.
300. **Hanson, J. P., Repke, D. J., Katz, A. M., and Aledort, L. M.,** Calcium ion control of platelet thrombosthenin ATPase activity, *Biochim. Biophys. Acta*, 314, 382, 1973.
301. **Thornes, S., Schaub, M. C., and Lüscher, E. F.,** A calcium-sensitizing system from human platelets and its activity on muscle and platelet actomyosin, *Experientia*, 29, 349, 1973.
302. **Collins, J. H.,** Structure and evolution of troponin C and related proteins, in *Calcium in Biological Systems*, Vol. 30, Cambridge University Press, Cambridge, 1976, 303.
303. **Adelstein, R. S.,** Myosin phosphorylation, cell motility and smooth muscle contraction, *TIBS*, 3, 27, 1978.
304. **Ebashi, S., Mikawa, T., Hirata, M., Toyooka, T., and Nonomura, Y.,** Regulatory proteins of smooth muscle, in *Excitation-Contraction Coupling in Smooth Muscle*, Casteels, R., Godfraind, T., and Rüegg, J. C., Eds., Elsevier/North-Holland, Amsterdam, 1977, 325.
305. **Mikawa, T., Nonomura, Y., and Ebashi, S.,** Does phosphorylation of myosin light chain have direct relation to regulation in smooth muscle?, *J. Biochem.*, 82, 1789, 1977.
306. **Mikawa, T., Nonomura, Y., Hirato, M., Ebashi, S., and Kakiuchi, S.,** Involvement of an acidic protein in regulation of smooth muscle contraction by the tropomyosin-leiotonin system, *J. Biochem.*, 84, 1633, 1978.
307. **Mikawa, T.,** ''Freezing'' of the calcium-regulated structures of gizzard thin filaments by glutaraldehyde, *J. Biochem.*, 85, 879, 1979.
308. **Cohen, J., Kaminski, E., and DeVries, A.,** Actin-linked regulation of the human platelet contractile system, *FEBS Lett.*, 34, 315, 1973.
309. **Muszbek, L., Kuznicki, J., and Drabikowski, W.,** Ca^{2+} regulation of bovine thrombosthenin, *Thromb. Haemost.*, 38, 80, 1977.
310. **Dabrowska, R. and Hartshorne, D. J.,** A Ca^{2+}- and modulator-dependent myosin light chain kinase from non-muscle cells, *Biochem. Biophys. Res. Commun.*, 85, 1352, 1978.
311. **Hathaway, D. R. and Adelstein, R. S.,** Human platelet myosin light chain kinase requires the calcium binding protein calmodulin for activity, *Proc. Natl. Acad. Sci. U.S.A.*, 76, 1653, 1979.
312. **Adelstein, R. S. and Conti, M. A.,** Phosphorylation of platelet myosin increases actin-activated myosin ATPase activity, *Nature (London)*, 256, 597, 1975.
313. **Lebowitz, E. A. and Cooke, R.,** Contractile properties of actomyosin from human blood platelets, *J. Biol. Chem.*, 253, 5443, 1978.

314. **Daniel, J. L., Holmsen, H., and Adelstein, R. S.,** Thrombin-stimulated myosin phosphorylation in intact platelets and its possible involvement in secretion, *Thromb. Haemostas.*, 38, 984, 1977.
315. **Nashikawa, M., Tanaka, T., and Hidaka, H.,** Ca^{2+}-calmodulin-dependent phosphorylation and platelet secretion, *Nature (London)*, 287, 863, 1980.
316. **Daniel, J. L., Molish, I. R., and Holmsen, H.,** Myosin phosphorylation in intact platelets, *J. Biol. Chem.*, 256, 7510, 1981.
317. **Daniel, J. L., Molish, I. R., Holmsen, H., and Salganicoff, L.,** Phosphorylation of myosin light chain in intact platelets: possible role in platelet secretion and clot retraction, in *Protein Phosphorylation, Cold Spring Harbor Conferences on Cell Proliferation*, Vol. 8, Rosen, D. M. and Krebs, E. G., Eds., Cold Spring Harbor Laboratory, Cold Spring Harbor, N.Y., 1981, 913.
318. **Fox, J. E. B. and Philips, D. R.,** Role of phosphorylation in mediating the association of myosin with the cytoskeletal structures of human platelets, *J. Biol. Chem.*, 257, 4120, 1982.
319. **Endo, T., Naka, M., and Hidaka, H.,** Ca^{2+}-phospholipid dependent phosphorylation of smooth muscle myosin, *Biochem. Biophys. Res. Commun.*, 105, 942, 1982.
320. **Gergely, P., Castle, A. G., and Crawford, N.,** Platelet phosphoprotein phosphatase activity. Its subcellular distribution and regulation, *Biochim. Biophys. Acta*, 611, 384, 1980.
321. **Hathaway, D. R., Eaton, C. R., and Adelstein, R. S.,** Regulation of human platelet myosin kinase by calcium-calmodulin and cyclic AMP, in *The Regulation of Coagulation*, Mann, K. and Taylor, R., Eds., Elsevier/North-Holland, Amsterdam, 1980, 271.
322. **Hathaway, D. R., Eaton, C. R., and Adelstein, R. S.,** Regulation of human platelet myosin light chain kinase by the catalytic subunit of cyclic AMP-dependent protein kinase, *Nature (London)*, 291, 252, 1981.
323. **Haslam, R. J. and Lynham, J. A.,** Relationship between phosphorylation of blood platelet proteins and secretion of platelet granule constituents. II. Effects of different inhibitors, *Thromb. Res.*, 12, 619, 1978.
324. **Muszbek, L. and Hársfalvi, J.,** Calmodulin binding proteins in platelet actomyosin, *Thromb. Haemost.*, 46, 172a, 1981.
325. **Scholey, J. M., Taylor, K. A., and Kendrick-Jones, J.,** Regulation of nonmuscle myosin assembly by calmodulin-dependent light chain kinase, *Nature (London)*, 287, 233, 1980.
326. **Suzuki, H., Onishi, H., Takahashi, K., and Watanabe, S.,** Structure and function of chicken gizzard myosin, *J. Biochem.*, 84, 1529, 1978.
327. **Scholey, J. M., Taylor, K. A., and Kendrick-Jones, J.,** Regulation of non-muscle myosin assembly by calmodulin-dependent light chain kinase, *Nature (London)*, 287, 233, 1980.
328. **Kakiuchi, S. and Sobue, K.,** Control of the cytoskeleton by calmodulin and calmodulin-binding proteins, *TIBS*, 8, 59, 1983.
329. **Sobue, K., Morimoto, K., Inui, M., and Kanda, K.,** Control of actin-myosin interaction of gizzard smooth muscle by calmodulin- and caldesmon-linked flip-flop mechanism, *Biomed. Res.*, 3, 188, 1982.
330. **Cote, G. P. and Smillie, L. B.,** The effects of platelet tropomyosin on the ATPase activities of muscle actomyosin subfragment 1 in the absence and presence of troponin and its components, and calmodulin, *J. Biol. Chem.*, 256, 11999, 1981.
331. **Amphlett, G. W., Vanaman, T. C., and Perry, S. V.,** Effect of the troponin C-like protein from bovine brain (brain modulator protein) in the Mg^{2+} stimulated ATPase of skeletal muscle actomyosin, *FEBS Lett.*, 72, 163, 1976.
332. **DerTerossian, E., Pruliere, G., and D'Albis, A.,** Purification of a troponin I-like factor from pig platelet, *FEBS Lett.*, 152, 202, 1983.
333. **Walsh, P. N.,** Platelet-coagulant protein interactions, in *Hemostasis and Thrombosis*, Colman, R. W., Hirsh, J., Marder, V. J., and Salzman, E. W., Eds., Lippincott, Philadelphia, 1982, 404.
334. **Ware, A. G., Falcey, J. L., and Seegers, W. H.,** Platelet extracts, fibrin formation and interaction of purified prothrombin and thromboplastin, *Am. J. Physiol.*, 154, 140, 1948.
335. **Seligmann, M., Goudemand, B., Janin, A., Bernard, J., and Grabar, P.,** Etudes immunochimiques sur la presence de fibrinogene dans des extraits de plaquettes humaines lavees et dans certains extraits leucocytaires, *Rev. Hematol.*, 12, 302, 1957.
336. **Grette, K.,** Studies on the mechanism of thrombin-catalyzed haemostatic reactions in blood platelets, *Acta Physiol. Scand.*, 56(Suppl. 195), 5, 1962.
337. **Day, H. J. and Solum, N. O.,** Fibrinogen associated with subcellular platelet particles, *Scand. J. Haematol.*, 10, 136, 1973.
338. **Lopaciuk, S., Lovette, K. M., McDonagh, J., Chuang, H. Y. K., and McDonagh, R. P.,** Subcellular distribution of fibrinogen and factor XIII in human blood platelets, *Thromb. Res.*, 8, 453, 1976.
339. **Davey, M. G. and Lüscher, E. F.,** Release reactions of human platelets induced by thrombin and other agents, *Biochim. Biophys. Acta*, 165, 490, 1968.
340. **Rosiek, O., Wegrzynowicz, A., Sawicki, A., and Kopec, M.,** Fibrinogensynthese in Blutplattchen, *Folia Haematol.*, 92, 553, 1969.
341. **James, H. L., Ganguly, P., and Jackson, C. W.,** Characterization and origin of fibrinogen in blood platelets. A review with recent data, *Thromb. Haemostas.*, 38, 939, 1977.

342. **Nachman, R., Levine, R., and Jaffe, E.**, Synthesis of actin by cultured guinea pig megakaryocytes. Complex formation with fibrin, *Biochim. Biophys. Acta,* 543, 91, 1978.
343. **Chesney, C. M., Pifer, D. P., and Colman, R. W.**, Factor V coagulant activity of human platelets generated by collagen, *Circulation,* 58, 209, 1978.
344. **Osterud, B., Rapaport, S. I., and Lavine, K. K.**, Factor V activity of platelets: evidence for an activated factor V molecule and for a platelet activator, *Blood,* 49, 819, 1977.
345. **Kane, W. H., Lindhout, M. J., Jackson, C. W., and Majerus, P. W.**, Factor V_a-dependent binding of factor Xa to human platelets, *J. Biol. Chem.*, 255, 1170, 1980.
346. **Buluk, K.**, An unknown function of blood platelets, *Pol. Tyg. Lek.*, 10, 191, 1955.
347. **Lüscher, E. F.**, Ein fibrinstabilisierender Faktor aus Thrombozyten, *Schweiz. Med. Wochenschr.*, 87, 1220, 1957.
348. **Bohn, H.**, Isolierung und Charakterisierung des fibrinstabilisierenden Faktors aus menschlichene Thrombozyten, *Thromb. Diath. Haemorrh.*, 23, 455, 1970.
349. **Muszbek, L. and Laki, K.**, Interaction of thrombin with proteins other than fibrinogen (thrombin-susceptible bonds). Activation of Factor XIII, in *The Thrombin,* Machovich, R., Ed., CRC Press, Boca Raton, Fla., 1984, 84.
350. **Kisselbach, T. H. and Wagner, R. H.**, Demonstration of factor XIII in human megakaryocytes by a fluorescent antibody technique, *Ann. N.Y. Acad. Sci.*, 202, 318, 1972.
351. **Ádány, R., Kiss, A., and Muszbek, L.**, Factor XIII of blood coagulation: a marker of mono- and megakaryocytopoesis, *Br. J. Haematol.*, in press.
352. **Broekman, M. J., Handin, R. J., and Cohen, P.**, Distribution of fibrinogen and platelet factor 4 and XIII in subcellular fractions of human platelets, *Br. J. Haematol.*, 31, 51, 1975.
353. **Joist, H. J. and Niewiarowski, S.**, Retention of platelet fibrin stabilizing factor during the platelet release reaction and clot retraction, *Thromb. Diath. Haemorrh.*, 679, 29, 1973.
354. **Cohen, J., Blankenberg, T. A., Borden, D., Kahn, D. R., and Veis, A.**, Factor XIIIa catalyzed cross-linking of platelet and muscle actin, *Biochim. Biophys. Acta,* 628, 365, 1980.
355. **Cohen, I., Young-Bandala, L., Blankenberg, T. A., Siefring, G. E., and Bruner-Lorand, J.**, Fibrinoligase-catalyzed cross-linking of myosin from platelet and skeletal muscle, *Arch. Biochem. Biophys.*, 192, 100, 1979.
356. **Asyee, G., Sturk, A., Kappelmayer, J., and Muszbek, L.**, Platelet vinculin, a substrate for activated Factor XIII, *Thromb. Haemost.*, 54, 63a, 1985.
357. **Muszbek, L., Asyee, G., Kappelmayer, J., and Sturk, A.**, Platelet vinculin, a substrate for activated Factor XIII of blood coagulation, submitted.
358. **Özsuylu, S. and Hicsönmez, G.**, Platelet aggregation in congenital Factor XIII deficiency, *Acta Haematol.*, 56, 314, 1976.
359. **Muszbek, L., Ádány, R., Szegedi, G., Polgár, J., and Kávai, M.**, Factor XIII of blood coagulation in human monocytes, *Thromb. Res.*, 37, 401, 1985.
360. **Ádány, R., Belkin, A., Vasilevskaya, T., and Muszbek, L.**, Identification of Factor XIII in human peritoneal macrophages, *Eur. J. Cell Biol.*, 38, 171, 1985.
361. **Ádány, R., Nemes, Z., Thomázy, V., and Muszbek, L.**, Identification of FXIII in macrophages invading lymph nodes with Hodgkin's disease, in *Hemostasis and Cancer,* CRC Press, Boca Raton, Fla., 1987, 115.
362. **Elödi, S. and Elödi, P.**, Surface-governed molecular regulation of blood coagulation, *Mol. Aspects Med.*, 6, 291, 1983.
363. **Walsh, P. N.**, Platelet coagulant activities and haemostasis: a hypothesis, *Blood,* 43, 597, 1974.
364. **Walsh, P. N. and Griffin, J. H.**, Contributions of human platelets to the proteolytic activation of blood coagulation factors XII and XI, *Blood,* 57, 106, 1981.
365. **Lipscomb, M. S. and Walsh, P. N.**, Human platelets and factor XI. Localization in platelet membranes of factor XI-like activity and its distinction from plasma factor XI, *J. Clin. Invest.*, 63, 1006, 1979.
366. **Walsh, P. N.**, The effects of collagen and kaolin on the intrinsic coagulant activity of platelets. Evidence for an alternative pathway in intrinsic coagulation not requiring factor XII, *Br. J. Haematol.*, 22, 393, 1972.
367. **Walsh, P. N.**, Different requirements for intrinsic factor Xa forming activity and factor 3 activity and their relationship to platelet aggregation and release, *Br. J. Haematol.*, 40, 311, 1978.
368. **Cox, C. A., Inyangetor, P., Esman, C. T., and White, B. N.**, The effect of aggregation and release on platelet prothrombin-converting activity, *Blood,* 54, 659, 1979.
369. **White, J. G. and Krivit, W.**, The ultrastructural localization and release of platelet lipids, *Blood,* 27, 167, 1966.
370. **Wolf, P.**, The nature and significance of platelet products in human plasma, *Br. J. Haematol.*, 13, 269, 1967.
371. **Horowitz, H. I. and Papayoanou, M. F.**, Release of nonsedimentable platelet factor 3 during coagulation, *J. Lab. Clin. Med.*, 69, 1003, 1967.

372. **Elödi, S., Váradi, K., and Vörös, E.,** Kinetics of formation of Factor IXa-Factor VIII complex on the surface of the platelets, *Thromb. Res.*, 21, 695, 1981.
373. **Váradi, K. and Elödi, S.,** Protection of platelet surface bound Factors IXa and VIII against specific inhibitors, *Thromb. Haemost.*, 47, 32, 1982.
374. **Tracy, P. B., Peterson, J. M., Nesheim, M. E., McDuffie, F. C., and Mann, K. G.,** Interaction of coagulation factor V and factor Va with platelets, *J. Biol. Chem.*, 254, 10354, 1979.
375. **Tollefson, D. M., Jackson, C. M., and Majerus, P. W.,** Binding of the products of prothrombin activation to human platelets, *J. Clin. Invest.*, 56, 241, 1975.
376. **Miletich, J. P., Majerus, D. W., and Majerus, P. W.,** Patients with congenital factor V deficiency have decreased factor Xa binding sites on their platelets, *J. Clin. Invest.*, 62, 824, 1978.
377. **Stenflo, J. and Dahlback, B.,** Activation of prothrombin by factor Xa on the surface of platelets, in *The Regulation of Coagulation,* Mann, K. G. and Taylor, F. B., Eds., Elsevier, Amsterdam, 1980, 225.
378. **Ong, T. C. and Esnouf, J.,** Protein cofactors, in *The Regulation of Coagulation,* Mann, K. G. and Taylor, F. B., Eds., Elsevier, Amsterdam, 1980, 133.
379. **Schick, P. K., Kurica, K. B., and Chacko, G. K.,** Location of phosphatidylethanolamine and phosphatidylserine in the human platelet plasma membrane, *J. Clin. Invest.*, 57, 1221, 1976.
380. **Chap, H. J., Zwaal, R. F. A., and Van Deenen, L. L. M.,** Action of highly purified phospholipases on blood platelets: evidence for an asymmetrical distribution of phospholipids in the surface membrane, *Biochim. Biophys. Acta,* 467, 146, 1977.
381. **Schick, P. K.,** The organization of aminophospholipids in human platelet membranes. Selective changes induced by thrombin, *J. Lab. Clin. Med.*, 91, 802, 1978.
382. **Zwaal, R. F. A., Comfurius, P., and Van Deenen, L. L. M.,** Membrane asymmetry and blood coagulation, *Nature (London),* 268, 358, 1977.
383. **Zwaal, R. F. A., Rosing, J., Tans, G., Bevers, E. M., and Hemker, H. C.,** Topological and kinetic aspects of phospholipids in blood coagulation, in *The Regulation of Coagulation,* Mann, K. G. and Taylor, F. E., Eds., Elsevier, Amsterdam, 1980, 95.
384. **Bevers, E. M., Comfurius, P., Van Rijn, J. L. M., Hemker, H. C., and Zwaal, R. F. A.,** Generation of prothrombin-converting activity and the exposure of phosphatidylserine at the outer surface of platelets, *Eur. J. Biochem.*, 122, 429, 1982.
385. **Brox, J. H. and Osterud, B.,** Evidence for appearance of lysis independent procoagulant activities in collagen or thrombin stimulated platelets, *Thromb. Res.*, 30, 449, 1983.
386. **Brox, J. H. and Osterud, B.,** Platelet factor 3 assay and the availability of platelet factor 3 in collagen or thrombin stimulated platelets, *Thromb. Res.*, 33, 555, 1984.
387. **Hársfalvi, J., Muszbek, L., Stadler, I., and Fésüs, L.,** Inhibition of platelet factor 3 availability by prostacyclin, *Prostaglandins,* 20, 935, 1980.
388. **Comfurius, P., Bevers, E. M., and Zwaal, R. F. A.,** The involvement of cytoskeleton in the regulation of transbilayer movement of phospholipids in human blood platelets, *Biochim. Biophys. Acta,* 815, 143, 1985.
389. **Szabó, O. and Muszbek, L.,** unpublished observation.

Chapter 7

INTERACTION OF PLATELETS AND LEUKOCYTES WITH ENDOTHELIAL CELLS

Elisabetta Dejana and Lucia Raffaella Languino

TABLE OF CONTENTS

I. INTRODUCTION

It has been generally assumed that in normal conditions the endothelial surface is not reactive to circulating cells like platelets or leukocytes. In recent years, however, evidence has been collected that there is a relationship between endothelial cells, platelets, and leukocytes in different pathophysiological conditions.

One of the initial and crucial events in the acute inflammatory response is direct adhesion of polymorphonuclear leukocytes (PMNs) to the endothelial lining of the blood vessels. Substances produced by these cells, such as oxygen radicals, platelet-activating factor (PAF), and proteases, could greatly modify several endothelial cell properties.

Monocyte adhesion to endothelial cells has been described in conditions such as hypercholesterolemia or tissue ischemia. This event is considered an important step in the development of endothelial cell damage and further proliferative alterations of the vessel wall.

Several interactions are now known between platelets and endothelial cells. Platelets appear to be important for the maintenance of vascular integrity in vivo, and when activated they can release a series of substances that interfere with endothelial cell functions.

This short review summarizes some of the characteristics of the interaction of leukocytes and platelets with endothelial cells, considering both direct adhesion of circulating cells to the endothelium and release of active agents that can reciprocally modulate cellular functions.

II. PLATELET ADHESION TO ENDOTHELIAL CELLS

It is a widely held belief that platelets do not adhere to intact endothelial cells. We still do not know the mechanisms of this nonreactivity. It is probably not a passive property, but a complex of different cellular functions. Several endothelial properties have been considered as responsible for their nonthrombogenicity. First, it appears that the endothelial cell membrane negative charges help repel platelets. Further, unlike vascular smooth muscle cells, the subendothelial matrix proteins which are mainly responsible for encouraging platelet deposition, such as collagen type I and III, fibronectin, and thrombospondin, are secreted and organized in the basal lamina by endothelial cells but not exposed on the outer part of the membrane in contact with the bloodstream.[1,2]

Prostacyclin, one of the most powerful inhibitors of platelet activation,[3] has been widely studied in the last few years as a possible factor responsible for endothelial cell nonthrombogenicity. Indeed, endothelial cells can produce more prostacyclin than the other cells of the vessel wall.[4-6] From several observations, however, it appears that prostacyclin is not responsible for the lack of platelet adhesion to endothelial cells. Aspirin treatment of the endothelium to prevent prostacyclin production does not result in platelets adhering to it.[7,8] Thus, though prostacyclin may contribute to limiting platelet activation in some pathological conditions it is not essential for preventing platelet adhesion to endothelial cells.

There is little information available regarding pathophysiological primary alterations of the endothelium that might promote platelet interactions with the vascular wall and therefore contribute to the pathogenesis of thrombosis and atherosclerosis. In vivo platelet adhesion to endothelial cells is rarely observed even in conditions of endothelial cell damage. Most reports describe vascular injury accompanied by vacuolation and retraction of endothelial cells. Platelets appear mostly to adhere to the subendothelium exposed at intercellular junctions.

In vitro adhesion of platelets to endothelial cells has been described in some experimental conditions. Thrombin treatment of rabbit thoracic aorta induced platelet accumulation on the surface.[9] Morphological examinations showed, however, that the platelets were not adhering to endothelial cells but to the subendothelial surface exposed at intercellular junctions. Czervionke et al.[10] showed that in the presence of thrombin platelet aggregates adhere to endothelial cells in culture. This was evident only when the endothelium was pretreated with aspirin in order to block prostacyclin production by the cells. The mechanism of this interaction is still obscure. Thrombin can bind to endothelial cells and activate platelets, thus promoting platelet aggregation and adhesion in the absence of prostacyclin. Activated platelets can release fibrinogen, which in turn might be converted to fibrin by thrombin. Fibrinogen and fibrin have been shown to bind to activated platelets and to endothelial cells.[11,12] They might therefore act as adhesive proteins for the platelet-endothelium interaction. Whatever the mechanism, this observation has been obtained in vitro, in the absence of flow, in conditions where the local thrombin concentration was very high and platelet aggregates could easily sediment on endothelial cells. It remains to be established whether the same phenomenon is also present in vivo.

A SV40-transformed cultured endothelial cell line has been found to have increased reactivity to platelets. Platelets adhere to the surface of these cells, but the phenomenon does not appear to be related to decreased prostacyclin production by this cell type, nor is it completely suppressible by exogenous prostacyclin even at pharmacologically high doses.[13]

SV40-transformed endothelial cells appear to be morphologically different from normal endothelium. They are elongated, and the membrane is covered by ruffles. It might be that they have undergone structural changes in the cell membrane, becoming reactive to platelet deposition.

In summary, platelets do not adhere to normal endothelium in vitro, and morphological evidence of platelet adhesion to vascular endothelium in vivo is still lacking. We have mentioned a few experimental conditions involving increased platelet deposition on endothelial cells. These studies suggest that there might be situations where altered and dysfunctional endothelium becomes reactive to platelets. The potential pathophysiological consequences of such an interaction merit further study.

A. Secretion of Active Substances by Platelets Able to Modify Endothelial Cell Functions

Even if platelets do not adhere to endothelial cells in normal conditions, when activated by aggregating agents they may release substances that can modulate some endothelial cell properties.[14] There is evidence in vivo that vascular integrity is better preserved in the presence of normal numbers of platelets than in thrombocytopenic states.[15] Capillaries from animals made thrombocytopenic present marked thinning with vesicles that bridge the endothelial thickness. In addition to these morphological changes in the endothelium of thrombocytopenic animals, there is evidence of altered function, such as increased vascular permeability.

In addition to the studies in whole animals, the effect of platelets on endothelial cells in culture has also been examined. Maca et al.[16] showed that the migration and proliferation of cultured endothelial cells was significantly increased in the presence of platelets in the culture medium.

The mechanism of the effects of platelets on endothelial cell structure and function is unknown, but it is possible that some platelet product has a trophic effect on endothelial cells.

It has been recently described that platelets can release a growth factor able to induce endothelial cell proliferation.[17] This peptide differed from the well-characterized platelet-derived growth factor (PDGF) known specifically to stimulate vascular smooth muscle cells and fibroblast proliferation. It was very heat labile and stimulated growth in endothelial cells more than in fibroblasts.

In vitro evidence indicates that platelets can also modulate prostacyclin production by endothelial cells. PDGF has been described as stimulating endothelial cells to produce prostacyclin.[18] This effect needed several hours of incubation to be apparent and lasted for several hours. 5-Hydroxytryptamine (5HT), which is also released by platelets during activation, appeared greatly to amplify the effect of PDGF on prostacyclin production.[19] β-thromboglobulin, released from platelet granuli, reportedly inhibits prostacyclin production by endothelial cells,[20] but this observation was obtained only on cultured endothelial cells and could not be reproduced by other authors.[21]

There are conflicting results regarding the possibility that activated platelets can stimulate prostacyclin synthesis by releasing endoperoxides during conversion of arachidonic acid to thromboxane A_2. This effect indeed seems to be evident only in vitro when a very large number of platelets are activated and incubated with endothelial cells.[22] The role of platelet endoperoxides in stimulating endothelial prostacyclin production might be amplified if in vitro platelet thromboxane synthesis is blocked by specific inhibitors, thus leading to accumulation of unconverted endoperoxides in platelets, available for conversion to prostacyclin by endothelial cells.[22] However, FitzGerald et al.[23] demonstrated that in man administration of thromboxane synthesis inhibitors did not increase 6-keto-PGF1 and 2,3-dinor-6-keto-PGF1 (stable prostacyclin metabolites) in the urine.

Aggregated platelets have been recently shown to release substances that induce coronary vessel contraction. Among these, 5HT appears to be one of the most active in inducing vascular contraction.[24] Several authors have shown that 5HT-induced vascular contraction was counteracted by the presence of endothelial cells on the vascular surface.[25,26] 5HT-stimulated endothelial cells do in fact release a still unidentified substance, termed endothelial cell relaxant factor (EDRF), that relaxes contracted vessels in vitro.[27,28]

Another aspect of the platelet-endothelial cell interaction is the binding to the endothelium of platelet factor 4 (PF4) contained in the granuli of platelets together with PDGF and β-thromboglobulin.[29] Different authors have shown that PF4 binds to endothelial cells in vitro and in vivo and that bound PF4 can be displaced by addition of various glycosaminoglycans. Heparin was the most potent displacer, followed by heparan sulfate and dermatan sulfate. Treatment of endothelial cells with heparatinase, which degrades heparan sulfate, prevents PF4 binding to the cells, thus strongly suggesting that PF4 binds to heparan sulfate on the cell surface. Binding of PF4 to heparan sulfate may be important in modulating the interaction of thrombin and antithrombin III, which is dramatically enhanced by the presence of endothelial cells, presumably due to the action of heparan sulfate on the cell surface.[30] PF4 binding to heparan sulfate would prevent the antithrombin III interaction with the glycosaminoglycan and would thus prevent enhancement of the rate of thrombin inactivation.

These examples illustrate some of the substances released during platelet activation which might modulate endothelial cell functions. Many of the observations reported have been obtained in vitro and require confirmation in vivo. The examples are by no means exhaustive, but they suggest the possibility of a complex interaction between platelets and endothelial cells.

III. LEUKOCYTE ADHESION TO ENDOTHELIAL CELLS

Attachment of PMNs to the endothelium is one of the initial events in the acute inflammatory response. In normal conditions PMNs flow freely through the vessel and adhere only momentarily to the endothelial surface. During acute inflammation the PMNs marginate and adhere locally along the vessel; then they migrate through the interendothelial junctions and accumulate at the site of injury.[31] We do not know what causes the PMNs to adhere to a particular location along the blood vessel near an injury or how they become attached. In vitro experiments using different types of cells in culture have indicated that PMNs adhere to endothelial cells rather than to vascular smooth muscle cells or fibroblasts.[31]

In vitro and in vivo experiments have indicated a number of factors involved in the attachment and localization of the PMN. These factors appear to mediate PMN adhesion by affecting the endothelium, the PMN, or both. Some groups have shown that divalent cations enhance the attachment of PMNs to endothelial cells, possibly by lowering the net surface charge of both cell types, thereby reducing the forces of repulsion caused by charge.[32,33]

Pearson et al.[34] showed that flavonoids increase adhesion by an effect on the endothelial cell surface, whereas agents that raise cAMP levels, including several prostaglandins, stimulated adhesion mainly by their effect on PMNs.

Some of the most important factors that control the attachment of PMN are chemotactic for these cells. In vivo chemotactic factors (e.g., complement factor 5 fragments and formylmethionyl-leucyl-phenylalanine [FMLP]) infused intravenously or generated intravascularly induce profound but transient neutropenia by increasing granulocyte adhesiveness and causing sequestration in the microvasculature.[35] In vitro studies showed that complement factor 5 fragments and FMLP promote PMN adhesion to cultured endothelial cells. This activity appears primarily due to stimulation of PMN by the chemotactic factors,[31,35,36] although some workers found that the endothelium had more than a passive role in this process. Indeed, endothelial cells appear to bind C5a fragments and FMLP, and pretreatment of the cells with these agents promote PMN adhesion.[31]

Leukotriene B4 (LTB4), a major product of the 5-lipoxygenase pathway in activated PMNs, also stimulates adhesion of these cells to the endothelium.[37,38] This effect appears to be selective for LTB4 compared with the other monohydroxy- and dihydroxyeicosatetraenoic acids tested. Hoover et al.[37] reported that LTB4-mediated increase in PMN adhesion to endothelial cells was selectively due to pretreatment of endothelial cells with this mediator. In contrast, treatment of PMNs with LTB4 did not enhance subsequent adhesion to an untreated monolayer of endothelial cells.

At present, however, there is no evidence of specific LTB4 receptors on vascular endothelium, although both low- and high-affinity LTB4 binding sites have been characterized in human PMN; and LTB4 is a very active stimulus for PMN activation and aggregation.[39,40] Further studies will be required to characterize the target cell receptor and the contribution of LTB4 to the endothelial-PMN interaction.

Another agent which has been described as increasing PMN adhesion to endothelial cells is platelet-activating factor (PAF, 1-alkyl-2-acetyl-*sn*-glycero-3-phosphocholine).[41] This compound has potent biological effects on both inflammatory and noninflammatory cells. It causes the activation of platelets, neutrophils, and monocytes. PAF, originally described as a product released from IgE-sensitized rabbit basophils,[42] is also produced by neutrophils, monocytes, and platelets.[43]

In contrast to the other chemotactic agents, PAF is also synthesized by endothelial cells. Camussi et al.[44] and McIntyre et al.[45] showed that thrombin, angiotensin II, histamine, bradykinin, and adenosine triphosphate stimulated endothelial cells to synthesize PAF. PAF also increased neutrophil adhesion to the endothelium at concentrations very close to those found in stimulated endothelial cell extracts or released by activated leukocytes.

Further studies are required to characterize PAF's pathophysiological role in vivo, but the evidence collected in vitro suggests that it might be one important contributor to increased endothelial cell reactivity to PMN.

Recently Harlan et al.[46] characterized a PMN membrane glycoprotein, GP-150 (M_r 150,000 daltons), which appeared to be essential for normal PMN adhesion to endothelial cells. The expression of this glycoprotein on the PMN surface is increased by stimulation with a series of chemoattractants and promotes PMN adhesion to the endothelium. GP-150 is lacking in patients with a congenital defect in neutrophil function characterized by an inability to form pus. These results point out the specific role of PMN activation in their interaction with endothelial cells. On the other hand, Bevilacqua et al.[47] showed that stimulation of endothelial cells with interleukin-1 (also discussed below) increases dramatically PMN adhesion to them. IL-1 appears to act selectively on endothelial cells without affecting PMN reactivity. These results indicate that PMN-endothelial cell interaction is a complex phenomenon mediated by a variety of agents which might selectively affect the endothelium, the PMN, or both.

Besides PMN, T-lymphocytes and monocytes and macrophages have been shown to adhere to vascular endothelium and migrate from the circulatory system to an extravascular compartment. Savion et al.[48] found in vitro that Concanavalin A and antigen-specific activated T-lymphocytes, as well as activated peritoneal macrophages, attached themselves to cultured endothelial cells and degraded the glycosaminoglycans of the subendothelial matrix. Di Corleto and de la Motte[49] showed that the human monocytic cell line U937 adhered to cultured endothelial cells of bovine, rat, and porcine origin. Much less binding was observed to either smooth muscle cells or fibroblasts from several species. In general while PMN adhesion to the endothelium is characteristic of acute inflammation, monocyte interaction with endothelial cells are observed in chronic inflammatory reactions.

Gerrity,[50,51] Faggiotto et al.,[52] and Faggiotto and Ross,[53] in morphological studies on the development of atherosclerotic lesions in chronic, diet-induced hypercholesterolemia in non-human primates, observed that one of the first events was monocyte adhesion to the endothelial surface. These cells appear to migrate subendothelially, accumulate lipids, and become lipid-laden macrophages (foam cells). After a few months lipid-laden macrophages seem to leave the intima and enter the circulation. This was accompanied by severe endothelial denudation, possibly due to increased tension on endothelial junctions during macrophage migration toward the bloodstream, and also possibly by these cells forming products toxic or lytic for endothelial cells.

Tissue ischemia is another in vivo condition in which the interaction of leukocytes with endothelial cells is increased. Mullane et al.[54] described invasion of leukocytes into and around a myocardial infarct. In dogs, PMNs and monocytes appeared to adhere to the endothelium of blood vessels within the ischemic area. Inhibitors of arachidonic acid conversion via lipoxygenase and cyclooxygenase in these cells attenuated leukocyte infiltration, infarct size, and cardiac arrhythmias. The authors proposed that migrating leukocytes contribute to the tissue injury accompanying myocardial ischemia, possibly releasing preinflammatory mediators such as lipoxygenase products.

In an experimental model of venous thrombosis mediated by stasis in the cat, Schaub et al.[55] showed that leukocytes adhere to endothelial cells in the early phase of thrombus formation. Platelets appeared to have only a secondary role and were seldom found at the vascular surface in the absence of adhering leukocytes.

These examples obviously do not cover all the experimental conditions of increased leukocytes adhesion to endothelial cells. However, it appears that this event is more frequent than platelet adhesion to the endothelium. Furthermore, adhesion of leukocytes to the endothelium is frequently accompanied by leukocyte and endothelial cell functional modifications. This process appears to play a very important role in inflammation and in the development of atherosclerotic plaques, cardiac ischemia, and venous thrombosis.

A. Secretion of Active Substances by Leukocytes Able to Modify Endothelial Cell Functions

There is increasing evidence that leukocytes produce and release substances that can modify endothelial cell function. Interaction of leukocytes with vascular endothelial cells can result in endothelial damage. Hydrogen peroxide, released during the respiratory burst associated with PMN activation, has been implicated in causing lethal damage to endothelial cells. On cultured endothelial cells exposed to H_2O_2, Ager and Gordon[56] measured K^+ efflux, prostaglandin production, and release of cytoplasmic purines from endothelial cells, and assessed cytotoxic effects by monitoring adenine uptake, ^{51}Cr release, and uptake of vital dye. The first three parameters of cell function listed above were all affected by H_2O_2 at concentrations 30 times lower than those causing lethal damage to the cells. In addition H_2O_2 exposure prevented endothelial cells from responding to vasoactive agents.

Other authors[57] have shown that activated neutrophils or H_2O_2 induced rapid, nonlytic release of prostacyclin from cultured endothelial cells. In contrast, Whorton et al.[58] reported that prostacyclin synthesis was greatly impaired by incubation of cultured endothelium with H_2O_2; they explain this discrepancy by the well-known effect of different peroxide tone, which can result in stimulation or inhibition of cyclooxygenase activity.

In addition to H_2O_2, Le Roy et al.[59] studied the effect on cultured endothelium of neutrophil elastase and cathepsin G, the major neutral proteases of neutrophils. They observed an increase in prostacyclin synthesis after cathepsin G stimulation and release of adenine nucleotides after elastase. After elastase treatment the cells became much less responsive to extracellular ATP or bradykinin-induced release of PGI_2.

Other mediators of cells of the immune system can affect endothelial cell properties. Pober et al.[60] observed that activated T-lymphocytes released products, including interferon, that mediated class II histocompatibility antigen (Ia antigen) expression by endothelial cells.

A number of experimental reports describe the effect of interleukin 1 (IL_1) on endothelial cell properties.[62,63] This protein, elaborated by activated monocytes and macrophages in response to a variety of stimuli, was originally defined as a stimulator of T-lymphocyte proliferation and differentiation. IL_1 acts on nonlymphoid target cells too, with multiple biological effects, including fever, generation of acute phase reactants, and fibroblast proliferation.[61]

Bevilacqua et al.[62] showed that cultured human endothelial cells were stimulated by IL_1 to produce a tissue factor-like procoagulant activity that required several hours to be apparent, was transiently expressed, and was blocked by protein synthesis inhibitors. IL_1 also induced prostacyclin synthesis by endothelial cells with characteristics very similar to the expression of procoagulant activity.[63] It required several hours to be detected, lasted a few hours before decaying, and required protein synthesis. Furthermore, Bevilacqua et al.[47] noted that after addition of IL_1, endothelial cells became dramatically reactive to leukocyte adhesion on their membrane.

All these functional modifications induced by IL_1 on endothelial cells require further studies. Efforts are needed to characterize the mechanism of action of this mediator and the relevance in vivo of the phenomena observed in vitro. However, the IL_1-endothelial cell interaction is a good example of a mediator of the immune system able to interact with the endothelium and induce multiple modifications of cellular function.

IV. CONCLUSIONS

The aim of this review was to describe briefly some of the mechanisms of interaction of platelets and leukocytes with endothelial cells, not only in terms of direct adhesion of the circulating cells to the endothelium but also in terms of release of active substances able to greatly modify the properties of endothelial cells. A general consideration is that platelet adhesion to endothelial cells is still a rare phenomenon, very difficult to substantiate in vitro and in vivo. Further studies are needed to point out the pathophysiological conditions that might induce this interaction or the stimuli that can mediate it.

Even if platelets do not directly adhere to the endothelium, they release during activation a series of substances that can modify endothelial cell activities. This should be taken into account, considering platelet function inhibitors. Indeed, the inhibition of platelet aggregation or release is an important goal not only in terms of thrombus formation but also in terms of the possible changes in vascular functions and reactivity induced by platelet activation.

In contrast to platelets, leukocytes have been described to adhere to endothelial cells in vitro and in vivo. During acute inflammation, PMNs marginate and adhere locally along the vessels; then they migrate through the interendothelial junctions and accumulate at the site of injury. Diet-induced hypercholesterolemia or tissue ischemia can be accompanied by monocyte adhesion to the endothelial surface. The mechanisms which regulate these interactions are still obscure. Different factors have been indicated as responsible for leukocytes attachment and localization.

The importance of leukocyte adhesion to endothelial cells is also related to the fact that they can release substances locally, such as hydrogen peroxide or lytic enzymes, that are able to affect endothelial functions and integrity. It is tempting to speculate that leukocyte interaction with the endothelium might be a first and important step in the development of vascular damage.

From a therapeutic point of view it appears that inhibitors of leukocytes functions might be the new and promising approach for vascular diseases.

In conclusion, the interaction of platelets and leukocytes with endothelial cells appears to be a field of major interest for a better understanding of the physiopathology of these cells. Additional studies might help better characterize the mechanisms at the basis of the development of vascular damage and immune responses.

ACKNOWLEDGMENTS

We thank Professor G. de Gaetano and Professor S. Garattini for fruitful discussion. This work was supported by the Italian National Research Council Progetto Finalizzato "Ingegneria Genetica e Basi Molecolari delle Malattie Ereditari" 84.00882.52. Lucia Raffaella Languino is a fellow of the PEPSICO Foundation.

Judith Baggott, Ivana Garimoldi, Antonella Bottazzi, and the staff of the G. A. Pfeiffer Memorial Library helped prepare the manuscript.

REFERENCES

1. **Bornstein, P., McPherson, J., and Sage, H.,** Synthesis and secretion of structural macromolecules by endothelial cells in culture, in *Pathobiology of the Endothelial Cell,* Nossel, H. L. and Vogel, H. J., Eds., Academic Press, New York, 1982, 215.
2. **Mosher, D. F., Doyle, M. J., and Jaffe, E. A.,** Synthesis and secretion of thrombospondin and fibronectin by cultured human endothelial cells, in *Pathobiology of the Endothelial Cell,* Nossel, H. L. and Vogel, H. J., Eds., Academic Press, New York, 1982, 201.
3. **Moncada, S. and Vane, J. R.,** Pharmacology and endogenous roles of prostaglandin endoperoxides, thromboxane A2 and prostacyclin, *Pharmacol. Rev.,* 30, 293, 1979.
4. **Moncada, S., Herman, A. G., Higgs, E. A., and Vane, J. R.,** Differential formation of prostacyclin (PGX or PGI_2) by layers of the arterial wall. An explanation for the antithrombotic properties of vascular endothelium, *Thromb. Res.,* 11, 323, 1977.
5. **Baenziger, N. L., Becherer, P. R., and Majerus, P. W.,** Characterization of prostacyclin synthesis in cultured human arterial smooth muscle cells, venous endothelial cells and skin fibroblasts, *Cell,* 16, 967, 1979.
6. **Dejana, E., Balconi, G., De Castellarnau, C., Barbieri, B., Vergara-Dauden, M., and de Gaetano, G.,** Prostacyclin production by human endothelial and bovine smooth muscle cells in culture. Effect of repeated stimulation with arachidonic acid, thrombin and ionophore A23187, *Biochim. Biophys. Acta,* 750, 261, 1983.
7. **Dejana, E., Cazenave, J.-P., Groves, H. M., Kinlough-Rathbone, R., Richardson, M., Packham, M. A., and Mustard, J. F.,** The effect of aspirin inhibition of PGI_2 production on platelet adherence to normal and damaged rabbit aortae, *Thromb. Res.,* 17, 453, 1980.
8. **Weksler, B. B., Ley, C. W., and Jaffe, E. A.,** Stimulation of endothelial cell. Prostacyclin production by thrombin, trypsin, and the ionophore A23187, *J. Clin. Invest.,* 62, 923, 1978.
9. **Dejana, E., Cazenave, J.-P., Hatton, M. W. C., Richardson, M., Groves, H. M., Kinlough-Rathbone, R. L., Packham, M. A., and Mustard, J. F.,** The effect of thrombin on platelet accumulation on the vessel wall. Influence of heparin and aspirin, *Thromb. Haemost.,* 50, 567, 1983.
10. **Czervionke, R. L., Hoak, J. C., and Fry, G. L.,** Effect of aspirin on thrombin-induced adherence of platelets to cultured cells from the blood vessel wall, *J. Clin. Invest.,* 62, 847, 1978.
11. **Marguerie, G. A., Plow, E. F., and Edgington, T. S.,** Human platelets possess an inducible and saturable receptor specific for fibrinogen, *J. Biol. Chem.,* 254, 5357, 1979.

12. **Dejana, E., Languino, L. R., Polentarutti, N., Balconi, G., Ryckewaert, J. J., Larrieu, M. J., Donati, M. B., Mantovani, A., and Marguerie, G.,** Interaction between fibrinogen and cultured endothelial cells. Induction of migration and specific binding, *J. Clin. Invest.*, 75, 11, 1985.
13. **Curwen, K. D., Gimbrone, M. A., Jr., and Handin, R. I.,** In vitro studies of thrombo-resistance. The role of prostacyclin (PGI_2) in platelet adhesion to cultured normal and virally transformed human vascular endothelial cells, *Lab. Invest.*, 42, 366, 1980.
14. **Kaplan, K. L.,** Interactions of platelets with endothelial cells, in *Pathobiology of the Endothelial Cell*, Nossel, H. L. and Vogel, H. J., Eds., Academic Press, New York, 1982, 339.
15. **Gimbrone, M. A., Jr., Aster, R. H., Cotran, R. S., Corkery, J., Jandl, J. H., and Folkman, J.,** Preservation of vascular integrity in organs perfused in vitro with a platelet-rich medium, *Nature (London)*, 221, 33, 1969.
16. **Maca, R. D., Fry, G. L., Hoak, J. C., and Loh, P. T.,** the effects of intact platelets on cultured human endothelial cells, *Thromb. Res.*, 11, 715, 1977.
17. **King, G. L. and Buchwaid, S.,** Characterization and partial purification of an endothelial cell growth factor from human platelets, *J. Clin. Invest.*, 73, 392, 1984.
18. **Coughlin, S. R., Moskowitz, M. A., Zetter, B. R., Antoniades, H. N., and Levine, L.,** Platelet-dependent stimulation of prostacyclin synthesis by platelet-derived growth factor, *Nature (London)*, 288, 600, 1980.
19. **Coughlin, S. R., Moskowitz, M. A., Antoniades, H. N., and Levine, L.,** Serotonin receptor-mediated stimulation of bovine smooth muscle cell prostacyclin synthesis and its modulation by platelet-derived growth factor, *Proc. Natl. Acad. Sci. U.S.A.*, 78, 7134, 1981.
20. **Hope, W., Martin, T. J., Chesterman, C. N., and Morgan, F. J.,** Human beta-thromboglobulin inhibits PGI_2 production and binds to a specific site in bovine aortic endothelial cells, *Nature (London)*, 282, 210, 1979.
21. **Poggi, A., Niewiarowski, S., Holt, J. C., Dall'Olio, A., Stewart, G. J., and Smith, J. B.,** Human platelet-secreted proteins (LA-PF4, BT4) do not modify prostacyclin (PGI_2) production by bovine aortic endothelial, *Thromb. Haemost*, 46, 37, 1981.
22. **Marcus, A. J., Weksler, B. B., Jaffe, E. A., and Broekman, M. J.,** Synthesis of prostacyclin from platelet-derived endoperoxides by cultured human endothelial cells, *J. Clin. Invest.*, 66, 979, 1980.
23. **FitzGerald, G. A., Brash, A. R., Oates, J. A., and Pedersen, A. K.,** Endogenous prostacyclin biosynthesis and platelet function during selective inhibition of thromboxane synthase in man, *J. Clin. Invest.*, 71, 1336, 1983.
24. **McGoon, M. D. and Vanhoutte, P. M.,** Aggregating platelets contract isolated canine pulmonary arteries by releasing 5-hydroxytryptamine, *J. Clin. Invest.*, 74, 828, 1984.
25. **Cohen, R. A., Sheperd, J. T., and Vanhoutte, P. M.,** 5-Hydroxytryptamine can mediate endothelium-dependent relaxation of coronary arteries, *Am. J. Physiol.*, 245, H1077, 1983.
26. **Cocks, T. M. and Angus, J. A.,** Endothelium-dependent relaxation of coronary arteries by noradrenaline and serotonin, *Nature (London)*, 305, 627, 1983.
27. **Furchgott, R. F.,** Role of endothelium in response of vascular smooth muscle, *Circ. Res.*, 53, 557, 1983.
28. **Griffith, T. M., Edwards, D. H., Lewis, M. J., Newby, A. C., and Henderson, A. H.,** The nature of endothelium-derived vascular relaxant factor, *Nature (London)*, 308, 645, 1984.
29. **Busch, C., Dawes, J., Pepper, D. S., and Wasteson, A.,** Binding of platelet factor 4 to cultured human umbilical vein endothelial cells, *Thromb. Res.*, 19, 129, 1980.
30. **Busch, C. and Owen, W. G.,** Identification in vitro of an endothelial cell surface cofactor for antithrombin III, *J. Clin. Invest.*, 69, 726, 1982.
31. **Hoover, R. L. and Karnovsky, M. J.,** Leukocyte-endothelial interactions, in *Pathobiology of the Endothelial Cell*, Nossel, H. L. and Vogel, H. J., Eds., Academic Press, New York, 1982, 357.
32. **Beesley, J. E., Pearson, J. D., Hutchings, A., Carleton, J. S., and Gordon, J. L.,** Granulocyte migration through endothelium in culture, *J. Cell Sci.*, 38, 237, 1979.
33. **Hoover, R. L., Briggs, R. T., and Karnovsky, M. J.,** The adhesive interaction between polymorphonuclear leukocytes and endothelial cells in vitro, *Cell*, 14, 423, 1978.
34. **Pearson, J. D., Carleton, J. S., Beesley, J. E., Hutchings, A., and Gordon, J. L.,** Granulocyte adhesion to endothelium in culture, *J. Cell Sci.*, 38, 225, 1979.
35. **Tonnesen, M. G., Smedly, L. A., and Henson, P. M.,** Neutrophil-endothelial cell interactions. Modulation of neutrophil adhesiveness induced by complement fragments C5a and C5a des arg and formyl-methionyl-leucyl-phenylalanine in vitro, *J. Clin. Invest.*, 74, 1581, 1984.
36. **Kirkpatrick, C. J. and Melzner, I.,** Alterations in the biophysical properties of the human endothelial cell plasma membrane induced by a chemotactic tripeptide: correlation with enhanced adherence of granulocytes, *J. Pathol.*, 144, 201, 1984.
37. **Hoover, R. L., Karnovsky, M. J., Austen, K. F., Corey, E. J., and Lewis, R. A.,** Leukotriene B_4 action on endothelium mediates augmented neutrophil/endothelial adhesion, *Proc. Natl. Acad. Sci. U.S.A.*, 81, 2191, 1984.

38. **Gimbrone, M. A., Jr., Brock, A. F., Schafer, A. I.,** Leukotriene B_4 stimulates polymorphonuclear leukocyte adhesion to cultured vascular endothelial cells, *J. Clin. Invest.*, 74, 1552, 1984.
39. **Pinchard, R. N.,** The new chemical mediators of inflammation, in *Current Topics in Inflammation and Infection,* Majno, G. and Cotran, R. S., Eds., Williams & Wilkins, Baltimore, 1982, 38.
40. **Samuelsson, B. and Paoletti, R., Eds.,** *Advances in Prostaglandins, Thromboxane, and Leukotriene Research,* Vol. 9, *Leukotrienes and Other Lipoxygenase Products*, Raven Press, New York, 1982.
41. **Zimmerman, G. A., McIntyre, T. M., and Prescott, S. M.,** Thrombin stimulates the adherence of neutrophils to human endothelial cells in vitro, *J. Clin. Invest.*, 76, 2235, 1985.
42. **Benveniste, J., Henson, P. M., and Cochrane, C. G.,** Leukocyte-dependent histamine release from rabbit platelets. The role of IgE, basophils, and a platelet-activating factor, *J. Exp. Med.*, 136, 1356, 1972.
43. **Snyder, F.,** Chemical and biochemical aspects of platelet activating factor: a novel class of acetylated ether-linked choline-phospholipids, *Med. Res. Rev.*, 5, 107, 1985.
44. **Camussi, G., Aglietta, M., Malavasi, F., Tetta, C., Piacibello, W., Sanavio, F., and Bussolino, F.,** The release of platelet-activating factor from human endothelial cells in culture, *J. Immunol.*, 131, 2397, 1983.
45. **McIntyre, T. M., Zimmerman, G. A., Satoh, K., and Prescott, S. M.,** Cultured endothelial cells synthesize both platelet-activating factor and prostacyclin in response to histamine, bradykinin, and adenosine triphosphate, *J. Clin. Invest.*, 76, 271, 1985.
46. **Harlan, J. M., Killen, P. D., Senecal, F. M., Schwartz, B. R., Yee, E. K., Taylor, R. F., Beatty, P. G., Price, T. H., and Ochs, H. D.,** The role of neutrophil membrane glycoprotein GP-150 in neutrophil adherence to endothelium in vitro, *Blood,* 66, 167, 1985.
47. **Bevilacqua, M. P., Pober, J. S., Wheeler, M. E., Cotran, R. S., and Gimbrone, M. A., Jr.,** Interleukin 1 acts on cultured human vascular endothelium to increase the adhesion of polymorphonuclear leukocytes, monocytes, and related leukocyte cell lines, *J. Clin. Invest.*, 76, 2003, 1985.
48. **Savion, N., Vlodavsky, I., and Fuks, Z.,** Interaction of T lymphocytes and macrophages with cultured vascular endothelial cells: attachment, invasion, and subsequent degradation of the subendothelial extracellular matrix, *J. Cell. Physiol.*, 118, 169, 1984.
49. **DiCorleto, P. E. and de la Motte, C. A.,** Characterization of the adhesion of the human monocytic cell line U937 to cultured endothelial cells, *J. Clin. Invest.*, 75, 1153, 1985.
50. **Gerrity, R. G.,** The role of the monocyte in atherogenesis. I. Transition of blood-bone monocytes into foam cells in fatty lesion, *Am. J. Pathol.*, 103, 181, 1981.
51. **Gerrity, R. G.,** The role of the monocyte in atherogenesis. II. Migration of foam cells from atherosclerotic lesions, *Am. J. Pathol.*, 103, 191, 1981.
52. **Faggiotto, A., Ross, R., and Harker, L.,** Studies of hypercholesterolemia in the nonhuman primate. I. Changes that lead to fatty streak formation, *Arteriosclerosis,* 4, 323, 1984.
53. **Faggiotto, A. and Ross, R.,** Studies of hypercholesterolemia in the nonhuman primate. II. Fatty streak conversion to fibrous plaque. *Arteriosclerosis,* 4, 341, 1984.
54. **Mullane, K. M., Read, N., Slamon, J. A., and Moncada, S.,** Role of leukocytes in acute myocardial infarction in anesthetized dogs: relationship to myocardial salvage by antiinflammatory drugs, *J. Pharmacol. Exp. Ther.*, 228, 510, 1984.
55. **Schaub, R. G., Simmons, C. A., Koets, M. H., Romano, P. J., II, and Stewart, G. J.,** Early events in the formation of a venous thrombus following local trauma and stasis, *Lab. Invest.*, 51, 218, 1984.
56. **Ager, A. and Gordon, J. L.,** Differential effects of hydrogen perioxide on indices of endothelial cell function, *J. Exp. Med.*, 159, 592, 1984.
57. **Harlan, J. M. and Callahan, K. S.,** Role of hydrogen peroxide in the neutrophil-mediated release of prostacyclin from cultured endothelial cells, *J. Clin. Invest.*, 74, 442, 1984.
58. **Whorton, A. R., Montgomery, M. E., and Kent, R. S.,** Effect of hydrogen peroxide on prostaglandin production and cellular integrity in cultured porcine aortic endothelial cells, *J. Clin. Invest.*, 76, 295, 1985.
59. **LeRoy, E. C., Ager, A., and Gordon, J. L.,** Effects of neutrophil elastase and other proteases on porcine aortic endothelial prostaglandin I_2 production, adenine nucleotide release, and responses to vasoactive agents, *J. Clin. Invest.*, 74, 1003, 1984.
60. **Pober, J. S., Gimbrone, M. A., Jr., Cotran, R. S., Reiss, C. S., Burakoff, S. J., Fiers, W., and Ault, K. A.,** Ia expression by vascular endothelium is inducible by activated T cells and by human γ interferon, *J. Exp. Med.*, 157, 1339, 1983.
61. **Dinarello, C. A.,** Interleukin-1 and the pathogenesis of the acute-phase response, *N. Engl. J. Med.*, 311, 1413, 1984.
62. **Bevilacqua, M. P., Pober, J. S., Majeau, G. R., Cotran, R. S., and Gimbrone, M. A., Jr.,** Interleukin 1 (IL-1) induces biosynthesis and cell surface expression of procoagulant activity in human vascular endothelial cells, *J. Exp. Med.*, 160, 618, 1984.
63. **Rossi, V., Breviario, F., Ghezzi, P., Dejana, E., and Mantovani, A.,** Prostacyclin synthesis induced in vascular cells by interleukin-1, *Science,* 229, 174, 1985.

Chapter 8

THE ROLE OF THE ENDOTHELIUM IN THE REGULATION OF THROMBIN AND PROTEIN C

Frederick J. Walker

TABLE OF CONTENTS

I. INTRODUCTION

The antithrombotic nature of the endothelial lining is thought to be key in the maintenance of blood fluidity. Investigation into the molecular nature of the antithrombotic properties of the endothelium has evolved from studies of plasma components involved in the regulation of thrombin. In particular, studies on the plasma proteins antithrombin III and protein C have become focal points for the examination of the role of the endothelium in the regulation of thrombin activity. This, along with the advent of improved technology for the growth of endothelial cells in culture that maintains their antithrombotic properties, has lead to a rapid advance in the understanding of the role of the endothelial cell in the regulation of blood coagulation.[1]

The purpose of this review is to examine recent studies into the role of the endothelium in the regulation of thrombin. This covers the role of the endothelium in the inactviation of thrombin, its role in the regulation of inhibitors of thrombin formation, and the potential role of the endothelium in the formation of thrombin.

II. WHAT IS THE NATURE OF THE THROMBIN INTERACTION WITH THE ENDOTHELIUM?

Studies of the interaction between proteins and cells are often beset by the uncertainty principle. In order to study the endothelium, it is necessary to alter the environment of the cell, leaving room for ambiguity in the results. In an attempt to capture the endothelial cell in a natural state, a number of experimental situations have been developed for the investigation of the interaction between the endothelium and thrombin. These include determination of binding in intact animals,[2] binding to isolated segments of vein,[3,4] binding in the Lagendorf-perfused heart preparation,[5] and binding of cells grown in tissue culture.[6-8]

Each method has various advantages and drawbacks. For example, binding in intact animals more closely represents a physiological reaction, but is not particularly convenient for experimental manipulation. At the other extreme, tissue culture cells are convenient for manipulation and biochemical analysis, although they lack the environment found in vivo. The variations observed in the measurement of thrombin binding suggest that somehow the cells differ from system to system. There are, however, several common features found in all experimental situations. One of these is the observation that thrombin binding to endothelial cells can be characterized by two types of interactions: reversible and irreversible.

A. Reversible Interactions between Thrombin and the Endothelial Cell

One of the tools used in a number of these studies is diisopropylphosphate-modified thrombin (DIP-thrombin). This is an analog of thrombin that has been inactivated with diisopropylfluorophosphate, which forms a covalent attachment with the active site serine. DIP-thrombin is useful because it maintains the native conformation of the enzyme while lacking the proteolytic activity. With this analog, it is possible to identify binding sites that do not require any proteolytic events catalyzed by the thrombin active site.

DIP-thrombin, injected into the circulation of a rabbit, was cleared within 1 min.[2] Analysis of the various tissues indicated that most was found in the lungs. However, when the point of injection was varied, thrombin was found in the vascular bed nearest the point of injection. Clearance of DIP-thrombin appeared to be reversible, since the addition of unlabeled DIP-thrombin would cause the release of the labeled protein.[2] Labeled thrombin, injected into the circulation, was cleared more slowly than DIP-thrombin and this took place predominantly in the liver. Electrophoretic analysis of plasma indicated that, at the earliest time measured, all of the thrombin existed in a complex with antithrombin III. DIP-thrombin inhibited the formation of the complex, suggesting that complex formation takes place when thrombin is bound to the high-affinity binding sites.[2]

Table 1
THROMBIN BINDING TO ENDOTHELIAL CELLS

Tissue[a]	Kd1	Kd2	No. of sites	Ref.
PAE	30 n*M*		30K	10
Rabbit	12 n*M*			2
RAE	26		580K	9
HUV	0.1	10	3K	8
Heart	2 n*M*			5
BCE			10K	7

[a] PAE, porcine aortic endothelium; RAE, rabbit aortic endothelium; HUV, human umbilical vein; and BCE, bovine corneal endothelium.

When the aortic surface from dogs and pigs was used, thrombin binding was also observed. Thrombin, bound to the aortic segment, retained activity toward chromogenic substrates;[3] however, the amount of activity recovered was less than that added to the cells. Additionally, when the experiment was performed in the presence of plasma, the inactivation of thrombin occurred rapidly.[4] When the thrombin interaction with endothelial cells was measured in the recirculating Langendorff heart preparation, reversible binding with a dissociation constant of 2 n*M* was observed.[5] Binding studies of thrombin to endothelial cells maintained in tissue culture revealed a site that had not been observed with the other methods. In tissue culture cells a small population of sites was observed with a dissociation constant of 0.1 n*M*.[8] In most other studies the high-affinity site had a dissociation constant in the range of 10 to 30 n*M*. Results from a number of binding studies are summarized in Table 1. Several studies[9,10] have indicated that heparin could inhibit thrombin binding. This could be expected, since thrombin is known to interact with heparin.[11,12]

B. Irreversible Binding

Following the rapid and reversible phase of thrombin binding to the endothelial cell, a slower and irreversible association has been observed. This nonequilibrium type of binding is characterized by a lack of effect of unlabeled DIP-thrombin on the process.[13] Irreversible binding is dependent upon the active site and is associated with the linkage of thrombin to a 30,000-M_r protein associated with the endothelial cell.[6,13] This complex was distinct from the thrombin-antithrombin III complex. It could be dissociated by treatment with hydroxylamine but not with high concentrations of salt.[7] Approximately 10,000 of the irreversible sites have been observed on the surface of corneal endothelial cells.[7] When thrombin is linked to this protein, it is internalized and degraded.[6,7]

The internalization process responds to the thrombin concentration, and can be up-regulated. That is, the number of irreversible binding sites appears to increase if cells are pretreated with thrombin prior to determination of the number of sites.[6,7] Irreversible thrombin binding was found to be specific for endothelial cells, as prothrombin was not internalized by endothelial cells, and when fibroblasts were used, thrombin was internalized extremely slowly.[6] Hence, it appears that thrombin can be inactivated by the endothelial cell via a mechanism by which it is taken up into the interior of the cell and degraded.

All binding studies indicate that thrombin can be rapidly and specifically bound with high affinity to endothelial cells. In the absence of plasma the only observed fate of thrombin is internalization and degradation by lysosomal enzymes. When binding is carried out in the presence of plasma, thrombin is rapidly inactivated by antithrombin III. The rapid formation of this complex suggests that the endothelium might also mediate the formation of this complex.

III. DOES THE ENDOTHELIAL CELL CATALYZE OR STIMULATE THE INACTIVATION OF THROMBIN BY ANTITHROMBIN III?

A. Heparin and the Thrombin-Antithrombin III Interaction

One of the principal inhibitors of thrombin is the plasma protease inhibitor antithrombin III. This protein can form a 1:1 molar complex with thrombin.[14] It is also capable of inactivating other proteases involved in the coagulation cascade, including factors XIIa(F-XIIa), IXa, Xa, and XIa.[15] The thrombin-antithrombin complex cannot be dissociated even with the use of denaturing agents,[14] although it can be dissociated with hydroxylamine.[16] The latter observation suggests that the binding is due to the formation of an ester bond between the active site of thrombin and antithrombin III.[16] When complexed, thrombin is unable to react with other substrates and to promote the formation of fibrin clots. Antithrombin III is also known as heparin cofactor, the plasma component that, with heparin, is a potent inhibitor of blood coagulation. The role of heparin was first recognized by Howell with the recognition that heparin worked with antithrombin to inhibit coagulation.[17] Antithrombin III is a slow inhibitor of thrombin; but in the presence of heparin the rate of thrombin inactivation is increased 2000-fold.[18]

A number of models to explain the effect of heparin on the rate of formation of the thrombin-antithrombin complex have been proposed. Most are based on either the interaction between heparin and antithrombin III, or the interaction between heparin and thrombin. Rosenberg and co-workers[18] have proposed that the effect of heparin can be mostly accounted for by formation of an antithrombin III-heparin complex, suggesting that the interaction between heparin and thrombin is not important. Owen[12] and Griffith[19] have concluded that heparin acts as a template, that is, binds both thrombin and antithrombin III simultaneously. This has recently been confirmed by Nesheim, who has derived a simple rate equation that describes the kinetics of the heparin-catalyzed interaction between thrombin and antithrombin III.[20]

Studies of the effects of heparin on the formation of the thrombin-antithrombin III complex have led to the question of whether the mucopolysaccharides found on the surface of the endothelial cell can act as thrombin receptors and catalyze the formation of the thrombin-antithrombin III complex in an analogous manner.

B. Does the Surface of the Endothelium Contain Heparin-Like Molecules?

The proposal that heparin-like material associated with the vascular lining is important in the thromboresistance of the endothelial cell lining was first proposed by Damus and co-workers.[21] Heparin is a mucopolysaccharide commercially derived from either porcine mucose or bovine lung. The commercially available preparations commonly consist of a number of molecular species that vary in size and charge density. Cultured endothelial cells are able to synthesize a mucopolysaccharide that is similar to heparin.[22] When these cells are treated with heparinase and heparitinase, an enzyme isolated from the bacteria *Flavobacterium heparinum*, sulfated sugars are released into the medium. This suggests that chains of heparitin sulfate are available on the surface of the endothelial cell.[23]

Two types of experiments have been conducted to determine if the mucopolysaccharides on the surface of the endothelium contain heparin-like activity. In the first experiment, mucopolysaccharides were isolated from human aorta.[24] These were fractionated and found to contain chondroitin 4-sulfate, chondroitin 6-sulfate, dermatan sulfate, heparan sulfate, and hyaluronic acid.[24] Of these, only heparan sulfate and dermatan sulfate could significantly increase the rate of thrombin inactivation by antithrombin III.[24,25] In the second type of experiment mucopolysaccharides were extracted from calf cerebral microvasculature and calf aorta.[26] The total mucopolysaccharide extract contained only small amounts of anticoagulant activity. When fractionated by its affinity to antithrombin III, it was found that 4.2% of the mass contained 75% of the anticoagulant activity. This suggested that the anticoagulant activity of the mucopolysaccharides is due to a small amount of material which behaves like heparin.[26] Mucopolysaccharides have also been examined in the microvasculature isolated from retina and cerebral gray matter from the calf. A heparin-like activity was detected that was precipitable with trichloroacetic acid and destroyed with *Flavobacterium* heparinase.[27] These experiments all tend to suggest that a subpopulation of the mucopolysaccharides found on the surface of endothelial cells contains components that function in a manner analogous to commercial heparin.

C. Do the Heparin-Like Molecules on the Cell Surface Act in a Manner Analogous to Soluble Heparin?

Even though mucopolysaccharides that have been extracted from the endothelium contain some heparin-like activity, it was unclear whether this activity was retained when the mucopolysaccharides were attached to the cell. There are several problems that need to be overcome in the design of the experiments to test this question. First, a system needs to be designed that can differentiate between soluble and cell surface reactions. If, in the experimental design, the cell has the capacity for a small amount of the available thrombin, it might not be possible to detect changes in the rate of inactivation due to surface phenomena. Second, one must be able to differentiate between thrombin inactivation by the endothelial cell and thrombin-antithrombin III formation. Therefore, it is important to measure the appearance of the thrombin-antithrombin complex rather than the disappearance of thrombin.

Two approaches have been used to determine if the endothelium is able to accelerate the formation of the thrombin-antithrombin III complex. One involves observing either thrombin inactivation or complex formation while perfusing thrombin through the tissue. The second type of experiment involves observing complex formation in the presence and absence of cultured endothelial cells.

Busch and Owen[28] have utilized the Lagendorff rat heart preparation through which thrombin has been perfused. They observed that platelet factor 4, protamine sulfate, and DIP-thrombin can inhibit the inactivation of circulating thrombin and the formation of the thrombin-antithrombin complex. The first two agents can inhibit heparin function. The effect of DIP-thrombin suggests a receptor-mediated event. Marcum and co-workers[29] used a similar approach, perfusing the rat hindquarters with thrombin and antithrombin III. They found that the endothelium enhanced the rate of thrombin inactivation as much as 19-fold over the uncatalyzed rate of reaction. Both platelet factor 4 or treatment of the vasculature with *Flavobacterium* heparinase reduced the rate to the control levels. Displacement of thrombin from the endothelium with DIP-thrombin reduced the amount of inactivation of thrombin. Modification of antithrombin such that it could not interact with heparin also caused the effect of the cells to be lost. Busch and Owen have also carried out similar experiments with endothelial cells in tissue culture. Their findings, similar to those with the perfused heart, revealed that endothelial cells in tissue culture can stimulate the formation of the thrombin-antithrombin complex[28]. A number of other groups have published findings that support this point, including the observation that antibodies made against heparin sulfate proteoglycans can abolish the anticoagulant activity of endothelial cells[30] or that protamine could abolish the cell-mediated inhibition of thrombin by antithrombin III.[30] These experiments support the hypothesis that the endothelium is able to enhance the rate of formation of the thrombin-antithrombin complex in a manner similar to that seen with soluble heparin.[29]

Lollar and co-workers[31] have come to somewhat different conclusions. They have found that the rate of thrombin inactivation by antithrombin III is the same for both bound and free thrombin. They have also observed that when an antithrombin III molecule is used that is modified such that it is unable to interact with heparin, there is no effect on the rate by cell-bound heparin. These experiments imply that the endothelium does not stimulate the inhibition of thrombin by antithrombin III.[30]

Most of the experiments reported support the hypothesis that mucopolysaccharides on the surface of endothelial cells catalyze the formation of the thrombin-antithrombin complex. The exception is the work of Lollar, in which the opposite result seems clear. This appears to be a question that needs further experiments for its resolution. In summary, the surface of the endothelial cell does contain mucopolysaccharides that can function in a manner similar to heparin. That this is their in vivo role remains unclear.

IV. THROMBOMODULIN, A MEDIATOR OF THE ANTICOAGULANT ACTIVITY OF THROMBIN

A. The Anticoagulant Activity of Protein C

Protein C is a vitamin K-dependent protein found in the blood plasma.[32] A number of enzymes have been observed that can convert protein C to a serine protease. These include trypsin,[33] thrombin,[34] and the F-X activator from Russell's viper venom.[35] My laboratory has also observed that the venom of *Agkistrodon contortrix contortrix* contains an activator of protein C.[84] Once a method of activating the protein was found, it became possible for Kisiel,[36] and subsequently Walker and co-workers,[35] to observe that the activated form of protein C was a potent inhibitor of blood coagulation through the selective inactivation of F-V.[35,37,38] Somewhat later it was observed that it could also inactivate factor VIII.[39,40] Activated protein C is identical to another inhibitor of coagulation, autoprothrombin IIa, which had been described by Mammen and co-workers.[41] Studies of the inactivation of F-Va by activated protein C have indicated that this reaction is similar to other reactions catalyzed by vitamin K-dependent serine proteases in that it requires the presence of calcium and phospholipids for maximum activity.[35]

It has been proposed by Walker[42] that a second vitamin K-dependent protein, protein S, acts as a cofactor for the anticoagulant activity of activated protein C. This has been confirmed by the observations that plasma that has been depleted of protein S is poorly anticoagulated by activated protein[42] and that the plasma from patients with protein S deficiencies lack cofactor activity for activated protein C.[43-45] Protein S is able to accelerate the inactivation of F-V[42,46] and VIII[47] by activated protein C. The effect of protein S appears to be to increase the binding of activated protein C to either phospholipid vesicles[46] or unstimulated platelets,[48] suggesting that its role is to facilitate the formation of a membrane-bound F-Va inactivation complex.

Protein S can also exist in plasma in several forms. It is able to form a complex with complement component C4-binding protein (C4bp).[49,50] When complexed with C4bp it is unable to participate as a cofactor in the inactivation of F-Va.[43] Protein S, which is a single chain protein,[51,52] can also exist as a two-chain protein. The latter form arises by thrombin-catalized proteolysis.[53-55] The two-chain form is without co-factor activity. It also has altered calcium-binding properties and is unable to interact with phospholipid vesicles.[54]

It has been suggested by Suzuki and co-workers and by Canfield and Kisiel that there exists a specific plasma inhibitor for activated protein C that is involved in the inactivation of this protease.[56,57]

All of the work carried out with protein C indicates that it is a potent inhibitor of blood coagulation. If this protein has a physiologically important role, then the mechanism of activation must be related to this role. This observation, first made by Esmon and Owen,[58] led to the discovery of thrombomodulin, a co-factor for the thrombin-catalyzed activation of protein C.

Table 2
PHYSICAL PROPERTIES OF THROMBOMODULIN

Species	Mol wt	Km Protein C (μM)	Km Thrombin (nM)	Ref.
Rabbit	68,000—74,000	0.72	0.48	60
Bovine	84,000	5.0	2.0	61, 62
Human	75,000—88,000	9.8	—	63, 64

B. Physiological Activators of Protein C

Initial studies by Kisiel and co-workers[34] and Mammen and co-workers[41] suggested that thrombin could convert protein C into an active protease.[34] Thrombin was observed to remove a tetradecapeptide from the amino terminal of the heavy chain of protein C.[34] However, the rate of activation was very slow and could be inhibited by calcium ions. This observation tended to suggest that thrombin was not the physiological activator. A role for endothelial cells in protein C activation was first reported by Esmon and Owen,[58] who observed that if thrombin and protein C were perfused through the myocardium, protein C would be activated at a rate approximately 20,000 times the rate observed with protein C and thrombin in the absence of the myocardium. They observed that DIP-thrombin could inhibit activation, suggesting that there may be a cell surface cofactor involved and that cultured endothelial cells could also stimulate the rate of protein C activation. This factor was observed to be present on the surface of endothelial cells from nearly every tissue, but not on smooth muscle cells or fibroblasts, suggesting that the factor was characteristic of endothelial cells. With respect to protein C activation, the cofactor has been observed to be saturable with respect to either protein C or thrombin. This factor can be inhibited with DIP-thrombin. These studies strongly suggest the presence of an endothelial cell surface protein that acts as a cofactor in the thrombin-mediated activation of protein C.[58,59]

To further test this hypothesis, purification of this factor, termed thrombomodulin, was attempted from rabbit lung. The strategy used for the purification was based on the observation that the observed K_m for thrombin with thrombomodulin was 0.48 nM.[60] This suggests that thrombomodulin would have a high affinity for thrombin. The isolation involved extraction of the cofactor from lung using detergents followed by chromatography on DIP-thrombin-agarose. The yield was 10 to 20%. The purified protein has a number of interesting properties. The single polypeptide chain appears to be an intrinsic membrane protein, as it requires detergents for both maintenance of the monomer structure and activity. The activity of thrombomodulin was found to be stable to SDS, urea, and guanidinium Cl upon boiling for 15 min and at pH from 2.0 to 10.0. However, either pepsin or beta-mercaptoethanol destroyed the activity. It has been noted that when the molecular weight of thrombomodulin was determined by SDS-polyacrylamide gel electrophoresis following reduction, it often appears to be greater than when run without reduction.[60] Thrombomodulin has now been isolated from several types of tissue, including rabbit lung,[60] bovine lung,[61,62] and the human placenta[63,64] (Table 2).

Thrombin-dependent activation of protein C has also been observed in vivo.[65] Infusion of thrombin into a dog led to an increase in a systemic anticoagulant activity. The formation of this activity was dependent on the presence of protein C in the plasma and the ability of thrombin to form a cell surface complex. These studies indicated that in vivo thrombin, at low concentrations, can be a potent activator of protein C.[65]

C. What Is the Effect of Thrombomodulin on the Activity of Thrombin?

Thrombin, the final serine protease produced in the coagulation cascade, appears to be able to cleave a number of proteins found in blood. Among these are fibrinogen, F-V, F-

VII, prothrombin, protein C, protein S, platelets, and endothelial cells. In addition it is able to interact with antithrombin III. A number of studies have been carried out to determine if thrombomodulin alters the activity either toward these macromolecular substrates or toward small-molecule synthetic substrates.

The isolated cofactor increases the rate of protein C activation approximately 1000-fold.[60] The expression of cofactor activity requires the presence of calcium ions or other divalent cations. Interestingly, this protein does not require the presence of a membrane bilayer for the expression of activity. This is a property that differs from other known cofactor proteins that participate in the process of blood coagulation.

The formation of the thrombin-thrombomodulin complex does not involve any changes in the primary structure of thrombin. However, there appears to be a profound change in the substrate specificity of thrombin when it is bound in this complex. Protein C, for example, is activated approximately 20,000 times more rapidly by endothelial cell-bound thrombomodulin than by soluble thrombin.[59] The purified thrombomodulin does not appear to be quite as effective, but it does enhance the rate substantially. On the other hand, the fibrinogen clotting activity of thrombin is entirely lost when it is in a complex with thrombomodulin.[66] However, if thrombin is displaced from thrombomodulin with DIP-thrombin, its clotting activity can be restored. The thrombin-thrombomodulin complex is unable to activate either F-V[66] or platelets.[67] The bovine thrombin-thrombomodulin complex has been reported to be unreactive with heparin co-factor II.[61] This finding appers not to be the case with preparations of human thrombomodulin prepared from placenta and partially purified from human lung.[64] The human thrombomodulin appeared to be an ineffective inhibitor of F-V activation, platelet activation, and the clotting of fibrinogen.[68] It was unclear, however, if this was a true species difference or due to the isolation of a partially degraded thrombomodulin. It has been reported that when thrombomodulin was isolated from bovine lung it was very sensitive to proteolysis during the extraction step.[61]

How does thrombomodulin alter the catalytic activity of thrombin? Two possibilities have been considered. The first is that thrombomodulin causes a change in the catalytic efficiency of the enzyme, resulting in an increased rate of hydrolysis of peptide bonds. The second possiblity is that substrate specificity has been altered. When thrombin is complexed with thrombomodulin, it appears to have an altered substrate specificity. That is, fibrinogen, F-V, and platelets become poor substrates, while protein C is preferred. For one protein substrate, antithrombin III, there does not appear to be an effect on specificity.[61] The rate of thrombin inactivation when complexed with thrombomodulin appears to be similar to that observed with the soluble thrombin. To test the possibility that there has been a change in the active site, the effects of rabbit lung thrombomodulin on TAME, BAEE, and S2238 have been examined. No effect was observed on the hydrolysis of either TAME or BAEE,[60] and a small stimulatory effect on S2238 has been observed. Others have observed that bovine thrombomodulin had no effect on the hydrolysis of S2238.[61] Since no substantial change in the hydrolysis of the small-molecule substrates is observed with the thrombin-thrombomodulin complex, it has been concluded that there has been no profound change in the conformation of the active site of thrombin by forming a complex with thrombomodulin. The findings tend to suggest that the major effect of thrombomodulin is on substrate specificity.

The activation of protein C by the thrombin-thrombomodulin complex is dependent upon the presence of divalent cations.[60] Of the divalent cations tested, calcium ions appeared to be the most effective.[60] Activation of protein C by thrombin-thrombomodulin complex using purified thrombomodulin was not affected by removal of the gamma-carboxyglutamic acid residues from protein C. Its activation, though still calcium dependent, proceeded at a normal rate. In contrast, Gla-domainless protein C was not activated at an appreciable rate over the surface of rabbit endothelial cells.[69] This suggests that on the surface of the endothelial cell there is a recognition site for the Gla residues of protein C. It also suggests that protein C may contain Gla-independent calcium binding sites. The latter suggestion has been confirmed by studies on the quenching of the intrinsic fluorescense of protein C by divalent cations. These studies have indicated that protein C, both in the presence and absence of its Gla domain, contains a high-affinity binding site for calcium (Kd, 0.062 m*M*).[70] The results of both the physical and functional studies tend to indicate that the high-affinity calcium-binding site on the protein C molecule is important for the interaction with the thrombin-thrombomodulin complex. Second, these studies have indicated that in addition thrombomodulin, the endothelial cell surface may contain another protein that is involved in the activation of protein C by thrombin.

D. The Role of Factor V in the Activation of Protein C

Is there a soluble system for the activation of protein C? Salem and co-workers[71] have reported that, during the coagulation of human blood, protein C is activated. Their studies have indicated that the light chain of activated F-V can stimulate thrombin-catalyzed activation of protein C 50-fold.[71] A comparison of the F-Va light chain with thrombomodulin indicated that thrombomodulin was at least 20 times more effective as a co-factor.[72] At high concentrations the light chain was able to inhibit protein C activation. Thrombin catalyzed protein C activation on human umbilical vein; endothelial cell was also observed to be enhanced by F-Va. Antibodies directed against thrombomodulin or against F-V could inhibit protein C activation. This suggests that F-V and thrombomodulin act in concert to activate protein C.[73]

V. CAN THROMBIN BE FORMED ON THE SURFACE OF THE ENDOTHELIAL CELL?

Though the endothelium is thought of as an antithrombin tissue, several investigators have ported that some of the reactions of the coagulation cascade can be supported on the surface of endothelial cells. Endothelial cells have been observed to contain at least two clotting factors — tissue factor and F-V — and endothelium binding sites for several others. These findings have raised the possibility that the endothelium may be involved in the formation of thrombin.

A. Do Endothelial Cells Promote Reactions Leading to Thrombin Formation?

Using isolated endothelial cells, studies have been carried out to determine if these cells contain any coagulation factors and whether the cells will support any of the reactions of the coagulation cascade. For the cases of F-IX and F-X, activation cells have been examined for specific binding sites.

Can endothelial cells express tissue factor activity? Neither bovine aortic nor human umbilical vein endothelium expresses significant amounts of tissue factor activity,[74] although it has been reported that freshly prepared endothelial cells from umbilical cord vein have weak tissue factor activity.[75] In the latter case, both endotoxin and thrombin were found to enhance this activity, as did the addition of platelets.[75] Maynard and co-workers[76] have reported that endothelial cells will produce tissue factor after being placed in culture; however, the cells needed to be broken for the expression of the activity. Treatment of endothelial cells with phorbol esters can cause the expression of a significant amount of tissue factor-like activity.[77] Though it appears that tissue factor can be synthesized by these cells, expression depends on specific environmental stimulus which does not appear to be well characterized.

Can endothelial cells support F-IX and F-X activation? The activation of F-IX on the surface of the endothelial cell has been observed under several sets of conditions. If tissue factor is first expressed in cells using phorbol ester, then F-IX can be activated by F-VIIa.[78] It is also possible for F-XI to be activated by exogenously added F-XIa.[77] Activated F-IX

Table 3
BINDING OF FACTORS IX, IXA, X, AND XA TO ENDOTHELIAL CELLS[a]

Factor	Kd1 (n*M*)	Kd2 (n*M*)	No. of sites/cell[b]	Cell type	Ref.
IX	4.1	240	280,000	BAE	80
IX	2.3			BAE	79
IXa	2.3		20,000	BAE	79
X	21	320	182,000	BAE	80
X	480		9,600,000	BAE	79

[a] BAE, bovine aortic endothelial cells.
[b] Sites for Kd1 binding.

has been observed to express procoagulant activity[77] and to activated F-X.[78] Several mechanisms of F-X activation have been observed. Activation of F-X by F-IXa required the addition of F-VIII but not phospholipid.[78] Following treatment of the cells with phorbol esters, F-X could be activated by F-VIIa and tissue factor.[77]

Can endothelial cells support prothrombin activation? Bovine endothelial cells, but not fibroblasts, corneal endothelial cells, or fetal lung cells, have been observed to support prothrombin activation.[74] The addition of F-V was not required, and antibodies directed against F-V were able to inhibit prothrombin activation.[74] The latter finding was also true for cells that were grown in a serum-free medium, suggesting that F-V might be synthesized in the endothelial cells. Pretreatment with thrombin did not stimulate activation. This suggests that the F-Va, rather than a surface-bound F-V, is expressed. However, some evidence has been presented that suggests that thrombin is required to obtain the maximum rates of prothrombin activation. It appeared that endothelial cells were comparable to platelets as a cellular surface for the activation of prothrombin.[79]

B. Do Endothelial Cells Have Receptors for Coagulation Factors?

The endothelial cell appears to have specific binding sites for a number of the factors involved in the production of thrombin. It appears that the binding sites, not unlike the thrombin sites, fall into two general classes. One class of sites appears to be specific for specific factors. The second class of sites appears to be specific for the active proteases.

The binding of F-IX[80,81] and IXa[80] to either bovine aortic or human umbilical vein endothelial cells was saturable, specific, and calcium dependent. Dissociation constants and number of sites are summarized in Table 3. Both IX and IXa competed for the same site. Neither prothrombin nor thrombin competed for the site, and F-IX remained active when bound.[80]

As with F-IX, F-X and Xa have been observed to exhibit calcium-dependent binding to endothelial cells.[80] It appears that F-IX and X bind to independent sites on the endothelial surface. F-IXa and Xa appear to bind to sites that are independent from the zymogen binding sites. It appears from in vivo studies that endothelial cells contain a protease-binding site that is capable of binding F-IXa and Xa, and thrombin. This site may be involved with the covalent attachment that has been observed between the endothelial cell and either F-Xa[78] or thrombin.[7,13]

C. Do Endothelial Cells Mediate the Inactivation of Coagulation Factors?

Once bound to the endothelial cell surface, F-IXa and Xa have several possible fates. In vivo F-IXa is rapidly cleared from the circulation. One fate is the formation of a complex with antithrombin III.[82] F-IXa is poorly inhibited by either α-2-macroglobulin or to α-1-proteinase inhibitor.[82] The addition of heparin causes all of F-IXa to become complexed with antithrombin III.[82] In vivo inactivation of F-IXa could be blocked by DIP-thrombin and DIP-F-Xa. F-Xa also appears to have several fates. When added to cultured endothelial cells, it is rapidly inactivated.[83] The inactivation appears to be due to irreversible binding to an endothelial cell component. In vivo studies indicated that the major in vivo inactivator of F-Xa is α-2-macroglobulin. In plasma, in the absence of cells, the predominant inhibitor is α-1-proteinase inhibitor.[83] Unlike thrombin, most of factor Xa in vivo is cleared in the liver as an α-2-macroglobulin complex.[83]

These studies have indicated that F-X and IX have specific binding sites on the surface of the endothelial cells. In their activated forms these factors are able to catalyze reactions that can lead to thrombin formation. In addition, it appears that the endothelial cell plays a role in the inactivation of these factors. The effect of the endothelium may not be the same for each protease. The endothelium stimulates the inactivation of F-IXa and thrombin by antithrombin III while it may play some role in the inactivation of F-Xa by α-2-macroglobulin. The nature of the cell surface receptor that mediates these reactions is still unclear. In addition, the importance of each of these reactions in the regulation of hemostasis remains to be determined.

VI. FUTURE TRENDS

Research into the role of the endothelium in the regulation of thrombin is relatively recent in origin. Besides the isolation of thrombomodulin and the characterization of cell surface glycosaminoglycans, little is known about the molecular constituents of the endothelial cell surface and their role in the maintenance of the antithrombotic properties of the endothelial linings. In the future, cell surface receptors for the various coagulation factors need to be characterized with respect to structure and function. In addition, little is known about factors, hormonal or otherwise, that may be involved in the regulation of the various procoagulant and anticoagulant activities of the endothelium. With the increased research interest in this tissue, one can expect an increase in an understanding of the molecular nature of the role of the endothelium in hemostasis.

ACKNOWLEDGMENTS

Frederick J. Walker is an Established Investigator of the American Heart Association with funds contributed, in part, from the Indiana Affiliate of the American Heart Association.

REFERENCES

1. **Jaffe, E. A., Nachmann, R. C., Becker, C. G., and Minick, C. K.,** Culture of human endothelial cells derived from unbilical veins, *J. Clin. Invest.*, 52, 2745, 1973.
2. **Lollar, P. and Owen, W. G.,** Clearance of thrombin from ciruclation in rabbits by high affinity binding sites on endothelium, *J. Clin. Invest.*, 66, 1222, 1980.
3. **Dryjski, M., Olsson, P., and Swedenborg, J.,** Uptake and inhibition of thrombin by the vascular wall, *Thromb. Res.*, 27, 467, 1982.
4. **Swedenborg, J., Dryjski, M., and Olsson, P.,** Inactivation of thrombin by the aortic endothelium, *Thromb. Haemost.*, 50, 635, 1983.
5. **Lollar, P., MacIntosh, S., and Owen, W. G.,** Interaction of thrombin with the vascular endothelium in a recirculating Lagendorff rabbit heart preparation, *Ann. N.Y. Acad. Sci.*, 82, 234, 1982.
6. **Savion, N., Isaacs, J. D., Gospodarowicz, D., and Shuman, M. A.,** Internalization and degradation of thrombin and up regulation of thrombin-binding sites in corneal endothelial cells, *J. Biol. Chem.*, 256, 4514, 1981.

7. **Isaacs, J. D., Savion, N., Gospodarowicz, D., Fenton, J. W., and Shuman, M. A.,** Covalent binding of thrombin to specific sites on corneal endothelial cells, *Biochemisty,* 20, 398, 1981.
8. **Awbrey, B. J., Hoak, J. C., and Owen, W. G.,** Binding of human thrombin to cultured human endothelial cells, *J. Biol. Chem.,* 254, 4092, 1979.
9. **Hatton, M. W. C., Dejana, E., Cazenave, J. P., Regoeczi, E., and Mustard, J.,** Heparin inhibits thrombin binding to rabbit thoracic aorta endothelium, *J. Lab. Clin. Med.,* 96, 861, 1980.
10. **Bauer, P. I., Machovich, R., Aranyi, P., Buki, K. G., Csonka, E., and Horvath, I.,** Mechanism of thrombin binding to endothelial cells, *Blood,* 61, 368, 1983.
11. **Machovich, R., Blaskó, G., and Palos, L. A.,** Action of heparin on thrombin-antithrombin reaction, *Biochim. Biophys. Acta,* 379, 193, 1975.
12. **Pomerantz, M. W. and Owen, W. G.,** A catalytic role for heparin: evidence for a ternary complex of heparin cofactor, thrombin and heparin, *Biochim. Biophys. Acta,* 535, 66, 1978.
13. **Lollar, P., Hoak, J. C., and Owen, W. G.,** Binding of thrombin to cultured human endothelial cells: nonequilibrium aspects, *J. Biol. Chem.,* 255, 10279, 1980.
14. **Rosenberg, R. and Damus, P.,** The purification and mechanism of action of human antithrombin-heparin cofactor, *J. Biol. Chem.,* 248, 6490, 1973.
15. **Rosenberg, R. D.,** Chemistry of the hemostatic mechanism and its relationship to the action of heparin, *Fed. Proc.,* 36, 10, 1977.
16. **Owen, W. G.,** Evidence for the formation of an ester between thrombin and heparin cofactor, *Biochim. Biophys. Acta,* 405, 380, 1975.
17. **Howell, W. H. and Holt, E.,** Two new factors in blood coagulation — heparin and pro-antithrombin, *Am. J. Phsiol.,* 47, 328, 1918.
18. **Jordon, R., Beeler, D., and Rosenberg, R.,** Fractionation of low molecular weight heparin species and their interaction with antithrombin, *J. Biol. Chem.,* 254, 2902, 1979.
19. **Griffith, M. J.,** Kinetics of the heparin-enhanced antithrombin III/thrombin reaction, *J. Biol. Chem.,* 257, 7360, 1982.
20. **Nesheim, M. E.,** A simple rate law that describes the kinetics of heparin-catalyzed reaction between thrombin and antithrombin III (1983), *J. Biol. Chem.,* 258, 14708, 1983.
21. **Damus, P. S., Hicks, M., and Rosenberg, R. D.,** Anticoagulant action of heparin, *Nature (London),* 246, 355, 1973.
22. **Buonassisi, V.,** Sulfated mucopolysaccharide synthesis and secretion in endothelial cell cultures, *Exp. Cell Res.,* 76, 363, 1973.
23. **Colburn, P. and Buonassisi, V.,** Anti-clotting activity of endothelial cell cultures and heparan sulfate proteoglycans, *Biochem. Biophys. Res. Commun.,* 104, 220, 1982.
24. **Nakazawa, K. and Murata, A.,** Acidic glycosaminoglycans in three layers of human aorta: their different constitution and anticoagulant function, *Arterial Wall,* 2, 203, 1975.
25. **Hatton, M. W. C., Berryk, L. R., and Regoeczi, E.,** Inhibition of thrombin by antithrombin III in the presence of certain glycosaminoglycans found in mammalian aorta, *Thromb. Res.,* 13, 655, 1978.
26. **Marcum, J. A. and Rosenberg, R. D.,** Anticoagulantly active heparin-like molecules from vascular tissue, *Biochemistry,* 23, 1730, 1984.
27. **Marcum, J. A., Fritze, L., Galli, S. J., Karp, G., and Rosenberg, R. D.,** Microvascular heparinlike species with anticoagulant activity, *Am. J. Physiol.,* 245, H725, 1983.
28. **Busch, C. and Owen, W. G.,** Identification *in vitro* of an endothelial cell surface cofactor for antithrombin III: parallel studies with isolated perfused rat hearts and microcarrier cultures of bovine endothelium, *J. Clin. Invest.,* 69, 726, 1982.
29. **Marcum, J. A., McKenney, J. B., and Rosenberg, R. D.,** Acceleration of thrombin-antithrombin complex formation in rat hindquarters via heparin-like molecules bound to the endothelium, *J. Clin. Invest.,* 74, 341, 1984.
30. **Dryjski, M., Larsson, R., Olsson, P., and Swedenborg, F.,** Effect of glycosaminoglycans and antithrombin III on uptake and inhibition of thrombin by the vascular wall, *J. Thromb. Res.,* 32, 355, 1983.
31. **Lollar, P., MacIntosh, S. C., and Owen, W. G.,** Reaction of antithrombin III with thrombin bound to the vascular endothelium: analysis in a recirculating perfused rabbit heart preparation, *J. Biol. Chem.,* 259, 4335, 1984.
32. **Stenflo, J.,** A new vitamin K-dependent protein: purification from bovine plasma and preliminary characterization, *J. Biol. Chem.,* 251, 355, 1976.
33. **Esmon, C. T., Stenflo, J., Suttie, J. W., and Jackson, C. M.,** A new vitamin K-dependent protein: a phospholipid-binding zymogen of a serine esterase, *J. Biol. Chem.,* 251, 3052, 1976.
34. **Kisiel, W., Ericsson, L. H., and Davie, E. W.,** Proteolytic activation of protein C from bovine plasma, *Biochemistry,* 15, 4893, 1976.
35. **Walker, F. J., Sexton, P. W., and Esmon, C. T.,** The inhibition of blood coagulation by activated protein C through the selective inactivation of activated factor V, *Biochim. Biophys. Acta,* 571, 333, 1979.

36. **Kisiel, W., Canfield, W. M., Ericsson, L. H., and Davie, E. W.,** Anticoagulant properties of bovine plasma protein C following activation by thrombin, *Biochemistry,* 16, 5824, 1977.
37. **Marlar, R. A., Kleiss, A. J., and Griffin, J. G.,** Mechanism of action of human activated protein C, a thrombin-dependent anticoagulant enzyme, *Blood,* 59, 1067, 1982.
38. **Suzuki, K., Stenflo, J., Dahlback, B., and Teodorsson, B.,** Inactivation of human coagulation factor V by activated protein C, *J. Biol. Chem.,* 258, 1914, 1983.
39. **Fay, P. J., Chavin, S. I., Schroeder, D., Young, F. E., and Marder, V. J.,** Purification and characterization of a highly purified human factor VIII consisting of a single type of polypeptide chain, *Proc. Natl. Acad. Sci. U.S.A.,* 79, 7200, 1982.
40. **Vehar, G. A. and Davie, E. W.,** Preparation and properties of bovine factor VIII (antihemophilic factor), *Biochemistry,* 19, 401, 1980.
41. **Mammen, E. F., Thomas, W. R., and Seegers, W. H.,** Activation of purified prothrombin to autoprothrombin I or autoprothrombin II (platelet cofactor II) or autoprothrombin II-a, *Thromb. Diath. Haemorrh.,* 5, 218, 1960.
42. **Walker, F. J.,** The regulation of activated protein C by a new protein: a possible function for bovine protein S, *J. Biol. Chem.,* 255, 5521, 1980.
43. **Comp, P. C., Nixon, R. R., Cooper, R., and Esmon, C. T.,** Familial protein S deficinecy is associated with recurrent thrombosis, *J. Clin. Invest.,* 74, 2082, 1984.
44. **Schwartz, H. P., Fischer, M., Hopmeier, P., et al.,** Plasma protein S deficiency in familial thrombotic disease, *Blood,* 64, 1297, 1984.
45. **Comp, P. C. and Esmon, C. T.,** Recurrent venous thromboembolism in patients with a partial deficiency of protein S, *N. Engl. J. Med.,* 311, 1525, 1984.
46. **Walker, F. J.,** Regulation of activated protein C by protein S: the role of phospholipid in factor Va inactivation, *J. Biol. Chem.,* 256, 11128, 1981.
47. **Lawrence, J. E., Batard, M. A., Berridge, C. W., and Fulcher, C. A.,** Protein S enhances the inactivation of factor VIII by activated protein C, *Thromb. Haemost.,* 54, 83, 1985.
48. **Harris, K. W. and Esmon, C. T.,** Protein S is required for bovine platelets to support activated protein C binding and activity, *J. Biol. Chem.,* 260, 2007, 1985.
49. **Dahlback, B. and Stenflo, J.,** High molecular weight complex in human plasma between vitamin K-dependent protein S and complement component C4b-binding protein, *Proc. Natl. Acad. Sci. U.S.A.,* 78, 2512, 1981.
50. **Dahlback, B.,** Purification of human C4b-binding protein and formation of its complex with vitamin K-dependent protein S, *Biochem. J.,* 209, 847, 1983.
51. **DiScipio, R. G. and Davie, E. W.,** Characterization of protein S, a gamma-carboxyglutamic acid containing protein from bovine and human plasma, *Biochemistry,* 18, 899, 1979.
52. **Stenflo, J. and Jonsson, M.,** Protein S, a new vitamin K-dependent protein from bovine plasma, *FEBS Lett.,* 101, 377, 1979.
53. **Dahlback, B.,** Purification of human vitamin K-dependent protein S and its limited proteolysis by thrombin, *Biochem. J.,* 209, 837, 1983.
54. **Walker, F. J.,** Regulation of vitamin K-dependent protein S: inactivation by thrombin, *J. Biol. Chem.,* 259, 10335, 1984.
55. **Suzuki, K., Nishioka, J., and Hashimoto, S.,** Regulation of activated protein C by thrombin-modified protein S, *J. Biochem.,* 94, 699, 1983.
56. **Suzuki, K., Nishioka, J., and Hashimoto, S.,** Protein C inhibitor, purification from human plasma and characterization, *J. Biol. Chem.,* 258, 163, 1983.
57. **Canfield, W. M. and Kisiel, W.,** Evidence of normal functional levels of activated protein C inhibitor in combined factor V/VIII deficiency disease, *J. Clin. Invest.,* 70, 1260, 1972.
58. **Esmon, C. T. and Owen, W. G.,** Identification of an endothelial cell cofactor for thrombin-catalyzed activation of protein C, *Proc. Natl. Acad. Sci. U.S.A.,* 78, 2249, 1981.
59. **Owen, W. G. and Esmon, C. T.,** Functional properties of an endothelial cell cofactor for thrombin-catalyzed activation of protein C, *J. Biol. Chem.,* 256, 5532, 1981.
60. **Esmon, N. L., Owen, W. G., and Esmon, C. T.,** Isolation of a membrane-bound cofactor for thrombin catalyzed activation of protein C, *J. Biol. Chem.,* 257, 859, 1982.
61. **Jakubowski, H. V. and Owen, W. G.,** Effect of bovine thrombomodulin on thrombin specificity, *Thromb. Haemost.,* 54, 119, 1985.
62. **Suzuki, K., Kusumoto, H., and Hashimoto, S.,** Isolation and characterization of thrombomodulin from bovine lung, *Thromb. Haemost.,* 54, 83, 1985.
63. **Kurosawa, S. and Aoki, N.,** Preparation of thrombomodulin from human placenta, *Thromb. Res.,* 37, 353, 1985.
64. **Salem, H. H., Maruyama, I., Ishii, H., and Majerus, P. W.,** Isolation and characterization of thrombomodulin from human placenta, *J. Biol. Chem.,* 259, 12246, 1984.

65. **Comp, P. C., Jacocks, R. M., Ferrell, G. L., and Esmon, C. T.,** Activation of protein C in vivo, *J. Clin. Invest.*, 70, 127, 1982.
66. **Esmon, C. T., Esmon, N. L., and Harris, K. W.,** Complex formation between thrombin and thrombomodulin inhibits both thrombin-catalyzed fibrin formation and factor V activation, *J. Biol. Chem.*, 257, 7944, 1982.
67. **Esmon, N. L., Carroll, R. C., and Esmon, C. T.,** Thrombomodulin blocks the ability of thrombin to activate platelets, *J. Biol. Chem.*, 258, 12238, 1983.
68. **Maruyama, I., Salem, H. H., Ishii, H., and Majerus, P. W.,** Human thrombomodulin is not an efficient inhibitor of procoagulant activity of thrombin, *J. Clin. Invest.*, 75, 987, 1985.
69. **Esmon, N. L., DeBault, L. E., and Esmon, C. T.,** Proteolytic formation and properties of gamma-carboxyglutamic acid domainless protein C, *J. Biol. Chem.*, 258, 5548, 1983.
70. **Johnson, A. E., Esmon, N. L., Laue, T. M., and Esmon, C. T.,** Structural changes required for activation of protein C are induced by Ca^{2+} binding to a high affinity site that does not contain gamma-carboxyglutamic acid, *J. Biol. Chem.*, 258, 5554, 1983.
71. **Salem, H. H., Broze, G. J., Miletich, J. P., and Majerus, P. W.,** Human coagulation factor Va is a cofactor for the activation of protein C, *Proc. Natl. Acad. Sci. U.S.A.*, 80, 1584, 1983.
72. **Salem, H., Esmon, N. L., Esmon, C. T., and Majerus, P. W.,** Effects of thrombomodulin and coagulation factor Va-light chain on protein C activation *in vitro, J. Clin. Invest.*, 73, 968, 1984.
73. **Maruyama, I., Salem, H. H., and Majerus, P. W.,** Coagulation factor Va binds to human umbilical vein endothelial cells and accelerates protein C activation, *J. Clin. Invest.*, 74, 224, 1984.
74. **Rogers, G. M., Greenberg, C. S., and Shuman, M. A.,** Characterization of the effects of cultured vascular cells on the activation of blood coagulation, *Blood*, 61, 1155, 1983.
75. **Brox, J. H., Osterud, B., Bjorklid, E., and Fenton, J. W.,** Production and availability of thromboplastin in endothelial cells: the effects of thrombin, endotoxin and platelets, *Br. J. Haematol.*, 57, 239, 1984.
76. **Maynard, J. R., Dreyer, B. E., Stemerman, M. E., and Pitlick, F. A.,** Tissue factor coagulant activity of cultured human endothelial and smooth muscle cells and fibroblasts, *Blood*, 50, 387, 1977.
77. **Stern, D. M., Drillings, M., Kisiel, W., Nawroth, P., Nossel, H. L., and LaGamma, K. S.,** Activation of factor IX bound to cultured bovine aortic endothelial cells, *Proc. Natl. Acad. Sci. U.S.A.*, 81, 913, 1984.
78. **Stern, D. M., Nawroth, P. P., Kisiel, W., Handley, D., Drillings, M., and Bartos, J.,** A coagulation pathway on bovine aortic segments leading to generation of factor Xa and thrombin, *J. Clin. Invest.*, 74, 1910, 1984.
79. **Rogers, G. M. and Shuman, M. A.,** Prothrombin is activated on vascular endothelial cells by factor Xa and calcium, *Proc. Natl. Acad. Sci. U.S.A.*, 80, 7001, 1983.
80. **Stern, D. M., Drillings, M., Nossel, H. L., and Hurlet-Jensen, J.,** Binding of factor IX and IXa to cultured vascular endothelial cells, *Proc. Natl. Acad. Sci. U.S.A.*, 80, 4119, 1983.
81. **Heimark, R. L. and Schwartz, S. M.,** Binding of coagulation factors IX and X to the endothelial cell surface, *Biochem. Biophys. Res. Commun.*, 111, 723, 1983.
82. **Fuchs, H. E., Trapp, H. G., Griffith, M. J., Roberts, H.,** Regulation of factor IXa *in vitro* in human and mouse plasma and *in vivo* in the mouse: role of the endothelium and the plasma proteinase inhibitors, *J. Clin. Invest.*, 73, 1696, 1984.
83. **Fuchs, H. E. and Pizzo, S. V.,** Regulation of factor Xa *in vitro* in human and mouse plasma and *in vivo* in mouse, *J. Clin. Invest.*, 72, 2041, 1983.
84. **Walker, F. J.,** unpublished observations.

Chapter 9

REGULATION OF VASCULAR FIBRINOLYSIS

Laurence A. Erickson

TABLE OF CONTENTS

I. INTRODUCTION

The hemostatic system, consisting of components in both the vessel wall and blood, is responsible for maintaining proper circulation, and thus ensuring adequate delivery of cells, nutrients, proteins, and other necessary molecular constituents to various body tissues. Evidence gathered from several different experimental approaches indicates that an intact vascular endothelium provides for unimpeded blood flow by preventing activation of the procoagulant molecules found in blood.[1-3] When perturbed, however, the endothelium and the exposed underlying layers of cells provide effective surfaces for activating such factors. In fact, these tissues are themselves rich sources of procoagulant molecules.[4] Injury-induced activation of components of the coagulation cascade culminates in the formation of thrombin. Thrombin not only converts fibrinogen to fibrin but also activates blood cells, which then adhere to the perturbed sites of the vessel wall.[5,6] Hemostasis is ultimately achieved by the formation of a fibrin-cellular thrombus, which stems the flow of blood and helps to initiate the early events of wound healing. A number of additional components function to ensure that the thrombus does not unduly restrict the flow of blood and thus compromise vessel patency for an extended period of time. These components collectively constitute the vascular thrombolytic system.[7,8] The coordinated regulation of thrombus formation (coagulation) and dissolution (thrombolysis) is of utmost importance to the maintenance of a proper hemostatic balance. In this chapter, the mechanisms involved in the transition from blood clot stabilization to thrombolysis is discussed. Particular emphasis is placed on those components that contribute to the initiation of vascular fibrinolysis.

II. THE INTERFACE BETWEEN THROMBUS FORMATION AND DISSOLUTION

Certain findings suggest that under normal conditions fibrin may be continually deposited on and removed from the endothelial lining of blood vessels.[9,10] However, other evidence indicates that fibrin formation and its subsequent dissolution occur only after vessel wall injury.[11] Because the extent to which such injury normally occurs has not been determined, it is not known whether the coagulation and vascular fibrinolytic systems are constantly active or quiescent in physiologic situations. In either case, platelets and other cells in the blood normally circulate in the presence of a high concentration of fibrinogen (10 μM) without apparent clot formation. Both the conversion of fibrinogen to fibrin and the activation of blood cells seem to be required for thrombus formation.[12] A key step in this process is the proteolytic conversion of the inactive zymogen, prothrombin, into the active protease, thrombin. This conversion is initiated by a prothrombinase complex assembled on the surface of platelets, which consists of coagulation factors Va (F-Va) and Xa, Ca^{2+} ions, and the membrane or phospholipid surface itself.[13] The assembly and activity of the prothrombinase complex has been extensively examined, and comprehensive reviews of the results of such studies have been published.[14,15] Another chapter under this title provides a detailed description of the interactions between activated prothrombin (thrombin) and the vessel wall. One such interaction involves the association of thrombin with thrombomodulin at the endothelial cell surface. When bound to thrombomodulin, thrombin has an increased capacity to activate protein C, which subsequently neutralizes F-Va and VIIIa.[16] As such, this mechanism constitutes an important pathway in the feedback inhibition of coagulation. Moreover, additional evidence suggests that thrombin-activated protein C is also involved in the initiation of vascular fibrinolysis.[17-20] The specific role of activated protein C (PCa) in the initiation of vascular fibrinolysis is discussed later (see Section IV.B.). Thus, thrombin not only initiates fibrin formation and cellular activation, but also serves a pivotal role in the transition between thrombus formation and the initiation of vascular fibrinolysis.

III. BASIC MECHANISMS OF VASCULAR FIBRINOLYSIS

The generation of the active fibrin-degrading enzyme, plasmin, and the actual dissolution of fibrin constitute the two most basic elements of the vascular fibrinolytic system. Following a brief discussion of these features, I focus on the interactions between molecules in the blood and components in the vessel wall as they pertain to the expression of vascular fibrinolytic activity.

A. Plasmin Formation

Although other enzymes have the capacity to degrade fibrin,[21,22] the primary fibrinolytic enzyme in the blood is plasmin.[23] Normally, the blood contains little, if any, active plasmin. Rather, it contains the inactive zymogen, plasminogen. Plasminogen is cleaved at Arg_{560}-Val_{561} by specific serine proteases termed plasminogen activators (PAs), resulting in the formation of active, two-chain plasmin.[24] Effective vascular fibrinolysis requires that the cleavage of plasminogen occurs only at specific localized sites of fibrin deposition. This ensures that other plasma proteins susceptible to proteolysis by plasmin are not consumed. Such localization is achieved by a complex set of interactions among several components present in blood.[25] One essential feature of this process is the binding of plasminogen and tissue plasminogen activator (tPA) to fibrin, which results in the formation of a cyclic ternary complex.[26] The mechanisms of localizing vascular fibrinolysis initiated by urokinase-like PA (uPA) or the so-called intrinsic PAs are not yet clear. However, it has been proposed that plasma contains a competitive inhibitor of single-chain uPA that restricts its ability to cleave plasminogen in the absence of fibrin.[27] It has been suggested further that the major unidentified intrinsic PA in plasma also has affinity for fibrin.[28] These interactions are certainly influenced in vivo by blood flow and by cell surfaces present in the vasculature that have not been accounted for in in vitro studies. Nevertheless, plasmin thus formed in association with fibrin is strategically located to commence the process of fibrin dissolution.

B. Fibrin Degradation

The initial breakdown of fibrin is characterized by cleavage of its α-polymer chains by plasmin. Subsequent proteolysis of the coiled coils in the protofibrils of fibrin leads to progressive clot lysis.[8,29] This results in the production of distinct fibrin degradation products that are released into the circulation and serve to depress the activity of the coagulation system.[30] Additional studies have demonstrated that the activation of native glu-plasminogen is enhanced by partially degraded fibrin. This enhancement appears to be mediated by the exposure of binding sites on fibrin that induce a conformational change in the zymogen.[31] Thus, degraded fibrin functions to limit the further deposition of fibrin as well as to perpetuate fibrinolysis via a positive feedback mechanism. On the other hand, fibrin dissolution is restricted by α_2-antiplasmin, which competes with fibrin(ogen) for lysine-binding sites on plasmin(ogen)[32] and also covalently binds to fibrin through the action of F-XIIIa.[33] In addition, although plasmin bound to fibrin is relatively resistant to α_2-antiplasmin, this inhibitor rapidly neutralizes plasmin that is released into the circulation.[34] Thus, when fibrinolysis is complete, α_2-antiplasmin prevents excess plasmin-mediated proteolysis. Concurrently, the actual generation of plasmin may also be restricted by factors that modulate the availability and the activity of circulating PAs. This concept emphasizes the importance of the endothelium in regulating fibrinolysis in the vicinity of a forming or degrading thrombus.

IV. REGULATION OF FIBRINOLYSIS BY THE VESSEL WALL

The molecular interactions discussed above are critical to the localization, progression, and termination of plasmin-associated fibrinolytic activity. In comparision to our knowledge of these mechanisms, the events associated with the initiation of vascular fibrinolysis are not well defined. The following sections outline our current understanding of the major contributions of the vessel wall, and associated components in the blood, to this latter process.

A. Plasminogen Activator

Since plasminogen is normally present in the circulation at a relatively high concentration (2.2 μM),[35] the initiation of fibrinolytic activity in the blood is primarily dependent upon the availability of active PA. Although other blood-borne cells produce PA,[36] endothelial cells appear to be the major source of vascular PA.[37] Therefore, the endothelium probably constitutes the primary site for regulating PA-mediated vascular fibrinolysis. However, the specific factors that control the expression of PA by endothelial cells, both in vitro and in vivo, are not known. Many compounds affect the fibrinolytic activity of these cells, but their specific mechanisms of action have not been elucidated.[38] Alterations of fibrinolytic potential induced by such compounds may result from (1) changes in the production of PA (i.e., an effect on gene expression and/or protein synthesis), (2) alterations in the rate of PA release, or (3) modulation of the activity of PA molecules already present (i.e., through an effect on plasminogen activator inhibitors, or PAIs). Few studies have been designed to distinguish between these various possibilities. In this context, it is important to appreciate that molecular probes for PA antigen[39] and mRNA[40] have been developed only recently. Prior to the utilization of such reagents, a rapid increase of extracellular PA activity was attributed to an effect on the secretory process of the cells, whereas a delayed increase was thought to be due to an effect on PA synthesis. With these points in mind, certain aspects of the expression of endothelial cell-mediated fibrinolysis at each of these levels of control are discussed.

1. Synthesis

Although the endothelium was believed to be the primary source of vascular PA based on histochemical studies, the fact that endothelial cells could actually synthesize PA was demonstrated only within the last several years. Such studies became possible when the conditions for maintaining these cells in culture were defined.[41] By studying endothelial cells in vitro, investigators were able to establish that these cells in fact have the capacity to produce PA.[42,43] Under certain conditions, they synthesize both urokinase-like PA and tissue-type PA.[43] Moreover, it was demonstrated that these two types of PA are regulated differentially by various compounds, including Ca^{2+} ionophore, dexamethasone, and thrombin.[38,44] Again, in these studies specific measurements of PA antigen and mRNA were not made, leaving open the question of whether or not such fluctuations of PA activity actually correlated with changes in PA production.

The foundation for directly examining the regulation of PA synthesis by endothelial cells has been derived from studying the production of PAs by other cells more amenable to in vitro culture conditions. The results obtained from these studies have been extensively reviewed[45] and suggest that the cellular expression of PA is multifaceted, since many different types of compounds affected the fibrinolytic potential of the cells. Although initial studies in this area were not designed to distinguish between effects on PA synthesis or activity, recent investigations of this type have employed specific reagents to measure fluctuations of PA antigen and mRNA that occur under different conditions. From these studies it seems clear that molecules such as epidermal growth factor,[46] phorbol ester,[47] and calcitonin[48] actually modulate the cellular expression of PA at the level of transcription. In similar studies, glucocorticoids[49] and sitosterol[50] were shown to affect the production of PA by endothelial cells. However, it is not yet clear whether these compounds act through a common pathway or through different mechanisms. Moreover, the in vivo correlates to these effector molecules have not been identified. Thus, numerous investigators are now attempting to

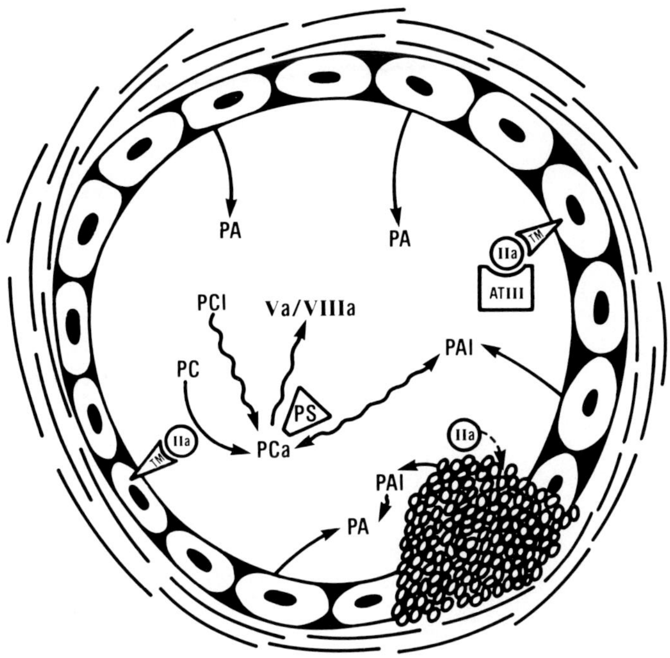

FIGURE 1. Regulation of vascular fibrinolysis. This schematic diagram portrays the primary factors that regulate vascular PA activity. The text contains a description of the components and interactions shown in this figure. (PA, plasminogen activator; TM, thrombomodulin; IIa, thrombin; ATIII, antithrombin III; PC, protein C; PCa, activated protein C, PCI, protein C inhibitor; Va, activated factor V; VIIIa, activated factor VIII; PS, protein S; PAI, PA inhibitor.)

identify the specific factors that control the physiologic cellular expression of PA, with particular emphasis on the endothelium. In this context, Tiku and Tomasi[51] have recently shown that lymphokines enhance the synthesis of PA by porcine aortic endothelial cells.

2. Secretion

Clearly, PA derived from the endothelium[52] must be released into the circulation to initiate vascular fibrinolysis (Figure 1). Elucidation of the mechanisms of PA secretion by endothelial cells thus is of fundamental importance to understanding the regulation of vessel wall-mediated thrombolysis. Endothelial cells not only synthesize PAs in vitro, they also release them into the surrounding culture medium.[53,54] Factors that affect this process can thus be examined under controlled conditions. For example, by using such a system, it has been demonstrated that thrombin induces the release of tPA by human umbilical vein endothelial cells.[53,55] This process is dependent upon protein synthesis and requires active thrombin. This observation emphasizes the important role that thrombin plays in the transition from thrombus formation to the initiation of fibrinolysis. Other molecules that affect the release of PA by endothelial cells include colchicine,[38] serum components,[56] and heparinoids.[57] These studies have provided some important insights into the process of PA secretion by endothelial cells, but it is not yet clear to what extent these findings are relevant to in vivo conditions.

Many compounds have the capacity to induce the release of tPA from endothelium in vivo. These factors include vasopressin and its analogs,[58,59] bradykinin,[60,61] and platelet activating factor.[62,63] Venous occlusion[64] and physical exercise[65] also increase the amount

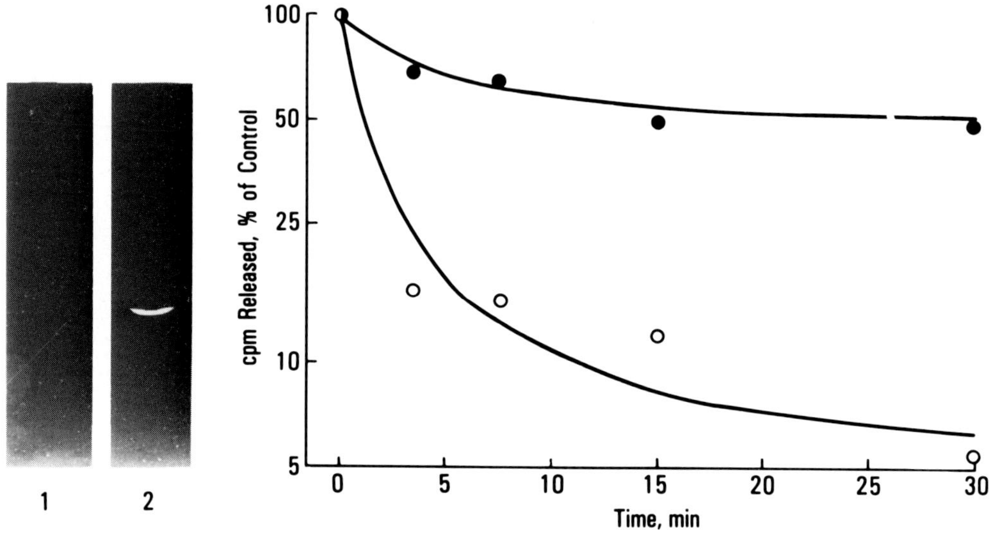

FIGURE 2. Measurement of PAI activity in human serum. The left panel shows the PAI detected in human serum by using reverse fibrin autography. (Lane 1) Serum derived from platelet-poor plasma; (lane 2) serum derived from platelet-rich plasma. The PAI detected has a M_r of about 50,000. The right panel displays the antifibrinolytic activity of these samples against tPA as determined by using the ^{125}I-fibrin plate assay. (●, platelet-poor serum; ○, platelet-rich serum.) The rapid decline of PA-mediated fibrinolysis in the platelet-rich sample indicates the presence of elevated PAI. See reference 74 for methodological details.

of tPA released into the circulation. Again, the specific mechanisms of such enhanced release have not been elucidated. Moreover, it has been demonstrated recently that the relationship between the amount of tPA antigen released into the circulation and the associated plasma tPA activity varies depending on the level of PAI present.[66-68] This finding suggests that an important consideration in these studies is the form of PA released. Is it free (uncomplexed) and already active (i.e., able to activate plasminogen), or is it bound to other molecules in the culture fluid or in blood that render it inactive? Both free and complexed PA have been detected in cells and in blood;[69,70] however, to what extent these forms of PA represent the forms that actually exist in vivo is not yet apparent. That is, the generation of free, active PA may result, at least partially, from the dissociation of PA-inhibitor complexes either in vivo or during sample collection and processing. Alternatively, the formation of PA-inhibitor complexes may occur in vitro after the release of these components by cells[53] or during the processing of blood samples. This distinction is an important one to appreciate if the nature of the interaction between these molecules in vivo is to be understood. Regardless, it is clear that after PAs are released into the circulation their activities may be affected by other components present in the blood.

3. Modulation of Activity

As stated earlier, α_2-antiplasmin efficiently inactivates plasmin that is not associated with fibrin. Therefore, the perpetuation of fibrinolysis beyond the clot surface is precisely regulated. Conceptually, PAIs also present may serve to prevent the premature initiation of fibrinolysis by effectively neutralizing the activity of clot-associated PAs. The PAIs in endothelial cells[71-73] and platelets[74,75] may be released during the formation of a thrombus and create a local environment that is quite inhibitory to fibrinolysis. This potential difference between a ''plasma like'' milieu and a ''serum like'' one is depicted in Figure 2. This figure shows that serum derived from platelet-rich plasma is much more inhibitory against tPA than is serum obtained from platelet-poor plasma. Although such results suggest that circulating PAs may be effectively neutralized by endogenous PAIs[76,77] the exact mechanisms of action of the PAIs have not been elucidated. These inhibitors may exhibit their activity in vivo by interacting with PAs at cell surfaces, in the circulation, and/or in association with a thrombus. For example, it is conceivable that PA may be associated with a specific inhibitor on the surface of the endothelium. After the release of such PA-PAI complexes into the circulation, they may bind to fibrin, release the inhibitor, and in the process allow the PA to activate plasminogen in the vicinity of the clot. This hypothesis suggests that a reversible interaction between enzyme and inhibitor would provide for a readily available pool of active PA in proximity to a formed thrombus. However, it is not yet apparent how complexes between PA and PAI interact with fibrin and other thrombus-associated molecules, or how other components in the blood affect complex formation. The fact that both the endothelial cell-derived PAI and the platelet-derived PAI can exist as either active or latent molecules[78-80] suggests that additional components in the blood may function to enhance or restrict the activity of the PAI itself.

B. Thrombomodulin

In addition to elaborating PA and PAI, endothelial cells may express thrombomodulin on their luminal surface (see Figure 1).[81,82] This component can bind thrombin and convert it from a prothrombotic molecule to a profibrinolytic one. Although antithrombin III can still inhibit thrombin that is bound to thrombomodulin, the interaction of these two components enables thrombin to cleave protein C in preference to fibrinogen.[16,83] This results in the generation of activated protein C, which not only depresses coagulation by inactivating F-Va and VIIIa but also enhances vascular fibrinolysis.[17-20,84,85] Further, the ability of PCa to regulate these systems is enhanced by protein S and restricted by a PC-specific inhibitor. Recent studies in this area indicate that PCa exerts its profibrinolytic activity through an as yet undefined effect on the endothelium as well as by directly interacting with the PAI.[86-88] Imbalances in this system at the level of PA, PAI, thrombomodulin, and/or protein C may lead to a depressed fibrinolytic state, which may culminate in excessive thrombus formation.[89,90]

V. PERTUBATIONS OF THE HEMOSTATIC BALANCE

Elevated vascular procoagulant activity may predispose an individual to develop thrombotic occlusions.[91,92] As suggested above, a depression of the fibrinolytic activity of the blood may also lead to such a state.[89,93] Thus, alterations of PA and/or PAI activities may be related to the development of occlusive vascular disease. Such situations have been described. These include cases in which PA release is actually defective,[94,95] and others in which elevated PAI masks the activity of normally released PA.[66-68,96,97] However, the specific underlying defects in these cases have not been identified. For example, the elevated plasma PAI activity may result from an enhanced release of PAI from endothelial cells and/or platelets. Whether at the genetic, cellular, or molecular level, alterations that result in a depression of vascular fibrinolysis may be intimately associated with the occurrence of thrombotic events. In many of these situations, therapeutic intervention is required to restore vessel patency. One approach that is used to alleviate such conditions is the infusion of agents that initiate the process of fibrin degradation, and eventually cause thrombolysis.

VI. RESTORATION OF VESSEL PATENCY

A. Thrombolytic Therapy

Several comprehensive reviews of the treatment of thrombotic disorders by thrombolytic agents have been published.[98-101] Aspects of thrombolytic therapy that pertain to the subject of this chapter are the mechanisms of action of infused prourokinase (single-chain uPA) and tPA. Clearly, the ability of single-chain uPA or tPA to initiate thrombus-specific fibrinolytic activity is greater than either streptokinase or urokinase.[102] The efficacy of these agents has been demonstrated in controlled clinical studies. Presumably, the relative fibrin specificity of single-chain uPA is attributable to its affinity for fibrin-associated plasminogen.[103] In addition, the competitive inhibitor of uPA in plasma may restrict expression of its activity unless it is associated with a fibrin clot.[27] The in vivo thrombolytic efficacy of uPA also may be related to its resistance to endogenous inhibitors.[104] Similarly, tPA is a poor activator of plasminogen in the absence of fibrin. The enhancement of the activity of tPA by fibrin is well documented.[26] This in vitro observation has given rise to the concept that tPA released from the endothelium in vivo, or exogenously infused, is active only when bound to fibrin (i.e., when it is in association with a thrombus). However, other results indicate that tPA may also be activated by denatured proteins.[105] Thus, the in vivo fibrin-specificity of tPA may not be absolute. In addition, the short in vivo half-life of tPA,[106] as reflected by the high dosage needed to achieve effective thrombolysis, may limit its utilization in the treatment of occlusive vascular disorders. The presence of elevated PAI activity in plasma may also influence the effectiveness of exogenously administered tPA to induce thrombolysis.[107,108] An alternative to this approach of restorative therapy is the administration of agents that modulate endogenous vascular fibrinolytic activity by altering the balance between PA and PAI at the cellular level.

B. Stimulation of Endogenous Fibrinolysis

Most substances that elevate the fibrinolytic activity of blood are thought to be effective by enhancing the release of tPA from the vessel wall.[58] Although the specific mechanisms of action are not known, most of these agents cause a rapid (within 2 min) increase in the level of circulating tPA and an associated elevation of blood fibrinolytic activity, which rapidly disappears. Obviously, a prolonged elevation of vascular PA would be more conducive to the creation of a nonthrombogenic environment in the vasculature.[109,110] Such a long-lasting effect may be achieved by the administration of compounds that stimulate the endogenous production of PA, presumably by the endothelium, or that depress PAI activity.[111] It is critical to gain an understanding of the exact mechanisms of endothelial cell PA and PAI expression to enable the design of specific agents that might induce such effects. Thus, studies focusing on the cellular regulation of both PA and PAI have important implications for the evaluation and subsequent treatment of thrombotic disorders.

VII. SUMMARY

The localized cellular expression of vascular PA activity is critical to the overall maintenance and restoration of blood vessel patency. The factors that control the expression of this activity are just now beginning to be understood, and the details of their mechanisms of action are currently under investigation. Considerable progress has been made recently in understanding the cellular basis of plasminogen activation. For example, biological probes with which to explore in greater depth the expression of PA genes are now available. Also, the primary endogenous inhibitor of vascular PAs has been identified, and many of its biochemical properties have been described. As the complex set of interactions that contributes to the elaboration of vascular fibrinolytic activity is understood more fully, the role that this system plays in the development and prevention of occlusive vascular disease will become evident. As a consequence, more effective strategies for treating thrombotic disorders may be developed from the perspective of regulating the initiation of endogenous vascular fibrinolysis.

ACKNOWLEDGMENTS

The author thanks Jeanne L. Obreiter for excellent secretarial assistance.

REFERENCES

1. **Sixma, J. J.,** Role of blood vessel, platelet and coagulation interactions in haemostasis, in *Haemostasis and Thrombosis,* Bloom, A. L. and Thomas, D. P., Eds., Churchill Livingstone, Edinburgh, 1981, chap. 16.
2. **Owen, W. G.,** The control of hemostasis. Role of endothelium in the regulation of inhibitory and catabolic pathways, *Arch. Pathol. Lab. Med.,* 106, 209, 1982.
3. **Nawroth, P., Kisiel, W., and Stern, D.,** The role of endothelium in the homeostatic balance of haemostasis, *Clin. Haematol.,* 14, 531, 1985.
4. **Stern, D. M., Nawroth, P. P., Kisiel, W., Handley, D., Drillings, M., and Bartos, J.,** A coagulation pathway on bovine aortic segments leading to generation of factor Xa and thrombin, *J. Clin. Invest.,* 74, 1910, 1984.
5. **Wall, R. T. and Harker, L. A.,** The endothelium and thrombosis, *Ann. Rev. Med.,* 31, 361, 1980.
6. **Williams, W. J.,** Disorders of hemostasis-thrombosis, in *Hematology,* Williams, W. J., Beutler, E., Erslev, A. J., and Lichtman, M. A., Eds., McGraw-Hill, New York, 1983, chap. 160.
7. **Astrup, T.,** Cell-induced fibrinolysis: a fundamental process, in *Proteases and Biological Control,* Reich, E., Rifkin, D. B., and Shaw, E., Eds., Cold Spring Harbor Press, Cold Spring Harbor, N.Y., 1975, 343.
8. **Francis, C. W. and Marder, V. J.,** Mechanisms of fibrinolysis, in *Hematology,* Williams, W. J., Beutler, E., Erslev, A. J., and Lichtmam, M. A., Eds., McGraw-Hill, New York, 1983, chap. 138.
9. **Hjort, P. F. and Hasselback, R.,** A critical review of the evidence for a continuous hemostasis *in vivo, Thromb. Diath. Haemorrh.,* 6, 580, 1961.
10. **Stormorken, H.,** The thrombo-haemorrhagic balance, *Acta Med. Scand. Suppl.,* 642, 131, 1980.
11. **Marder, V. J. and Francis, C. W.,** Clinical aspects of fibrinolysis, in *Hematology,* Williams, W. J., Beutler, E., Erslev, A. J., and Lichtman, M. A., Eds., McGraw-Hill, New York, 1983, chap. 159.
12. **Ratnoff, O. D.,** Thrombosis and the hypercoagulable state, *Circulation,* 70(Suppl. 3), 72, 1984.
13. **van Rijn, J. L. M. L., Govers-Riemslag, J. W. P., Zwaal, R. F. A., and Rosing, J.,** Kinetic studies of prothrombin activation: effect of factor Va and phospholipids on the formation of the enzyme-substrate complex, *Biochemistry,* 23, 4557, 1984.
14. **Jackson, C. M. and Nemerson, Y.,** Blood coagulation, *Ann. Rev. Biochem.,* 49, 765, 1980.
15. **Jackson, C. M.,** Biochemistry of prothrombin activation, in *Haemostasis and Thrombosis,* Bloom, A. L. and Thomas, D. P., Eds., Churchill Livingstone, Edinburgh, 1981, chap. 10.
16. **Guinto, E. R. and Esmon, C. T.,** Loss of prothrombin and of factor Xa-factor Va interactions upon inactivation of factor Va by activated protein C, *J. Biol. Chem.,* 259, 13986, 1984.
17. **Zolton, R. P. and Seegers, W. H.,** Autoprothrombin II-A: thrombin removal and mechanism of induction of fibrinolysis, *Thromb. Res.,* 3, 23, 1973.
18. **Comp, P. C. and Esmon, C. T.,** Evidence for multiple roles for activated protein C in fibrinolysis, in *The Regulation of Coagulation,* Mann, K. G. and Taylor, F. B., Jr., Eds., Elsevier/North-Holland, New York, 1980, 583.
19. **Comp, P. C. and Esmon, C. T.,** Generation of fibrinolytic activity by infusion of activated protein C into dogs, *J. Clin. Invest.,* 68, 1221, 1981.
20. **Sakata, Y., Curriden, S., Lawrence, D., Griffin, J. H., and Loskutoff, D. J.,** Activated protein C stimulates the fibrinolytic activity of cultured endothelial cells and decreases antiactivator activity, *Proc. Natl. Acad. Sci. U.S.A.,* 82, 1121, 1985.
21. **Chen, L. B. and Buchanan, J. M.,** Plasminogen-independent fibrinolysis by proteases produced by transformed chick embryo fibroblasts, *Proc. Natl. Acad. Sci. U.S.A.,* 72, 1132, 1975.
22. **Sundsmo, J. S. and Fair, D. S.,** Relationships among the complement, kinin, coagulation, and fibrinolytic systems, *Springer Sem. Immunopathol.,* 6, 231, 1983.
23. **Landmann, H.,** Biochemistry of the factors of the fibrinolytic system, in *Fibrinolytics and Anti-fibrinolytics,* Markwardt, F., Ed., Springer-Verlag, New York, 1978, 3.
24. **Müllertz, S.,** Fibrinolysis: an overview, *Sem. Thromb. Hemost.,* 10, 1, 1984.
25. **Lijnen, H. R. and Collen, D.,** Interaction of plasminogen activators and inhibitors with plasminogen and fibrin, *Sem. Thromb. Hemost.,* 8, 2, 1982.
26. **Hoylaerts, M., Rijken, D. C., Lijnen, H. R., and Collen, D.,** Kinetics of the activation of plasminogen by human tissue plasminogen activator. Role of fibrin, *J. Biol. Chem.,* 257, 2912, 1982.

27. **Lijnen, H. R., Zamarron, C., Blaber, M., Winkler, M. E., and Collen, D.,** Activation of plasminogen by pro-urokinase. I. Mechanism, *J. Biol. Chem.*, 261, 1253, 1986.
28. **Kok, P. and Nilsson, T.,** Assay characteristics and fibrin affinity of plasminogen activators of the intrinsic fibrinolytic system, *Thromb. Res.*, 41, 197, 1986.
29. **Ogston, D.,** *The Physiology of Hemostasis,* Harvard University Press, Cambridge, Mass., 1983, chap. 4.
30. **Horwitz, B. H., Váradi, A., and Scheraga, H. A.,** Localization of a fibrin γ-chain polymerization site within segment Thr-374 to Glu-396 of human fibrinogen, *Proc. Natl. Acad. Sci. U.S.A.*, 81, 5980, 1984.
31. **Suenson, E., Lützen, O., and Thorsen, S.,** Initial plasmin-degradation of fibrin as the basis of a positive feed-back mechanism in fibrinolysis, *Eur. J. Biochem.*, 140, 513, 1984.
32. **Wiman, B. and Collen, D.,** On the kinetics of the reaction between human antiplasmin and plasmin, *Eur. J. Biochem.*, 84, 573, 1978.
33. **Sakata, Y. and Aoki, N.,** Cross-linking of α_2 plasmin inhibitor to fibrin by fibrin-stabilizing factor, *J. Clin. Invest.*, 65, 290, 1980.
34. **Wiman, B. and Collen, D.,** On the mechanism of the reaction between human α_2-antiplasmin and plasmin, *J. Biol. Chem.*, 254, 9291, 1979.
35. **Collen, D.,** Molecular biology of human plasminogen. II. Metabolism in physiological and some pathological conditions in man, *Thromb. Diath. Haemorrh.*, 34, 403, 1975.
36. **Gordon, S., Unkeless, J. C., and Cohn, Z. A.,** Induction of macrophage plasminogen activator by endotoxin stimulation and phagocytosis. Evidence for a two-stage process, *J. Exp. Med.*, 140, 995, 1974.
37. **Ljungnér, H., Holmberg, L., Kjeldgaard, A., Nilsson, I. M., and Åstedt, B.,** Immunological characterisation of plasminogen activators in the human vessel wall, *J. Clin. Pathol.*, 36, 1046, 1983.
38. **Levin, E. G. and Loskutoff, D. J.,** Regulation of plasminogen activator production by cultured endothelial cells, *Ann. N.Y. Acad. Sci.*, 401, 184, 1982.
39. **Rijken, D. C., Juhan-Vague, I., DeCock, F., and Collen, D.,** Measurement of human tissue-type plasminogen activator by a two-site immunoradiometric assay, *J. Lab. Clin. Med.*, 101, 274, 1983.
40. **Pennica, D., Holmes, W. E., Kohr, W. J., Harkins, R. N., Vehar, G. A., Ward, C. A., Bennett, W. F., Yelverton, E., Seeburg, P. H., Heyneker, H. L., Goeddel, D. V., and Collen D.,** Cloning and expression of human tissue-type plasminogen activator cDNA in *E. coli, Nature (London),* 301, 214, 1983.
41. **Gimbrone, M. A., Jr.,** Culture of vascular endothelium, in *Progress in Haemostasis and Thrombosis,* Vol. 3, Spaet, T. H., Ed., Grune & Stratton, New York, 1976, 1.
42. **Laug, W. E., Tokes, Z. A., Benedict, W. F., and Sorgente, N.,** Anchorage independent growth and plasminogen activator production by bovine endothelial cells, *J. Cell Biol.*, 84, 281, 1980.
43. **Levin, E. G. and Loskutoff, D. J.,** Cultured bovine endothelial cells produce both urokinase and tissue-type plasminogen activators, *J. Cell Biol.*, 94, 631, 1982.
44. **Loskutoff, D. J.,** Effect of thrombin on the fibrinolytic activity of cultured bovine endothelial cells, *J. Clin. Invest.*, 64, 329, 1979.
45. **Danø, K., Andreasen, P. A., Grøndahl-Hansen, J., Kristensen, P., Nielsen, L. S., and Skriver, L.,** Plasminogen activators, tissue degradation, and cancer, *Adv. Cancer Res.*, 44, 139, 1985.
46. **Lee, L.-S. and Weinstein, I. B.,** Epidermal growth factor, like phorbol esters, induces plasminogen activator in HeLa cells, *Nature (London),* 274, 696, 1978.
47. **Waller, E. K. and Schleuning, W.-D.,** Induction of fibrinolytic activity in HeLa cells by phorbol myristate acetate, *J. Biol. Chem.*, 260, 6354, 1985.
48. **Sudol, M.,** Hormonal regulation of protein synthesis in cultured kidney cells, *Mol. Cell. Endocrinol.*, 40, 245, 1985.
49. **Laug, W. E.,** Glucocorticoids inhibit plasminogen activator production by endothelial cells, *Thromb. Haemost.*, 50, 888, 1983.
50. **Hagiwara, H., Shimonaka, M., Morisaka, M., Ikekawa, N., and Inada, Y.,** Sitosterol-stimulative production of plasminogen activator in cultured endothelial cells from bovine carotid artery, *Thromb. Res.*, 33, 363, 1984.
51. **Tiku, M. L. and Tomasi, T. B.,** Enhancement of endothelial plasminogen activator synthesis by lymphokines, *Transplantation,* 40, 293, 1985.
52. **Kristensen, P., Larsson, L.-I., Nielsen, L. S., Grøndahl-Hansen, J., Andreasen, P. A., and Danø, K.,** Human endothelial cells contain one type of plasminogen activator, *FEBS Lett.*, 168, 33, 1984.
53. **Levin, E. G., Marzec, U., Anderson, J., and Harker, L. A.,** Thrombin stimulates tissue plasminogen activator release from cultured endothelial cells, *J. Clin. Invest.*, 74, 1988, 1984.
54. **Moscatelli, D.,** Urokinase-type and tissue-type plasminogen activators have different distributions in cultured bovine capillary endothelial cells, *J. Cell. Biochem.*, 30, 19, 1986.
55. **Gelehrter, T. D. and Sznycer-Laszuk, R.,** Thrombin induction of plasminogen activator-inhibitor in cultured human endothelial cells, *J. Clin. Invest.*, 77, 165, 1986.
56. **Levin, E. G. and Loskutoff, D. J.,** Serum-mediated suppression of cell-associated plasminogen activator activity in cultured endothelial cells, *Cell,* 22, 701, 1980.

57. **Delvos, U., Paul, J. E., and Müller-Berghaus, G.,** Effect of the heparinoid pentosan polysulphate (SP 54) on the functional properties of cultured bovine aortic endothelial cells, *Blut,* 51, 127, 1985.
58. **Cash, J. D.,** Control mechanism of activator release, in *Progress in Chemical Fibrinolysis and Thrombolysis,* Vol. 3, Davidson, J. F., Rowan, R. M., Samama, M. M., and Desnoyers, P. C., Eds., Raven Press, New York, 1978, 65.
59. **Juhan-Vague, I., Conte-Devolx, B., Aillaud, M. F., Mendez, C., Oliver, C., and Collen, D.,** Effects of DDAVP and venous occlusion on the release of tissue-type plasminogen activator and von Willebrand factor in patients with panhypopituitarism, *Thromb. Res.,* 33, 653, 1984.
60. **Emeis, J.,** Perfused rat hindlimbs. A model to study plasminogen activator release, *Thromb. Res.,* 30, 195, 1983.
61. **Smith, D., Gilbert, M., and Owen, W. G.,** Tissue plasminogen activator release in vivo in response to vasoactive agents, *Blood,* 66, 835, 1985.
62. **Emeis, J. J. and Kluft, C.,** PAF-acether-induced release of tissue-type plasminogen activator from vessel walls, *Blood,* 66, 86, 1985.
63. **Klöcking, H.-P., Markwardt, F., and Hoffmann, A.,** Release of tissue-type plasminogen activator by platelet-activating factor, *Thromb. Res.,* 38, 413, 1985.
64. **Stalder, M., Hauert, J., Kruithof, E. K. O., and Bachmann, F.,** Release of vascular plasminogen activator (v-PA) after venous stasis: electrophoretic-zymographic analysis of free and complexed v-PA, *Br. J. Haematol.,* 61, 169, 1985.
65. **Marsh, N. and Gaffney, P.,** Some observation on the release of extrinsic and intrinsic plasminogen activators during exercise in man, *Haemostasis,* 9, 238, 1980.
66. **Bergsdorf, N., Nilsson, T., and Wallén, P.,** An enzyme linked immunosorbent assay for determination of tissue plasminogen activator applied to patients with thromboembolic disease, *Thromb. Haemost.,* 50, 740, 1983.
67. **Brommer, E. J. P., Verheijen, J. H., Chang, G. T. G., and Rijken, D. C.,** Masking of fibrinolytic response to stimulation by an inhibitor of tissue-type plasminogen activator in plasma, *Thromb. Haemost.,* 52, 154, 1984.
68. **Nilsson, I. M., Ljungnér, H., and Tengborn, L.,** Two different mechanisms in patients with venous thrombosis and defective fibrinolysis: low concentration of plasminogen activator or increased concentration of plasminogen activator inhibitor, *Br. Med. J.,* 290, 1453, 1985.
69. **Levin, E. G.,** Latent tissue plasminogen activator produced by human endothelial cells in culture: evidence for an enzyme-inhibitor complex, *Proc. Natl. Acad. Sci. U.S.A.,* 80, 6804, 1983.
70. **Thorsen, S. and Philips, M.,** Isolation of tissue-type plasminogen activator-inhibitor complexes from human plasma, *Biochim. Biophys. Acta,* 802, 111, 1984.
71. **Esnard, F., Dupuy, E., Dosne, A. M., and Bodevin, E.,** Partial characterization of a fibrinolytic inhibitor produced by cultured endothelial cells derived from human umbilical vein, *Thromb. Haemost.,* 47, 128, 1982.
72. **van Mourik, J. A., Lawrence, D. A., and Loskutoff, D. J.,** Purification of an inhibitor of plasminogen activator (antiactivator) synthesized by endothelial cells, *J. Biol. Chem.,* 259, 14914, 1984.
73. **Sprengers, E. D., Verheijen, J. H., van Hinsbergh, V. W. M., and Emeis, J. J.,** Evidence for the presence of two different fibrinolytic inhibitors in human endothelial cell conditioned medium, *Biochim. Biophys. Acta,* 801, 163, 1984.
74. **Erickson, L. A., Ginsberg, M. H., and Loskutoff, D. J.,** Detection and partial characterization of an inhibitor of plasminogen activator in human platelets, *J. Clin. Invest.,* 74, 1465, 1984.
75. **Booth, N. A., Anderson, J. A., and Bennett, B.,** Platelet release protein which inhibits plasminogen activators, *J. Clin. Pathol.,* 38, 825, 1985.
76. **Wiman, B., Chmielewska, J., and Rånby, M.,** Inactivation of tissue plasminogen activator in plasma. Demonstration of a complex with a new rapid inhibitor, *J. Biol. Chem.,* 259, 3644, 1984.
77. **Colucci, M., Paramo, J. A., and Collen, D.,** Generation in plasma of a fast-acting inhibitor of plasminogen activator in response to endotoxin stimulation, *J. Clin. Invest.,* 75, 818, 1985.
78. **Hekman, C. M. and Loskutoff, D. J.,** Endothelial cells produce a latent inhibitor of plasminogen activators that can be activated by denaturants, *J. Biol. Chem.,* 260, 11581, 1985.
79. **Erickson, L. A., Hekman, C. M., and Loskutoff, D. J.,** The primary plasminogen-activator inhibitors in endothelial cells, platelets, serum, and plasma are immunologically related, *Proc. Natl. Acad. Sci. U.S.A.,* 82, 8710, 1985.
80. **Erickson, L. A., Hekman, C. M., and Loskutoff, D. J.,** Denaturant-induced stimulation of the β-migrating plasminogen activator inhibitor in endothelial cells and serum, *Blood,* 68, 1298, 1986.
81. **Owen, W. G. and Esmon, C. T.,** Functional properties of an endothelial cell cofactor for thrombin-catalyzed activation of protein C, *J. Biol. Chem.,* 256, 5532, 1981.
82. **Esmon, N. L., Carroll, R. C., and Esmon, C. T.,** Thrombomodulin blocks the ability of thrombin to activate platelets, *J. Biol. Chem.,* 258, 12238, 1983.

83. **Salem, H. H., Esmon, N. L., Esmon, C. T., and Majerus, P. W.,** Effects of thrombomodulin and coagulation factor V_a-light chain on protein C activation *in vitro, J. Clin. Invest.*, 73, 968, 1984.
84. **van Hinsbergh, V. W. M., Bertina, R. M., van Wijngaarden, A., van Tilburg, N. H., Emeis, J. J., and Haverkate, F.,** Activated protein C decreases plasminogen activator-inhibitor activity in endothelial cell-conditioned medium, *Blood,* 65, 444, 1985.
85. **Taylor, F. B., Jr. and Lockhart, M. S.,** A new function for activated protein C: activated protein C prevents inhibition of plasminogen activators by releasate from mononuclear leukocytes-platelet suspensions stimulated by phorbol diester, *Thromb. Res.*, 37, 155, 1985.
86. **Taylor, F. B., Jr. and Lockhart, M. S.,** Whole blood clot lysis: *in vitro* modulation by activated protein C, *Thromb. Res.*, 37, 639, 1985.
87. **de Fouw, N. J., Haverkate, F., Bertina, R. M., Koopman, J., van Wijngaarden, A., and van Hinsbergh, V. W. M.,** Human activated protein C (APC) accelerates blood clot lysis *in vitro, Thromb. Haemost.*, 54, 107, 1985.
88. **Sakata, Y., Griffin, J. H., and Loskutoff, D. J.,** Role of protein C in fibrinolysis, *Thromb. Haemostas.*, 54, 118, 1985.
89. **Korninger, C., Lechner, K., Niessner, H., Gossinger, H., and Kundi, M.,** Impaired fibrinolytic capacity predisposes for recurrence of venous thrombosis, *Thromb. Haemost.*, 52, 127, 1984.
90. **Horellou, M. H., Conard, J., Bertina, R. M., and Samama, M.,** Congenital protein C deficiency and thrombotic disease in nine French families, *Br. Med. J.*, 289, 1285, 1984.
91. **Pilgerman, L. O.,** Abnormalities in clotting and thrombolysis as a risk factor for stroke, *Thromb. Diath. Haemorrh.*, 31, 245, 1974.
92. **Davies, J. A. and McNicol, G. P.,** Blood coagulation in pathological thrombus formation and the detection in blood of a thrombotic tendency, *Br. Med. Bull.*, 34, 113, 1978.
93. **Aoki, N., Matsuda, M., and Yoshida, N.,** Abnormalities in the platelets and fibrinolytic system as predisposing factors to thrombosis, *Asian Med. J.*, 23, 382, 1980.
94. **Isacson, S. and Nilsson, I. M.,** Defective fibrinolysis in blood and vein walls in recurrent ''idiopathic'' venous thrombosis, *Acta Chir. Scand.*, 138, 313, 1972.
95. **Stead, N. W., Bauer, K. A., Kinney, T. R., Lewis, J. G., Campbell, E. E., Shifman, M. A., Rosenberg, R. D., and Pizzo, S. V.,** Venous thrombosis in a family with defective release of vascular plasminogen activator and elevated plasma factor VIII/von Willebrand's factor, *Am. J. Med.*, 74, 33, 1983.
96. **Brakman, P., Mohler, E. R., Jr., and Astrup, T.,** A group of patients with impaired plasma fibrinolytic system and selective inhibition of tissue activator-induced fibrinolysis, *Scand. J. Haematol.*, 3, 389, 1966.
97. **Jorgensen, M., Mortensen, J. Z., Madsen, A. G., Thorsen, S., and Jacobsen, B.,** A family with reduced plasminogen activator activity in blood associated with recurrent venous thrombosis, *Scand. J. Haematol.*, 29, 217, 1982.
98. **Sherry, S., Fletcher, A. P., and Alkjaersig, N.,** Rationale and limitations of the use of thrombolytic (fibrinolytic) agents in the treatment of thromboembolic disease, *Prog. Hematol.*, 3, 244, 1962.
99. **Collen, D. and Lijnen, H. R.,** New approaches to thrombolytic therapy, *Arteriosclerosis,* 4, 579, 1984.
100. **Duckert, F.,** Thrombolytic therapy, *Sem. Thromb. Hemost.*, 10, 87, 1984.
101. **Sherry, S. and Gustafson, E.,** The current and future use of thrombolytic therapy, *Ann. Rev. Pharmacol. Toxicol.*, 25, 413, 1985.
102. **Williams, D. O., Borer, J., Braunwald, E., Chesebro, J. H., Cohen, L. S., Dalen, J., Dodge, H. T., Francis. C. K., Knatterud, G., Ludbrook, P., Markis, J. E., Mueller, H., Desvigne-Nickens, P., Passamani, E. R., Powers, E. R., Rao, A. K., Roberts, R., Ross, A., Ryan, T. J., Sobel, B. E., Winniford, M., Zaret, B., et al.,** Intravenous recombinant tissue-type plasminogen activator in patients with acute myocardial infarction: a report from the NHLBI thrombolysis in myocardial infarction trial, *Circulation,* 73, 338, 1986.
103. **Lijnen, H. R., Zamarron, C., and Collen, D.,** Characterization of the high-affinity interaction between human plasminogen and pro-urokinase, *Eur. J. Biochem.*, 150, 141, 1985.
104. **Gurewich, V., Pannell, R., Louie, S., Kelley, P., Suddith, R. L., and Greenlee, R.,** Effective and fibrin-specific clot lysis by a zymogen precursor form of urokinase (pro-urokinase), *J. Clin. Invest.*, 73, 1731, 1984.
105. **Radcliffe, R. and Heinze, T.,** Stimulation of tissue plasminogen activator by denatured proteins and fibrin clots: a possible additional role for plasminogen activator?, *Arch. Biochem. Biophys.*, 211, 750, 1981.
106. **Jaffe, A. S. and Sobel, B. E.,** Thrombolysis with tissue-type plasminogen activator in acute myocardial infarction. Potentials and pitfalls, *JAMA,* 255, 237, 1986.
107. **Paramo, J. A., Colucci, M., and Collen, D.,** Plasminogen activator inhibitor in the blood of patients with coronary artery disease, *Br. Med. J.*, 291, 573, 1985.
108. **Hamsten, A., Wiman, B., de Faire, U., and Blombäck, M.,** Increased plasma levels of a rapid inhibitor of tissue plasminogen activator in young survivors of myocardial infarction, *N. Engl. J. Med.*, 313, 1557, 1985.

109. **Fox, K. A. A., Robison, A. K., Knabb, R. M., Rosamond, T. L., Sobel, B. E., and Bergmann, S. R.,** Prevention of coronary thrombosis with subthrombolytic doses of tissue-type plasminogen activator, *Circulation,* 72, 1346, 1985.
110. **Gold, H. K., Leinbach, R. C., Garabedian, H. D., Yasuda, T., Johns, J. A., Grossbard, E. B., Palacios, I., and Collen, D.,** Acute coronary reocclusion after thrombolysis with recombinant human tissue-type plasminogen activator: prevention by a maintenance infusion, *Circulation,* 73, 347, 1986.
111. **Fearnley, G. R.,** Pharmacological enhancement of fibrinolysis, in *Chemical Control of Fibrinolysis-Thrombolysis,* Schor, J. M., Ed., John Wiley & Sons, New York, 1970, chap. 7.

INDEX

A

B

C

D

E

F

G

H

I

J

K

L

M

Q

R

S

T

U

V

W